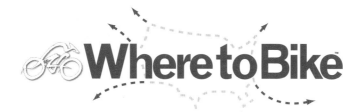

Where to Bike™

New York City

- Manhattan
- The Bronx
- Queens
- Brooklyn
- Staten Island
- Northern New Jersey

By J.P. Partland

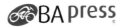
BA press

Where to Bike LLC

Email: mail@wheretobikeguides.com
Tel: +61 2 4274 4884 - Fax: +61 2 4274 0988
www.wheretobikeguides.com

First published in the USA in 2012 by Where to Bike
LLC.

Design and Layout - Justine Powell
Advertising - Phil Latz
Photography - Matt Wittmer
All additional photos taken by J.P. Partland unless
otherwise specified.
Mapping - Justine Powell, Bicycling Australia
Printed in China by RR Donnelley
Cover: Photo by Matt Wittmer

Library of Congress Control Number: 2011943161
Author: J.P. Partland
Title: Where to Bike New York City
ISBN: 978-0-9808587-8-5
          978-0-9808587-9-2

*The Cycling Kangaroo logo is a trademark of Lake
Wangary Publishing Company Pty Ltd.*

*Where to Bike is a proud sponsor of World Bicycle
Relief.*

*Where to Bike is a proud member of the Bikes
Belong Coalition, organizers of the People for Bikes
campaign; and the League of American Bicyclists.*

peopleforbikes.org

League of American Bicyclists

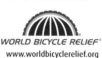

WORLD BICYCLE RELIEF®
www.worldbicyclerelief.org

www.bikeleague.org

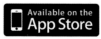

Available on the App Store

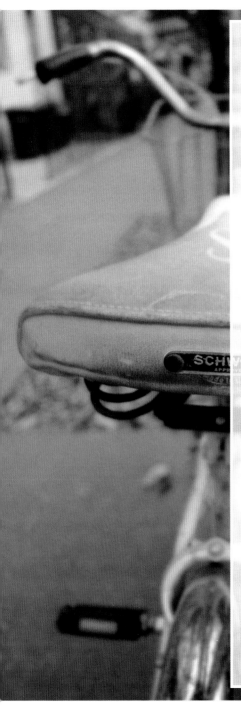

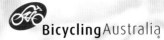

About us...

Cycling has many health and environmental benefits, but in addition to these it's a fun leisure time activity for all ages. Bike touring is also a great way to get up close and personal with a new destination. Where to Bike guides provide locals and tourists alike with advice on the best ride options for fun, exploration and relaxation on two wheels.

Most of our team are active cyclists; we love to ride and hope that we can inspire and motivate readers to join us on two wheels. We're committed to our vision of enhancing all aspects of cycling through these Where to Bike guides and our other publications.

Available in printed hard copy through bike shops and book stores, Where to Bike publications are also offered in digital format online. Check the iTunes store for an eBook version if you prefer a soft copy, or download the IOS App and we'll guide you along the route of each ride as you go!

Look out for other Where to Bike titles and the 'cycling kangaroo' logo in news stands and bookstores; it's your key to quality cycling publications.

We have made every effort to ensure the accuracy of the content of this book, but please feel free to contact us at feedback@wheretobikeguides.com to report any changes to routes or inconsistencies you may find.

For more information about *Where to Bike New York City* and other books in this series, visit **www.wheretobikeguides.com**.

Photo Matt Wittmer

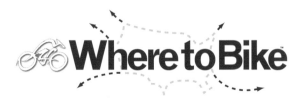

Where to Bike

New York City

Contents

Author's Note

I love this town. I love riding bicycles. I am an unapologetic booster of both. That I came to do this book, while not a foregone conclusion, was hardly a surprise.

I'm a native. I ride a bike nearly every day. Long before this book was even a glimmer in the eye of Bicycling Australia, I had visited all five boroughs on two wheels; I knocked that out in one day when I was twelve, on my first Five Boro Bike Tour. By the time I got around to writing this book, I had ridden and raced bicycles in every borough. I had ridden all but two of the bridges that join Manhattan to other land masses (the two remaining are off-limits to bikes). I had seen both the sunrise and sunset from the saddle while cruising over the Brooklyn Bridge. I had circumnavigated Manhattan, toured the Bronx, made my way to Queens and Long Island, knew countless routes around northern New Jersey.

And yet, I had never seen the entire city by bike. I hadn't ridden around all the edges, hadn't seen all the parks, hadn't sought out good riding in more than a few places in the city. Most of my city rides were rides to places, not rides where the point was to take a loop within a borough. It's a big world, but many don't stop to check out their own backyard, myself included.

So I took it all in. New York may be a small city in terms of square mileage, but with something like 6,000 miles of roads, it takes a while to ride it.

J.P. Partland
Author

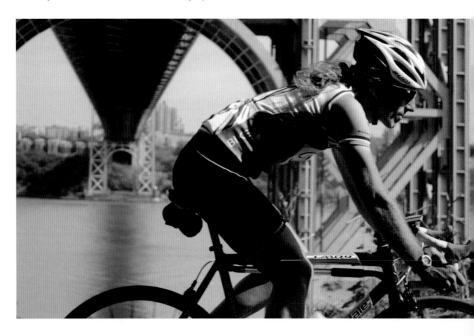

About the Author

J. P. Partland has been exploring the New York City metropolitan area by bicycle for as long as he can remember. He enjoys road, off-road, and track racing as well as daily commuting by bicycle. He served as editor in chief of *Cycling Times*, a regional publication for cyclists, and has covered bicycling for *the New York Times, New York magazine, Fitness, Outside,* and *Boys' Life*. His books include *Mountain Bike Madness, The World of BMX*, and *Tour Fever: An Armchair Cyclist's Guide to the Tour de France*. He dreams of a New York City with less car traffic.

Acknowledgments

Many people helped make this book possible. The folks on this side of the planet include: Jeannine Bardo, Hannah Borgeson, Andrew Burdess, Josh Caesar, Jason Chupick, Alice Dodds, Lester Freundlich, Lars Klove, Andrea Partland, Wojciech Plata, Meredith Sladek, Keith Snyder, Paul Steely White, and Matt Wittmer. And the people down under. They include Joanne David, Gary Hunt, Phil Latz and Justine Powell.

Dedication

To Oscar

Photography

Many thanks to **Matt Wittmer**, author and photographer of the inspiring *Where to Bike Washington, D.C.*, who assisted in creation of this book by capturing additional images to compliment those taken by JP Partland.

All photos Matt Wittmer

Introduction

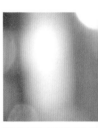

Νew York City is a great place to ride a bicycle. And it's getting better. I expect it will take some convincing for you to believe the above.

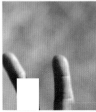

First, New York City is fairly flat, so you rarely have to concern yourself with steep hills to climb or descend.

Second, the city is fairly compact, so no matter where you are, it's easy to find places to ride.

Third, because of all the density and all the stuff going on, drivers often find it hard to speed. And speeding is one of the biggest dangers cars present. Yes, there are some distracted drivers, but really distracted driving is dangerous for drivers, and they respond. Non-cyclists look at a Manhattan avenue and they see chaos, but it's actually quite manageable. The cars have to cross a street every 1/20th of a mile and at every crossing they have to worry about pedestrians darting out. They have to worry about parked cars suddenly jumping out. They have to be ready for an SUVdriver to cut them off. They have to get a read on when the bus is going to stop. They can't see beyond the delivery truck in front of them. And there are pushcarts, potholes, horse-drawn carriages, and so on.

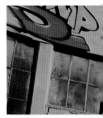

Fourth, there is a large and growing network of bike paths. And the city government has made a big commitment to re-imagining the city as being dominated by human-powered transport and mass transit. The changes are happening pretty fast: when I first tried my tri-borough route, they were just starting work on a bike path entry to the 59th Street bridge. By the third time, a few months later, the path was within days of completion.

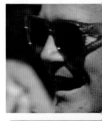

Fifth, there is incredible diversity in the city. Whether it's architecture, food, people, old stuff, new stuff, arcane stuff, it can be found. And cycling allows you to sample the diversity more easily than you can by any other mode of transport. You think you know what the city looks like? Think again. It's more than skyscrapers and suburbs.

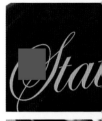

Sixth, the weather is conducive for riding. Yes, it can get pretty cold in the winter and pretty hot in the summer, but it's rarely below freezing for long and rarely above 90 degrees Fahrenheit for more than a short stretch or three. And we're not overwhelmed by precipitation any season of the year. In the winter, it snows, but rare is the storm that leaves roads snowy for more than a few days afterwards.

Seventh, because of all of the above, using a bike for commuting, visiting, errands, as well as exercise is easy. No need to get in a car when all you're doing is picking up some Chinese or dropping off a library book. Got a small kid? Put a seat on the back of your bike and take them with you. Riding is more fun than taking the subway and often faster than the bus.

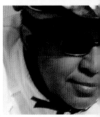

Take a quick scan of the rides. You'll see that many of them are on the edges of the city and in parks. This was a deliberate choice. Anyone can wheel onto a street or avenue and take it somewhere without a guidebook. I was more interested in creating rides that take you somewhere you might not otherwise go.

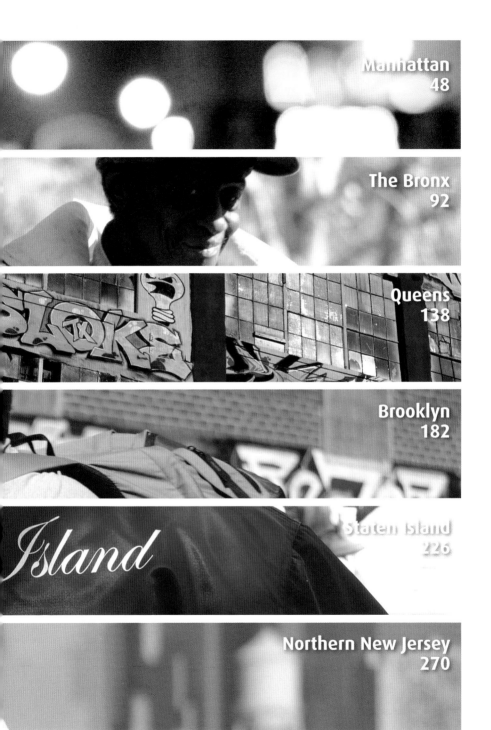

All photos Matt Wittmer

How to Use This Book

In *Where to Bike New York City* you will find 58 adult rides spread through five boroughs and just across the Hudson in New Jersey. We've broken down the rides into boroughs, with Jersey being effectively the sixth borough.

Within each section, the rides are identified as bike path, on-road, off-road or mountain bike, or any combination thereof. Most of the rides utilize bike paths; these are rides that are marked in some fashion and are separated from the road by anything from a painted line to a forest. This classification system is designed to make your initial selection quick and easy based on the terrain you're likely to encounter along the way.

Ride Scale

To help you better understand at a glance how difficult each ride might be, this book rates the rides using the Where to Bike rating scale that the publisher, Bicycling Australia, uses for all its cycling guidebooks. Each ride is assigned points based on the total distance covered, the elevation gain of the ride and the predominant road surface. Then the points are added up to determine the overall rating. The tables below show how these calculations are made.

You can find the Where to Bike rating on the introductory page of each ride; just look for the Bicycling Australia kangaroo symbols. They look like this:

The New York region has a wide variety of terrain and roads and wind. Some places, like Brooklyn, are pretty flat, but others are rather hilly. There is just about always wind coming off the water, so expect wind on any ride that runs along a river or bay or ocean.

The Where to Bike rating is only a guide. If you're new to cycling or not currently fit, start with level 1 and 2 rides. As your cycling skills and fitness improve, you will be able to advance to the higher levels.

While the maps have been produced with accurate GPS-collected data, they do not always show sufficient information or detail to allow you to navigate relying exclusively on them. That's where the ride logs opposite each map come in. Refer to the logs constantly as you ride, since they provide all the information and detail you'll need to get from start to finish.

There's also a chance that things have changed on particular roads and paths since I've been there last. Change in NYC can occur fast and places where there isn't a bike path today, there might be one tomorrow. A bike path designated with *sharrows* (share-the-road

	1 pt	2 pts	3 pts	4 pts	5 pts
Distance – Road (miles)	<12	12-19	19-25	25-37	>37
Distance – MTB (miles)	<6	6-9	9-16	16-25	>25
Climbing (feet)	<500	500 - 1,000	1,000 - 1,500	1,500 - 2,000	>2,000
Surface	Paved smooth	Paved rough	Unpaved smooth	Unpaved moderate	Unpaved rough

Accumulated Points	Riding Level/Grade	Suggested Suitability
3	1	Beginner
4-5	2	
6-7	3	Moderately fit
8-9	4	
10+	5	Experienced cyclist

rrows) today may be a protected path in a week.

And make sure you use the specifically designed nside front cover to keep you on the right page. This 'old-out flap also includes the key to the maps and ntroductory pages.

We hope all of these design features will ensure that you enjoy rides that are safe and carefree, informative and entertaining.

Ride Classifications

Ride Classifications are used to represent the distinct character of the ride itself and are usually a reflection of the environment or landscape the cyclist will enjoy as they travel the route.

In *Where to Bike New York City*, there are six classifications to look for on the ride At a Glance page:

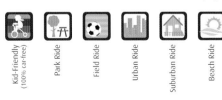

Kid-Friendly (100% car-free)   Park Ride   Field Ride   Urban Ride   Suburban Ride   Beach Ride

Ride Links

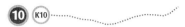

If you're partial to adding to your ride, or simply interested in other routes nearby, information on ride links can be found on both the ride At a Glance page, and on the maps.

At a Glance: Ride numbers included in the 'Links to' panel on the At a Glance page are considered direct links—rides that intersect with, or can be accessed with ease from the current route.

Maps: Each map includes easy to identify ride link icons at either the location of junction, or at the closest point the linked ride can be accessed from the current ride. The maps show all links, both direct and non-direct—and each link route is highlighted with an easy to identify orange dashed line.

Bike Shops and Rentals

Bike shops and bike rental outlets are marked upon each map with icons as above. Each icon carries a number which correlates to a comprehensive store listing on page 310. Here you'll find the name, number and web details of the stores that are an easy pedal from all of the rides. No spares? No worries.

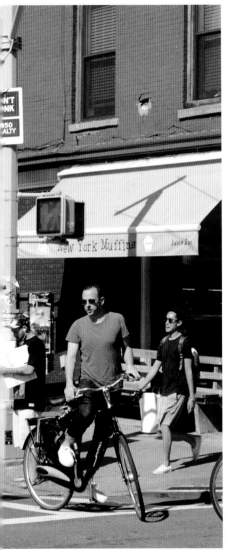

Photo Matt Wittmer

Ride Overview

Manhattan

Page	Ride	Ride Name	Start Location
52	1	Central Park Loops	Central Park, Manhattan
56	2	Highbridge MTB Trails	Highbridge Park, Manhattan
60	3	Upper Manhattan Loop	St. Nicholas Park, Manhattan
64	4	Upper West Side Loop	Riverside Park, Manhattan
68	5	Upper East Side Loop	120th Street and FDR Drive, Manhattan
72	6	Randall's Island Loop	Ward's Island Bridge, Manhattan
76	7	Lower Manhattan Loop	11th Avenue and 20th Street, Manhattan
80	8	Brooklyn & Manhattan Bridges	Sara D. Roosevelt Park, Manhattan
84	9	Governors Island Loop	Governors Island

The Bronx

Page	Ride	Ride Name	Start Location
96	10	Wave Hill Loop	Henry Hudson Memorial Park, The Bronx
100	11	Van Cortlandt Park Loop	Van Cortlandt Park, The Bronx
104	12	Woodlawn Loop	Mosholou Parkway Bike Path and Hull Avenue, The Bronx
108	13	Bronx Zoo Loop	Asia Gate of The Bronx Zoo, The Bronx
112	14	Pelham Parkway Loop	Boston Road and Pelham Parkway West, The Bronx
116	15	Orchard Beach Loop	Bartow-Pell Circle, The Bronx
120	16	City Island Loop	City Island, The Bronx
124	17	Yankee Stadium Loop	Yankee Stadium, The Bronx
128	18	Maritime College Loop	Monsignor Scanlan High School, The Bronx
132	19	Soundview Loop	Soundview Park, The Bronx

Queens

Page	Ride	Ride Name	Start Location
142	20	Fort Totten Ride	Brooklyn-Queens Greenway, Queens
146	21	Douglaston Loop	Douglaston LIRR Station, Queens
150	22	Cunninghamm Park MTB Trails	Cunningham Park Trailhead, Queens
154	23	Vanderbilt Motor Parkway Loop	73rd and Hollis Hills Terrace, Queens
158	24	Kissena Velodrome	Kissena Park, Queens
162	25	Flushing Meadows-Corona Park Loop	Flushing Meadows-Corona Park, Queens
166	26	Roosevelt Island Loop	Roosevelt Island, Queens
170	27	Three-Borough Loop	Underneath the Queensboro Bridge, Queens
174	28	Ridgewood Reservoir Ride	Highland Park, Queens
178	29	The Wind and the Rockaways Ride	Beach 67th Street and Rockaway Freeway, Queens

Terrain	Kid-Friendly	Distance (miles)	Elev. Gain (feet)	WTB Rating
On Road Lane / Path		6.7/1.9/1.4	560/149/157	
MTB		0.2/0.2/0.7	54/119/124	
On Road / On Road Lane / Path	partial	9.4	605	
On Road / Path	partial	6.5	372	
On Road / On Road Lane / Path	partial	4.9	126	
On Road / On Road Lane / Path	partial	5.4	213	
On Road / On Road Lane / Path	partial	9.6	110	
On Road / On Road Lane Protected On Road Lane/ Path	no	4.0	199	
On Road / Path		2.1/1.4/1.5	54/32/56	

Terrain	Kid-Friendly	Distance (miles)	Elev. Gain (feet)	WTB Rating
On Road		6.5	732	
On Road / Path / Off Road	partial	5.5	358	
On Road / Path	partial	6.3	392	
On Road / Path	partial	5.9	333	
On Road / Path	partial	7.1	250	
On Road / Path	partial	2.8	112	
On Road	no	3.3	114	
On Road / On Road Lane	no	2.5	188	
On Road	no	8.2	277	
On Road / On Road Lane Protected On Road Lane/ Path	partial	5.0	158	

Terrain	Kid-Friendly	Distance (miles)	Elev. Gain (feet)	WTB Rating
On Road / On Road Lane / Path	partial	8.7	427	
On Road	no	2.9	263	
MTB		2.1/6.5	185	
On Road / On Road Lane / Path	partial	5.8	404	
Path		0.3	0	
On Road / On Road Lane / Path	partial	4.9	62	
On Road / Path	partial	3.5	173	
On Road / On Road Lane Protected On Road Lane/ Path	no	10.8	344	
Path		2.2	83	
On Road / On Road Lane / Path	partial	20.3	136	

Ride Overview continued

Brooklyn

Staten Island

Northern New Jersey

Terrain		Kid-Friendly	Distance (miles)	Elev. Gain (feet)	WTB Rating
On Road Lane / Path			3.4/2.1/2.9	185/78/181	
On Road / On Road Lane / Path		partial	8.6	255	
On Road / On Road Lane / Path		partial	5.7	188	
On Road / On Road Lane / Path		partial	8.2	350	
On Road / On Road Lane / Path		partial	18.1	426	
On Road / On Road Lane / Path		partial	7.7	105	
Path			0.9	4	
On Road / Path		partial	6.6	121	
Path			2.3	9.3	
On Road / On Road Lane / Path		partial	9.6	98	

Terrain		Kid-Friendly	Distance (miles)	Elev. Gain (feet)	WTB Rating
On Road / Path		no	6.7	201	
On Road		no	7.5	410	
On Road / Path		partial	7.5	305	
On Road		no	2.5	259	
On Road / Path		partial	1.8	15	
On Road / Path		partial	3.4	45	
On Road Lane / MTB		partial	2.8	182	
On Road / Path		partial	1.8	64	
On Road / On Road Lane / Path		partial	3.8	196	
On Road / Path		partial	5.0	269	

Terrain		Kid-Friendly	Distance (miles)	Elev. Gain (feet)	WTB Rating
On Road		no	42.6	2248	
On Road / Path		no	16.6	1325	
On Road		no	20.9	1134	
On Road		no	42.7	2999	
On Road		no	4.9	340	
On Road / Path		partial	5.5	120	
On Road / Path		partial	3.2	49	
On Road / Path		partial	5.2	25	
Path			1.3	40	

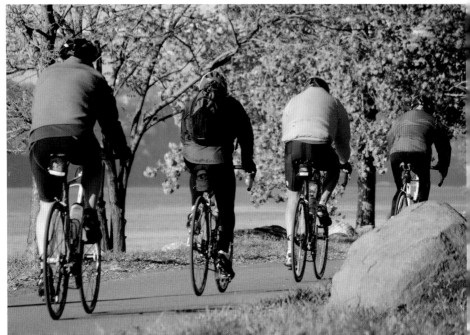

Photo Matt Wittmer

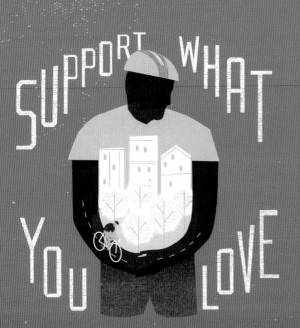

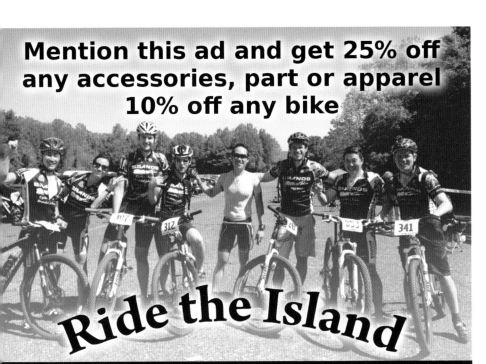
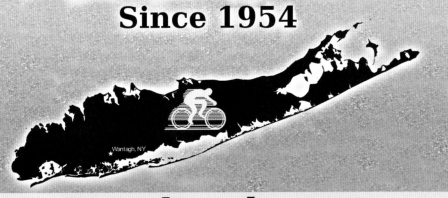

Terrain Guide

To help you understand what to expect on the route, terrain types are described on both the At a Glance page, and directly on the maps with easy to follow colored ride lines, as follows:

On-Road:

A *red ride line* depicts sections of the ride that are on-road. The cyclist shares the road with vehicular traffic, and is expected to abide by road rules and laws. These routes are either Class III Bike Routes, or are considered comparably safe for recommendation by the author.

On-Road Bike Lane:

A *green ride line* depicts sections of the ride where exclusive on-road bike lanes are provided. Here the cyclist is clearly separated from vehicular traffic by a traffic lane marked on an existing roadway that is restricted to cycle traffic. These routes are Class II Bike Routes, and are only indicated if such infrastructure is in place.

Protected On-Road Bike Lane:

A *blue ride line* depicts sections of the ride where exclusive, protected on-road bike lanes are provided. Here the cyclist is clearly separated from vehicular traffic by a physical barrier that is restricted to use by cycle traffic. Such barriers can consist of parked cars or painted curbs. These routes are also considered Class I Bike Routes, and are only indicated if such infrastructure is in place.

Designated Bike Path:

A *yellow ride line* depicts sections of the ride that are on smooth bike paths where the cyclist is completely separated from roads. The path can either be a sidepath (designated for use by cyclists) or a shared-use footway (for use by both cyclists and pedestrians). These routes are either Class I Bike Routes, or are considered comparably safe for recommendation by the author.

Off-Road:

A *brown ride line* depicts sections of the ride that are on wide, unpaved dirt trails, that are smooth enough for navigation by any type of bike.

MTB:

A *black ride line* depicts sections of the ride that are on narrower, more challenging dirt trails. Here the cyclist would generally be required to be riding a mountain bike designed to handle such conditions.

Kids' Rides

Riding with kids can be great fun. Problem is in the more urban areas of the city, riding with them on roads that are shared with cars can be harrowing for the adults and potentially dangerous for the kids. Riding in parks also presents difficulties, because even if you have a park down the street, chances are it doesn't have a road or path that's permissible for adults to ride on. And as many New Yorkers don't have cars, schlepping both an adult bike and a kid bike somewhere can be tough.

Riding bikes on sidewalks in New York City is only permissible when two criteria are met. The first is that the wheels must be less than 26 inches in diameter. The second is that the rider of the bicycle is 12 years of age or younger. Kids under 14 are also required to wear a helmet.

My recommendation is that if you want to get your kids to ride more, first take them to a quiet park or empty basketball court where you can help them learn to balance on their own and observe them practicing until they get the hang of it. If no one else is around, you can probably ride alongside them. Knowing how to start, stop, turn, ride a straight line, and signal are all essential skills. Then, take them to rides that are comprised entirely of off-street bike paths or just do the car-free segments of rides, like the Vanderbilt Motor Parkway in Queens, or Fort Wadsworth in Staten Island, or Bronx Park. Central Park, Prospect Park, the Marine Park Oval are obvious car-free selections, but any waterfront bike path can be great as well, and there are those in every borough. There are waterfront bike paths in New Jersey as well, and both Liberty State Park and Lincoln Park are also easy for kids.

I've been told that for kids under 10 years of age, riding up to 10 miles at a stretch is doable with a little training. All the same, probably shooting for five miles or fewer is more easily attainable.

Another interesting riding tip I heard was that a way for a parent to ride with their child on streets is

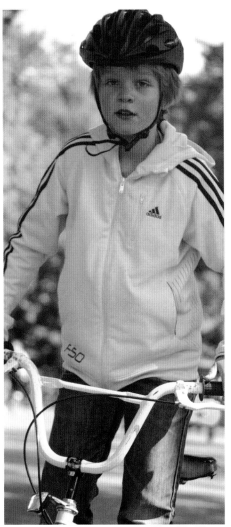

Photo Matt Wittmer

ride together but separately. Kid rides on the sidewalk while the parent rides parallel in the street. The parent accompanies them across the intersection. Then, if the road seems quiet, the kid shifts to riding on the street until the road seems to be getting busy with car traffic, then shifts back on the sidewalk.

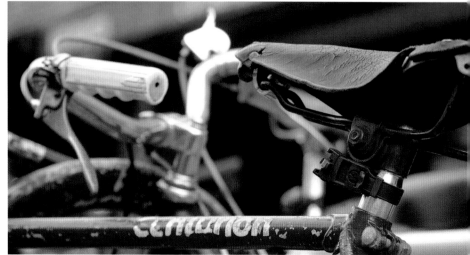

Beyond the Basics

I'm not a rules person. I'm more of a guidelines guy. I like to know ground rules, limitations, big dangers, big draws, and kind of feel my way for the rest. It helps make riding an adventure rather than following a textbook. I encourage you to use the book in this fashion.

All the same, I realize that if you're not 100% comfortable with your riding ability, or aren't confident in staying on route, or get spooked by traffic, you should probably pay more careful attention to the details. The newer you are to riding, the less comfortable you are in traffic, the more carefully you should pay attention to the book.

Most of the rides are loops. I prefer to do loops rather than out-and-back rides; I find loops more interesting. But owing to the scope and purpose to this book, there were several areas where loops were less than ideal and these are the areas where I have out-and-back rides as well as some one-way rides. The one-ways are pretty short, so you can either link to other rides or very easily ride back.

I list nearest train or ferry stops for all the rides, figuring that part of bike riding is living a car-free lifestyle. If you must drive, I've marked where there are parking lots in many areas; some are free, some you have to pay for. I also assume that if you're within up to several miles of a route, you'll ride to the start, probably joining the route where it's nearest to your starting point rather than the starting point I chose.

I also recommend that you pick up a copy of the free official NYC Bike Map. The publisher of this book tells me it's one of the best he's seen. I find it rather impressive. Take a look at the map, find where you live, and find where the ride is, and you can probably find bike routes that take you at least part of the way. You can find more copies of this map at just about every city bike shop. Get extras; they'll come in handy. Also pick up a new one every year; since miles of bike lanes get added each year, having a current one is always a good idea.

If you're a newer rider, I'd recommend looking for shorter routes that are either close to home or easy to get to. My feeling is master the familiar before venturing farther. Once you feel like you've got the familiar down, you're probably ready to go beyond.

With this book, without it, or beyond, my most basic recommendation is to think about starting small, getting comfortable with what's nearby, and then starting to branch out, and getting more adventurous.

How to Ride

You've heard "It's just like riding a bicycle" before. Maybe you've even said it. It's both true and hopelessly wrong.

It's true because the mental gymnastics it takes to balance on two spinning wheels as you're propelling a bicycle, once learned, never goes away. It's hopelessly wrong because riding well is the sum total of a huge bushel of skills and knowledge that no matter how much you read, you can always learn more and it's never the same as actually doing it.

Luckily, just about all the cycling knowledge you need is stuff you can pick up along the way. There is no shortage of books written on how to ride a bike. We don't have the space to go into everything here. But I will tell you a few things that stand out.

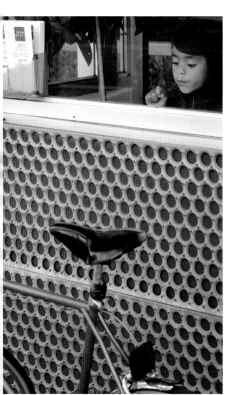

Photo Matt Wittmer

- One of the biggest misconceptions, and the one I feel is most dangerous, is the popular parental warning not to use your front brake for fear of endo-ing, aka flipping over your handlebars. Erase this misinformation from your head. Good, safe, fast braking requires the use of both front and rear brakes, with the front brake doing most of the work.
- Another has to do with pedal speed. Pedaling at walking pace is what most people do when they start riding. That's often 60 pedal revolutions per minute (rpm) or less. That's one pedal stroke a second. Turning your legs over at this rate is too slow; you should be pedaling faster (like 90rpm) as it's easier to respond to changes in terrain and the higher cadence results in less muscular strain on your body. Start with an in-between 75-80rpm and work your way up as your coordination and comfort level improves.
- If a hill seems hard, keep shifting into lower gears until it either feels easy or you run out of gears.
- Another has to do with soreness. Muscular soreness is fine. But a sore back, butt, or hands are things you should look into. A sore back might be a sign that your saddle isn't in a comfortable position or your stem is too short or too long. A sore butt might mean you need to stand on your pedals more during the ride. Sore hands might mean you need padded gloves or more padding on your handlebars. The difficulty is that some of this could just be from not being used to riding; note the aches and track them for a while. If they don't go away, a change might be in order.

Before You Go

It is cliché to tell you that before you start riding, there are two things you should do. But all the same, I must repeat. First, if you haven't been exercising, you should consult your doctor to make sure you're cleared for riding. Considering the health benefits of cycling, it's hard to imagine any doctor saying no, but all the same, check. Second, is to make sure your bike is in safe working condition.

If your bike has been sitting a while, it might be worthwhile to take it to your local shop for a tune-up. At the very least, you want to:

- Make sure your tires are whole, not cracking from age or rot, and inflated to the recommended air pressure (the number is found on the sidewalls).
- Make sure the brakes can stop the bike. Inspect the pads to make sure there is sufficient material on them.
- That the wheels spin true and don't rub against the frame or brakes.
- That the wheels are properly secured in the fork tips and dropouts.
- That the chain moves without squeaking. Ideally, it is clean and lubed.
- That the gears can shift without slipping.
- At home, it's good to have a floor pump to keep the tires at the proper pressure and some lube to make sure the chain doesn't get rusty.
- In terms of the bike itself, make sure it fits you and you can both reach the brakes and the shifters comfortably.

It's best to take care of most of these things in between rides, not the morning of a ride. Tire-pumping is for the morning of your ride. You'll find the recommended pressure range on the tire sidewalls.

Your best source of advice and help is a bike shop. While the most convenient one makes sense, it's good to have a decent relationship with the people working

at the shop you frequent as they can be a huge help—the better you know each other, the easier it is to help. Don't be afraid to check out different shops in search of good people.

What to Take

On all of the rides in this book, you're never far from civilization. What you take, and don't take, should depend on how far you're going and what hassles you're willing to put up with.

Here's what should be considered the minimum you should have for pretty much any ride:

- A bicycle helmet that fits properly and is adjusted correctly.
- Identification.
- Money.
- Information about any medical conditions.
- If there's any chance you'll be out after dark, and riding at night is relatively easy in NYC, have working front and rear lights. Lights after dark are the law. "Blinky" lights, aka flashing LED lights, are fine. Front blinky lights should be pointed not directly out, but so they hit the ground about 20 feet in front of you. Having lights on your bike in NYC is mostly about being seen; with the streetlights and ambient light, you probably won't need illumination for riding on streets. Night riding on bike paths may well be different: you may need a real light to show you where you're going.

It is de rigueur for any cycling guidebook to tell you to carry a repair kit and pump. It is true that you want to have the basics so you can take care of things like fixing a flat tire or tightening a loose bolt. Many cyclists carry these on just about all their rides, but at the same time, they often don't have them for errands or rides of a few miles. Don't feel you have to buy lots of gear just to ride a few miles from home. At worst, you'll walk back; three miles should take the average person about an hour to hoof. If that seems like a bad idea, then maybe you should be well-equipped for even your short rides.

Here's what you should have in either a bag or on your bike:

* Water. Have either a portable hydration system on your back or a bottle on your bike.
* An inner tube in the size that fits your tires, and a valve that fits your wheel.
* A sticker-style patch kit so you can repair a punctured tube if necessary.
* Tire levers to remove the tire(s) from your wheels.
* A pump or CO_2 cartridges and an inflator for putting air in tires.
* A multi-tool for tightening bolts. Usually, all you need are 4,5,6mm Allen keys and a small screwdriver, but having an 8mm key, a second screwdriver (so you have both slotted and Philips head), and a chain tool doesn't hurt.
* If your wheels have axle nuts instead of quick releases, a wrench to loosen the nuts.

All the same, I know that many people, even after they purchase these things and mount them on their bike, don't know how to use them. So, if you're the kind who doesn't and are going far, I suggest riding with the gear anyways, in case you're with someone who can, and also have this book handy because there are public transit maps and phone numbers of bike shops. You can always call a cab to take you to a shop. If this is your method of repair, it can take a long while and get expensive, but at least you'll get home.

If you are game for learning how to use the tools, there are books, videos on the internet, even classes from both bike clubs and bike shops. If you have a decent relationship with some bike shop folk, you

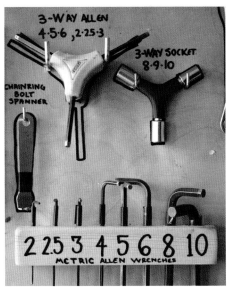

Photo Matt Wittmer

could probably just visit during a slow time and they might take the time to watch you struggle with changing a tire and offer advice on how to do it better.

On top of everything else, there are a few extras that can really make a difference for riding:

* It's a great idea to have a bike computer mounted to your handlebars or stem. You can have fun watching the speed and use the odometer feature to determine how far you've ridden. These can be very inexpensive.
* A lock. If you already leave your bike in a common room or storage area, you probably own a good one. When you're out for a ride, it's something you only need to bring if you're leaving your bike unattended. Most cable locks are only good for leaving a bike in a safe-seeming place for a short time. Otherwise, a burly lock is the way to go. There are heavy chains and U-type locks to fit this need; the U-type are easier to carry, but you need to lock at least both your frame and front wheel, if not your frame, front and rear wheels, if you're leaving it for a while.

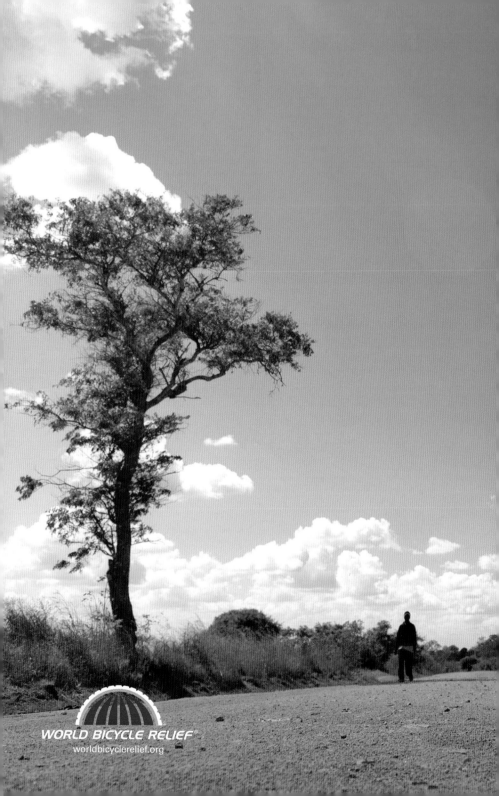

WORLD BICYCLE RELIEF®
worldbicyclerelief.org

teacher. doctor. engineer…

This bicycle is more than transportation;
it's a new beginning.
worldbicyclerelief.org/pages/newbeginning

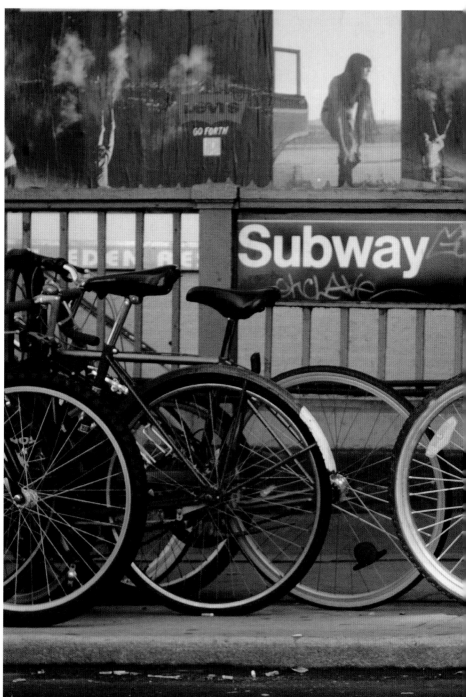

Photo Matt Wittmer

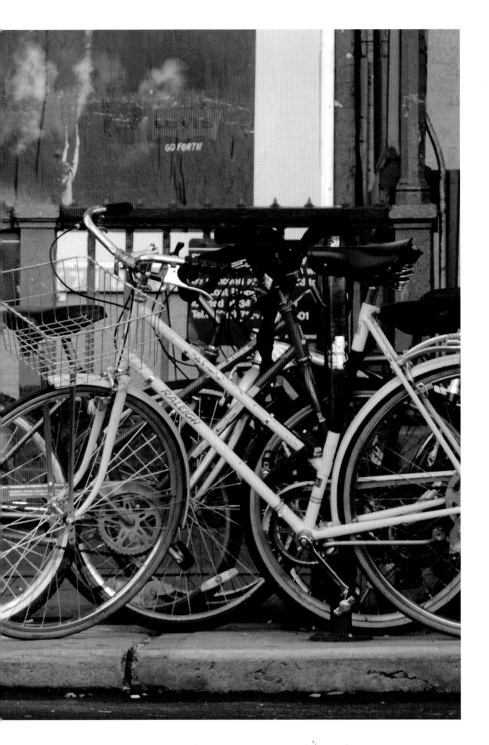

On the Road

There are lots of great things about riding, and I hope you get a feeling for some of them throughout these pages, but there is one thing that is forever an issue: the asymmetric relationship between cars and bikes. Cycling is a very safe activity, but the one thing that adds measurable risk to the sport is the reality of moving motorized vehicles, particularly of the car and truck kind. In a tangle with a car, a bike never wins. So ride like your life depends on it; if you think it's safer to break a traffic law, you might want to do that and accept the consequences of a ticket, rather than following the law and crashing or getting hit.

Cycling in New York is safe and getting safer. Part of it is a result of the NYCDOT doing a great job in recent years including cycling in the transit equation, part of it is the result of more cyclists on the road. But cars will always present a risk. Comparing crash stats between the United States and other countries where cycling is more popular seems to indicate that the more popular cycling is, the safer all cyclists are.

Non-cyclists overemphasize the importance of helmets; the first question that comes up when anyone is hit by a car is "was he wearing a helmet?" It's as if they think a bike helmet is some magical coat of armor. It isn't. All the same, wear a helmet when you ride. Good helmets these days can be pretty cheap, very comfortable, and if you hit your head, can save your life. The cost of wearing one is very little and the benefit for that one-in-a-million freak accident is huge. It will do you as much good on an abandoned dirt trail as it will on a bike path or on a busy street.

When you're riding, you want to be seen. Bright clothing isn't chic, but gets you noticed. Having "blinky" lights for the front and back of your bike is also great insurance. These things are cheap, small, mount unobtrusively, and can flash for hours on end. Some people I know even have them on during daylight hours.

Since **safety is paramount**, I'd like to offer some advice as sometimes this sort of knowledge isn't intuitive.

- Know how to properly use the quick release levers on your wheels. They are the little levers that help secure your wheels into your fork and frame.
- Know the traffic laws. We have them in this book. But just because you know them doesn't mean anyone else does. Non-cyclists, even those in public-safety jobs, often don't.
- Signal before you turn and look before moving into what could be a car's way. You'll find commonly-used hand signals in the NYC Bike Map, available at your local bike store.
- Don't think that just because you're riding in a bike lane that drivers or pedestrians will treat the bike lane with deference or respect. Some drivers think a bike lane is for parking and passing and some pedestrians believe that bike lanes are for walking with luggage. Use your judgment as to whether or not you should use the lane. If you think it's too dangerous use the road and the law backs you up.
- Use your voice to be noticed; even a good bell is hard for most people to hear. Loud but polite is the way to go. Thank pedestrians and drivers, even when they're in the wrong.
- Try to ride out far enough from parked cars so that you're not surprised by a sudden opening of a car door. Getting hit this way is known as being "doored" and it hurts. The law allows you to ride 3-4 feet away from parked cars, a safe range to avoid dooring.
- Because of the dooring phenomenon, make a point of riding on the left side of most one-way streets, as drivers drive on the left and exit their cars on the sidewalk. So long as the street is 40-feet wide, as measured from curb to curb, cyclists can ride on either the right or left side of the road. Certain

places, like the separated sections of Queens Boulevard or Manhattan's Fifth Avenue along Central Park, riding on the right is safer.

- If you feel unsafe on busy streets with a bike lane, try to find quieter streets that run parallel.
- Ride predictably. This includes riding with the flow of traffic, whether it's a shared road or an exclusive bike lane, and following at least the spirit of the law. When in traffic, using signals helps. But it's more than signaling. It's about not swerving, not weaving (except when car traffic is stopped), not leaving others to think that you're turning when you're not.
- Pedestrians, especially those with dogs, can be the hardest to read. They're not held by any regulation, they're moving slowly, but can move in any direction fast. Don't try to squeeze behind them thinking they won't see you. You know what it's like being a pedestrian, so think about what you'd do in their shoes.
- Assume that when you see pedestrians starting to cross a street or a car nudging out from the driveway or side street that the person hasn't seen you.
- Try to make eye contact with people who appear to be poised to cross in front of you. People typically react better to having someone look at them.
- Assume that pedestrians and drivers are lousy at estimating how fast you're going.
- For smaller potholes, all you need to do is lift your butt off your saddle. Go right over the bump/crack/ small hole in the pavement. If your tires are inflated to their recommended pressure, the tires, wheels, and frame will absorb the bump. Bigger holes you need to go around, but take a smooth line rather than a sudden swerve.
- There is a common assumption that cyclists should ride as far over to the side of the road as possible. This is incorrect. You only need to ride as far over

as is safe. On one-lane roads, you can take the lane if you deem the side of the road unsafe.

- Acknowledge other cyclists. If you're going the opposite direction on a road or bike path, wave. If you're overtaking another cyclist, let them know you're coming without surprising them. Yelling out "passing on your left," or whatever seems appropriate. If you see a cyclist stopped with a mechanical or another that has crashed, stop to make sure they're okay.
- Most cyclists start out hesitant in traffic and do their best to stay out of the way of cars and trucks. It's an intuitive survival strategy. All the same, most cyclists who ride daily ride assertively. They make their presence known on the street and are not worried about forcing drivers to slow down for them. Experienced cyclists, when concerned about their safety, often take up a traffic lane because if they're in the middle of traffic, they can't be doored and the cars behind them won't be tempted to squeeze between them and another car. The law generally protects this behavior. At the same time, experienced cyclists know when to squeeze toward the side of the road. As Kenny Rogers sang, "know when to hold 'em/Know when to fold 'em".

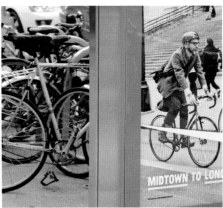

Photo Matt Wittmer

Off the Road

We have three off-road rides in this book. They are the three official mountain bike (mtb) trails in NYC. No where else in NYC is riding off-road legal.

Many of the guidelines that apply to road riding apply to off-road riding. Make sure your bike is safe to operate before going into the woods. Use both brakes. Wear a helmet. Recognize that you're sharing the trail with other users. Ride responsibly.

Many people new to mountain biking might believe, from looking at the bikes sold and the images that adorn magazines, that mountain biking is all about aggro' riding. It isn't. Most people don't get big air or need body armor for riding. And you definitely don't need armor or a big-hit bike to ride the trails detailed here. These are beginner trails and you should be able to ride them comfortably and safely with just about any knobby-tired bike.

The International Mountain Bicycling Association (IMBA) has their Rules of the Trail that are appropriate to reprint here.

1. Ride open trails.
2. Leave no trace.
3. Control your bicycle.
4. Yield appropriately.
5. Never scare animals.
6. Plan ahead.

You can learn more at **www.imba.com**.

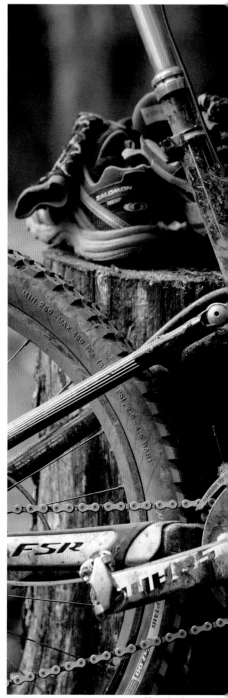

Photo Sterling Lorence

You, Your Bike and Transport in the New York Metro Area

I prefer riding from my door rather than getting in a car or taking public transit, and all of the rides are accessible by public transportation and are so noted. A big part of cycling is about time efficiency and maximizing riding time and calories burned, but a small part is feeling the absurdity of using heavy, polluting equipment to ride. Still, there are reasons to take your bike on public transit before you ride, even if in NYC, you're probably riding to that public transit before taking it to ride more.

If you take a look at the NYC Bike Map included with this book, you'll find the info you need there.

Here are some highlights:

The NYC subways are great for cyclists. While bikes are always allowed on, they're discouraged during rush hours. Regional train service is not quite so kind: non-folding bikes are definitely not allowed for the busy side of rush hour (like inbound to NYC in the morning rush and outbound on the evening rush) and some holidays and a few other things. The LIRR, for example, doesn't allow non-folding bikes on the train the day of The Montauk Century.

For Metro-North and LIRR regional trains, both require the same $5 pass, which is good for life. NJ Transit doesn't require it. Metro-North doesn't permit bikes going inbound weekday 5 a.m.- 10 a.m. and outbound weekday 4 p.m.- 8:15 p.m. The LIRR doesn't allow it weekday inbound from 6 a.m.- 10 a.m. Weekday outbound is not permitted from 3 p.m.- 8 p.m. NJ Transit doesn't permit weekday inbound 6 a.m.- 10 a.m. and doesn't permit weekday outbound from 4 p.m.- 7 p.m.

- PATH trains, the line that goes under the Hudson to Hoboken, Jersey City, and Newark, bikes are allowed on at all times save weekday rush hours. Rush hours are defined as 6:30 a.m.- 9:30 a.m. and 3:30 p.m.- 6:30 p.m. weekdays. Folding bikes are allowed on, folded, during rush hours.
- Local ferries allow bikes on at all times. The Staten Island, New York Water Taxi, and Governor's Island ferries are all free. NY Waterways charges $1 and Sea Streak is $5.
- Folding bicycles are permitted aboard local and limited buses at all times. Please fold your bike before boarding and don't block the aisle or doors. Folding bikes are not allowed on express buses. All other bicycles are prohibited.
- Amtrak is a hard one to make sense of. There's no one policy. You can take a folder on as one of your two carry-on items. Some lines have bike racks, but not in the Northeast. You can check a bike, but it needs to be in a bike box, and you can only put it on and take it off at a station that is considered "staffed." New York, Philadelphia, Boston, and Washington are all staffed. The box can have the maximum dimensions of 69 inches by 41 inches by 8.5 inches. It will cost $15.
- For regional travel in the northeast, lots of people have come to like the "Chinatown buses." This is Bolt and the like that have cheap fares and a cargo hold where they typically take a bike for free. I haven't heard of anyone having to put their bike in a bag or box, but many have a thin nylon bag to minimize the chances of scratching bike parts.

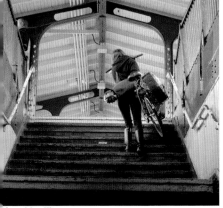

Photo Matt Wittmer

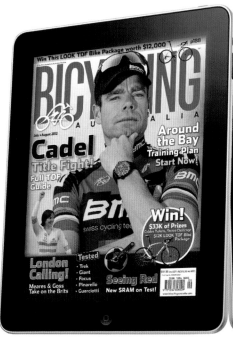
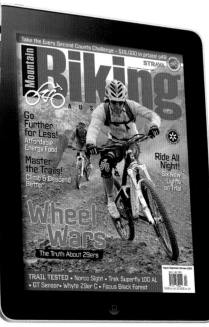
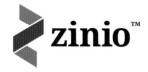

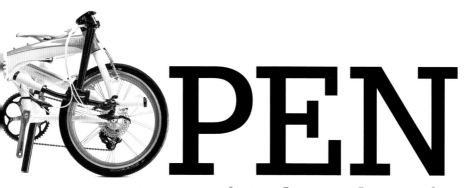

OPEN

source your inter-borough transit.

ternbicycles.com/us

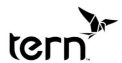

tern™

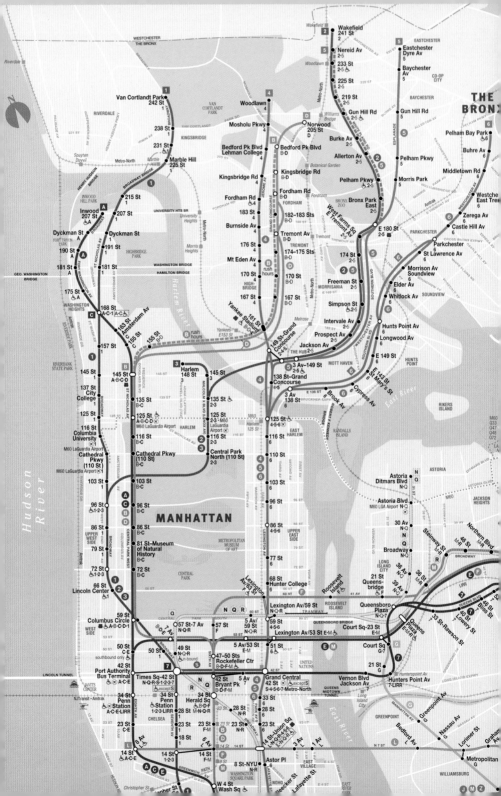

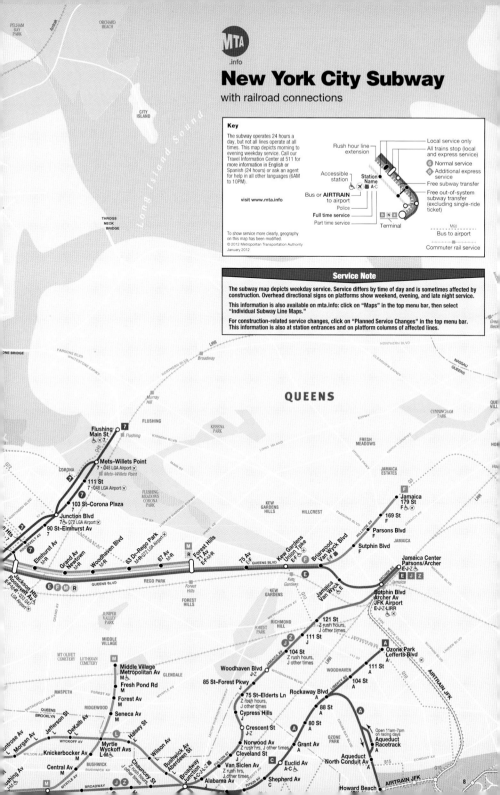

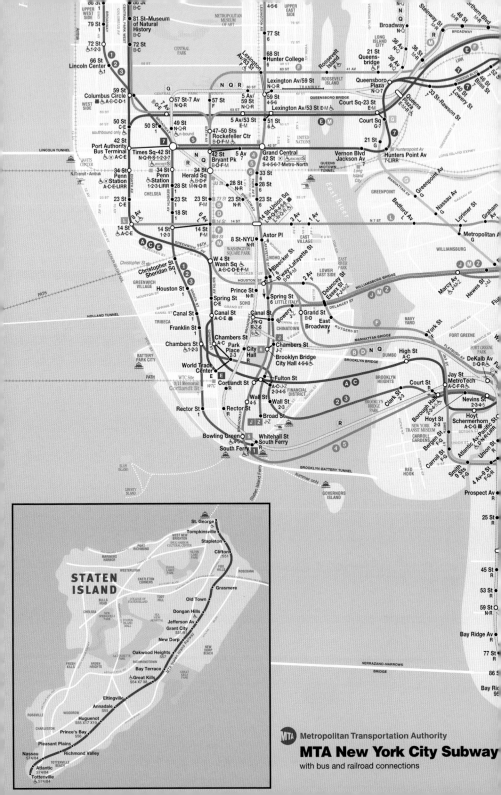

MTA Metropolitan Transportation Authority

MTA New York City Subway

with bus and railroad connections

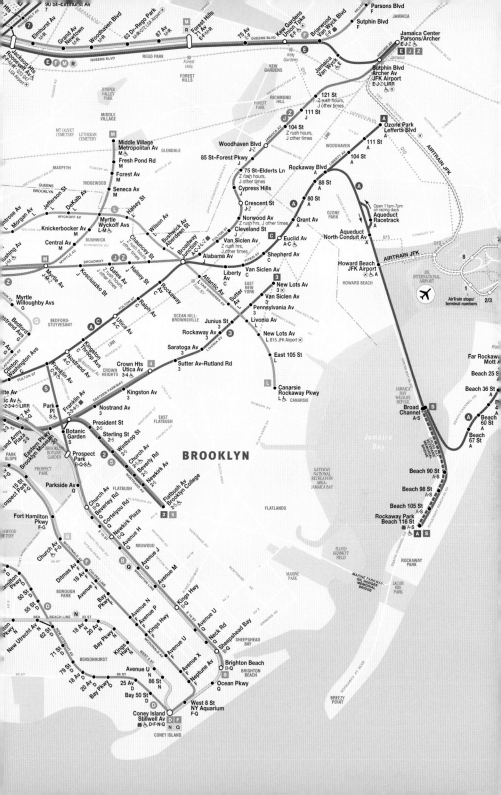

MTA New York City Railroads

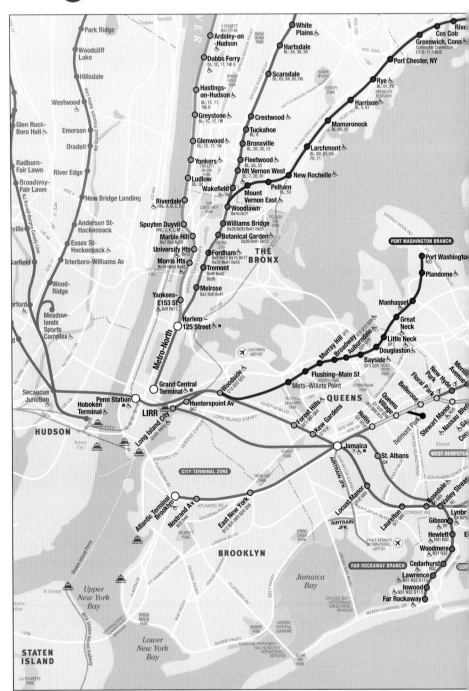

For More Information

As this book is aimed at a fairly broad intended audience, from beginners contemplating buying their first bike to cyclists with years of experience, there was no way I could provide detailed information on subjects ranging from buying a bike to training for racing. I can, however, point you to places on the web where such information can be found.

City Resources

Probably the first place to go for more information is **Transportation Alternatives'** website. They're the leading advocacy group in the city. Their site has information on most basic cycling in New York City queries. Advice on general stuff like locking your bike safely, commuting, riding in various weather conditions, what to do if you get a ticket while riding and much more. They also have advice on creating a bike room in your building.
www.transalt.org

Bike New York, the organization that runs the Five Boro Bike Tour, has an extensive list of classes. They also have a pretty comprehensive advice section, where they offer advice on things like buying a bike, fitting a helmet, assessing your own bicycles.
www.bikenewyork.org

Time's Up, a direct action environmental organization, offers interesting rides and classes as well as a bike co-op.
www.times-up.org

A number of **city bike shops** offer classes on all manner of bike repair. Check in with your local shop to see what, if anything, they offer. Two that I know of are Bicycle Habitat in downtown Manhattan and Mod Squad Cycles in Harlem.

Clubs

Bicycle clubs are a way that many people who are developing an interest in riding find not only like-minded people, but more rides and more learning. There are clubs for all interests in New York City.

One method for finding local clubs that share or promote your interests is through the **BNY and TA sites**. But you can probably find more comprehensive listings by finding national umbrella organizations and looking for area clubs through the organization

The League of American Bicyclists, aka LAB, is the oldest and largest advocacy group in the country. Their website is pretty comprehensive, but if you're looking for local clubs and organizations, go to their "Find It" page.
www.bikeleague.org or **www.members.bikeleague. org/members_online/members/findit.asp**.

Adventure Cycling Association is the bike touring organization in the U.S. It has info on solo touring, group tours, resources for traveling cyclists, Cyclists' Yellow Pages, even a companion finder resource.
www.adventurecycling.org

For people who have a yen to do more with mountain biking, the most comprehensive online resource is from the **International Mountain Bike Association, IMBA**. They're at **www.imba.com**. Locally, the New York City Mountain Bike Association is also a great resource.
www.nycmtb.com

If bike racing interests you, find a racing-oriented club. **USA Cycling** is the governing body for bike racing in the United States. Racing includes BMX, cyclocross, mountain biking, road riding, and track. If you're looking for a local club, use their "Clubs" page.
www.usacycling.org or **www.usacycling.org/clubs/**

If triathlons interest you, start with the **International Triathlon Union, ITU**.
www.triathlon.org

NYC/NY State and NJ Traffic Rules and Regulations

Source: NYCDOT and NJ DOT website

N.Y.C. Traffic Rules and Regulations

4-01 (b) - Definitions

A bicycle is defined as every two- or three- wheeled device upon which a person or persons may ride, propelled by human power through a belt, a chain or gears, with such wheels in a tandem or tricycle, except that it shall not include a device having solid tires and intended for use only on a sidewalk by pre-teenage children.

4-02 (a) - Compliance with and Effect of Traffic Rules

The provisions of N.Y.C. Traffic Rules are applicable to bicycles and their operators.

4-07 (c)(3) - Restrictions on crossing sidewalks

No driving bikes on sidewalks unless sign allows or wheels are less than 26 inches in diameter and rider is twelve years or younger. See also *Administrative Code §19-176.*

4-08 (e)(9) - Stopping, standing and parking prohibited in specified places

No parking, standing or stopping vehicles within or otherwise obstructing bike lanes.

4-12 (e) - Driver's hand on steering device

Driver of a bicycle must have hand on steering device or handlebars.

4-12 (h) - Reporting accidents by drivers of other than motor vehicles

Rider involved in accident resulting in death or injury to person or damage to property must stop and give name, address, insurance information, etc., and must report to Police Department.

4-12 (o)(1) - Use of Roadways

Bicycles are prohibited on expressways, drives, highways, interstate routes, bridges and thruways, unless authorized by signs.

4-12 (p) - Bicycles

Bicycle riders must use bike path/lane, if provided, except for access, safety, turns, etc. Other vehicles shall not drive on or across bike lanes except for access, safety, turns, etc. Bicyclists may use either side of a 40-foot wide one-way roadway.

4-14 (c) - Restricted areas of parks

No person shall ride a bicycle in any park, except in places designated for bike riding; but persons may push bikes in single file to and from such places, except on beaches and boardwalks.

N.Y.C. Administrative Code

10-157 - Bicycles used for commercial purposes

- Business must be identified on the bike by name and identification number.
- Operator must wear upper body apparel with business' name and operator's number on the back.
- Business must provide operator with a helmet according to A.N.S.I. or Snell standards.
- Operator shall wear a helmet provided by business.
- Operator must carry and produce on demand a numbered ID card with operator's photo, name, home address and business' name, address and phone number.
- Business must maintain log book that includes the name, identification number and place of residence of each bicycle operator; and the date of employment and discharge. The log book must also include information on daily trips, identifying the bicycle operator's identification number and name; and name and place of origin and destination.
- Owner of business must file an annual report with the Police Department identifying the number of bicycles it owns and the identification number and identity of any employees.

19-176 - Bicycles operation on sidewalks prohibited

Bicycles ridden on sidewalks may be confiscated and riders may be subject to legal sanctions. See also *N.Y.C. Traffic Rules and Regulations §4-07 (c).*

New York State Vehicle And Traffic Law

102-a – Definition of Bicycle Lane
A portion of the roadway which has been designated by stripping, signing and pavement markings for the preferential or exclusive use of bicycles.

102-b – Definition of Bicycle Path
A path physically separated from motorized vehicle traffic by an open space or barrier and either within the highway right–of-way or within an independent right-of-way and which is intended for the use of bicycles.

375(24-a) - Equipment
Rider cannot wear more than one earphone attached to radio, tape player or other audio device while riding.

1231 - Traffic Laws Applicable to Persons Riding Bicycles
Bicyclists are granted all rights and subject to all duties applicable to operator of vehicle except where not applicable.

1232 - Riding on Bicycles
- Must ride on a permanent seat;
- Feet must be on pedals;
- Bike must carry only number of persons for which it is designed and equipped.

1233 - Clinging to vehicles
No attaching bike or person to another vehicle being operated on the roadway.

1234 - Riding on roadways, shoulders, bicycle lanes and bicycle paths
- Must ride bicycle on the right side of the roadway (some conditions and exceptions apply - see also *N.Y.C. Traffic Rules and Regulations Section 4-12* above)
- No more than two abreast. *1235 - Carrying articles*. Rider must keep at least one hand on handlebars when carrying packages.

1236 - Lamps and other equipment
- White headlight and red taillight must be used from dusk to dawn.
- Bell or other audible signal (not whistle) required
- Working brakes required
- Reflective tires and/or other reflective devices required.

1237 - Hand and arm signals

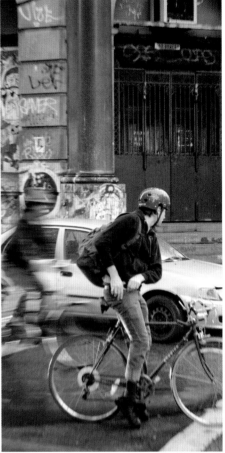

Photo Matt Wittmer

- Bicyclists are required to use hand signals to turn left and right and to stop or decrease speed
- Rider can use either hand to signal a right turn.

1238 - Helmets and carrying children
- A child under age one is not permitted to ride on a bicycle.
- A child one or more years of age but less than five years of age must wear an approved helmet and be carried in a properly affixed child carrier.
- A child five or more years of age but less than fourteen years of age must wear an approved helmet.

NYC/NY State and NJ Traffic Rules and Regulations continued

New Jersey Cycling Regulations

Bicycling in New Jersey is regulated under Title 39 of the Motor Vehicles and Traffic Regulation laws.

39:4-14.5 Definition

"Bicycle" means any two wheeled vehicle having a rear drive which is solely human powered and having a seat height of 25 inches or greater when the seat is in the lowest adjustable position.

39:4-10 Lights on Bicycles

When in use at nighttime every bicycle shall be equipped with: 1) A front headlamp emitting a white light visible from a distance of at least 500 feet to the front; 2) A rear lamp emitting a red light visible from a distance of at least 500 feet to the rear; 3) In addition to the red lamp a red reflector may be mounted on the rear.

39:4-11 Audible Signal

A bicycle must be equipped with a bell or other audible device that can be heard at least 100 feet away, but not a siren or whistle.

39:4-11.1 Brakes

A bicycle must be equipped with a brake that can make wheels skid while stopping on dry, level, clean pavement.

39:4-12 Feet and Hands on Pedals and Handlebars; Carrying Another Person

Bicyclists should not drive the bicycle with feet removed from the pedals, or with both hands removed from the handlebars, nor practice any trick or fancy driving in a street. Limit passengers to only the number the bicycle is designed and equipped to carry (the number of seats it has).

39:4-14 Hitching on Vehicle Prohibited

No person riding a bicycle shall attach themselves to any streetcar or vehicle.

39:4-14.1 Rights and Duties of Persons on Bicycles

Every person riding a bicycle on a roadway is granted all the rights and subject to all of the duties of the motor vehicle driver.

39:4-14.2, 39:4-10.11 Operating Regulations

Every person riding a bicycle on a roadway shall ride as near to the right roadside as practicable exercising due care when passing a standing vehicle or one proceeding in the same direction. A bicyclist may move left under any of the following conditions: 1) To make a left turn from a left turn lane or pocket; 2) To avoid debris, drains, or other hazardous conditions on the right; 3) To pass a slower moving vehicle; 4) To occupy any available lane when traveling at the same speed as other traffic; 5) To travel no more than two abreast when traffic is not impeded, but otherwise ride in single file. Every person riding a bicycle shall ride in the same direction as vehicular traffic.

In New Jersey, the law states a bicyclist must obey all state and local automobile driving laws. A parent may be held responsible for the child's violation of any traffic law.

Helmet Law

Title 39:4-10.1

In New Jersey, anyone under 17 years of age that rides a bicycle or is a passenger on a bicycle, or is towed as a passenger by a bicycle must wear a safety helmet.

On August 1, 1998 this helmet law was extended to include roller and inline skates and skateboards. Roller skates means a pair of devices worn on the feet with a set of wheels attached, regardless of the number or placement of those wheels and used to glide or propel the user over the ground.

The definition of bicycle with reference to the helmet legislation is a vehicle with two wheels propelled solely by human power and having pedals, handle bars and a saddle-like seat. The term shall include a bicycle for two or more persons having seats and corresponding pedals arranged in tandem.

All helmets must be properly fastened and fitted. Bicycle helmets must meet the federal standards de-

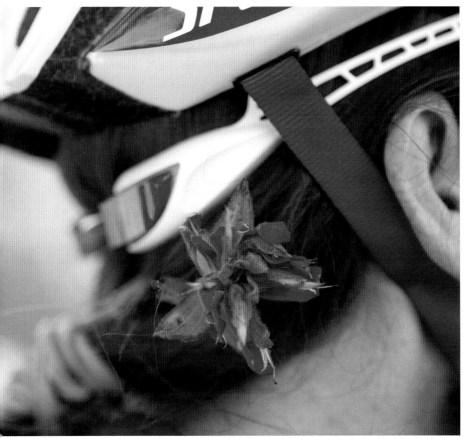

veloped by the Consumer Product Safety Commission (CPSC) effective March 10, 1999 that ensure the best head protection and strong chin straps to keep the helmet in place during a fall or collision. Also acceptable are helmets meeting the Snell Memorial Foundation's 1990 Standard for Protection Headgear.

Exemptions from the helmet requirement are persons who operate or ride a bicycle (as a driver or a passenger) on a roadway closed to motor traffic; on a trail, route, course, boardwalk, path or area set aside only for the use of bicycles. These exemptions do not apply if the areas of operation are adjacent to a roadway and not separated from motor vehicle traffic by a barrier that prevents the bicycle from entering the roadway. Bicyclists or passengers operating in an area where helmets are not required who need to cross a road or highway should walk with the bicycle.

Initial violators of the helmet law will receive warnings. For minors, the parent or legal guardian may be fined a maximum of $25 for the first offense and a maximum of $100 for subsequent offense(s), if lack of parental supervision contributed to the offense.

Bicycle salespersons and rental agents must display a sign at least 15 inches long and eight inches wide at the point where the transaction is completed when they sell or rent a bicycle. This sign should read: "STATE LAW REQUIRES A BICYCLE RIDER UNDER 17 YEARS TO WEAR A HELMET." In the case of bicycle rentals, the salesperson/rental agent must provide a helmet, if necessary, for a fee.

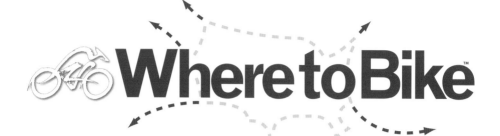

Where to Bike™

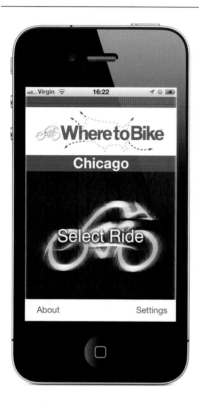

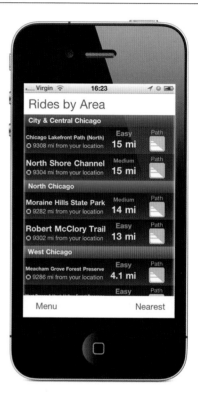

Getting Started

Step 1. Download the *Where to Bike* app for your city on the iTunes App Store. Once you load the app, you'll see this main page where you can select your ride, learn more about us, or configure settings. In the settings menu you can choose between miles and km, whether you want to display your speed, and whether you'd like a fixed or rotating map.

Select Your Ride

Step 2. Tap 'select ride' from the main screen and you will arrive at this page, where you will see a list of great rides organized into sections. These are the same as you will find in your *Where to Bike* book guide. In the bottom right-hand corner you will also see an option to arrange the rides based on their proximity to your current location.

www.**where**to**bike**guides**.com**

Our *Where to Bike* apps are the perfect companion for your next ride. Don't leave home without it!

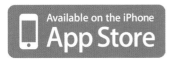 **+** **=**

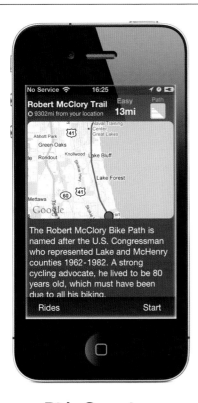

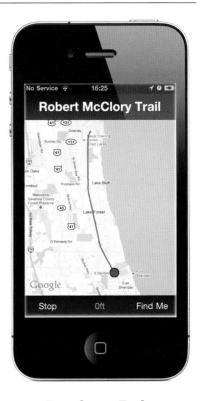

Ride Overview

Step 3. Once you select a ride, you'll be taken to this ride overview screen. Here you'll see a thumbnail map of the route, and a short description of the ride. You will also see important information such as ride difficulty, total distance, as well as how far you currently are from start of the ride. When you are ready, tap the 'Start' button to commence the ride.

Ready to Ride

Step 4. Now you are ready to ride, it really is that simple! Your current position will be displayed by the red dot icon. You can slide your finger to scroll anywhere on the map, and if you lose your place, simply tap 'Find Me' to return to the ride route. If you feel like taking a break, simply tap the 'stop' button and you can continue again whenever you like. Have fun!

Find us on the iTunes App Store!

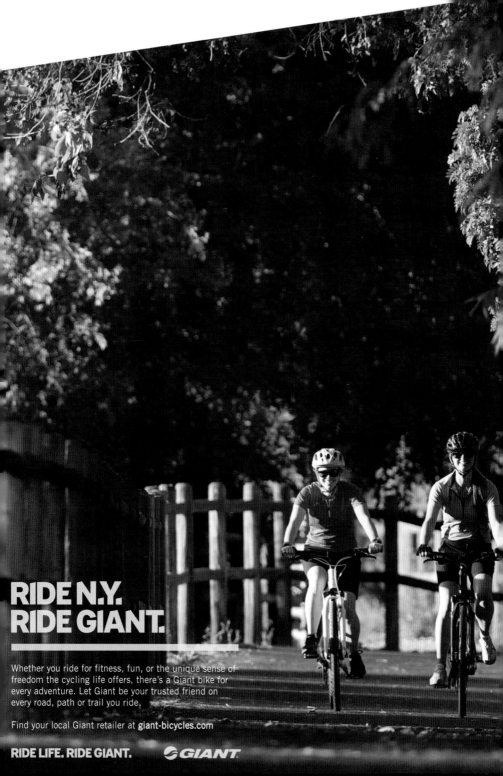

RIDE N.Y.
RIDE GIANT.

Whether you ride for fitness, fun, or the unique sense of freedom the cycling life offers, there's a Giant bike for every adventure. Let Giant be your trusted friend on every road, path or trail you ride.

Find your local Giant retailer at **giant-bicycles.com**

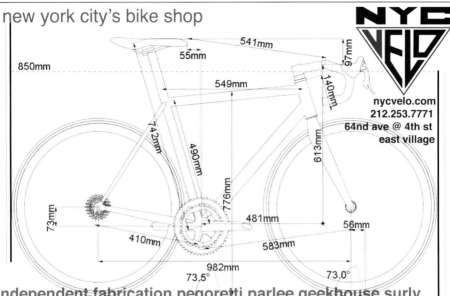
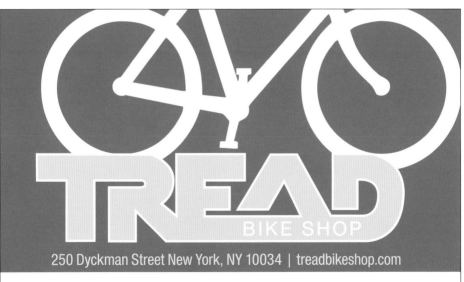

Manhattan

While New York might have the most diverse population of any city in the world, it is not immune to the lures of provincialism. As Manhattan is my home province, I hope my location hasn't clouded my judgment. It's a great place to ride. Hyper-urban it is, but it's also very flat and dense and actually very easy for cyclists. In my estimation, the easiest borough to ride in.

It's striking that the most urban borough also has the longest car-free bike paths in the city. Part of the reason is luck; Central Park was built before cars and has been taken over by New Yorkers keen on creating a real separation from the hyper-urban environment just outside of the park walls. The other is that it was here in Manhattan where the idea of creating a greenway that rings the island between the roads and the rivers first took root.

Because the greenway is effectively near just about everyone in Manhattan – it is a long narrow island – just about all the rides make their way to the water and travel alongside it for at least a short stretch. Rides that take you to the water have other advantages; no cars to contend with and relatively few pedestrians, as it's much harder for them to get to the water than it is for cyclists. And for the more popular sections of the West Side path, there are separated pedestrian walkways that mean fewer worries.

Because of the density, this is the first borough amongst equals where riding to the ride is a good idea. As a result, you're going to be doing some street riding regardless of what you take in. The seeming chaos can be overwhelming, but taken in small doses, you can experience it, start seeing patterns, and learn how to safely surf the sea of traffic and distractions that occur on the road.

There is so much to see and do in Manhattan; I had trouble even making a small selection of non-bike activities. My bias for rides is to ride first, experience the city from the saddle, and save museums, performance halls, and the like for times when your purpose is to drink in indoor culture.

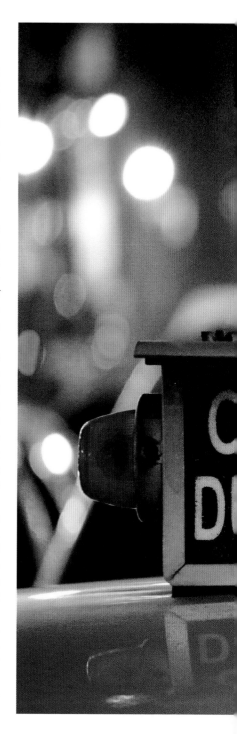

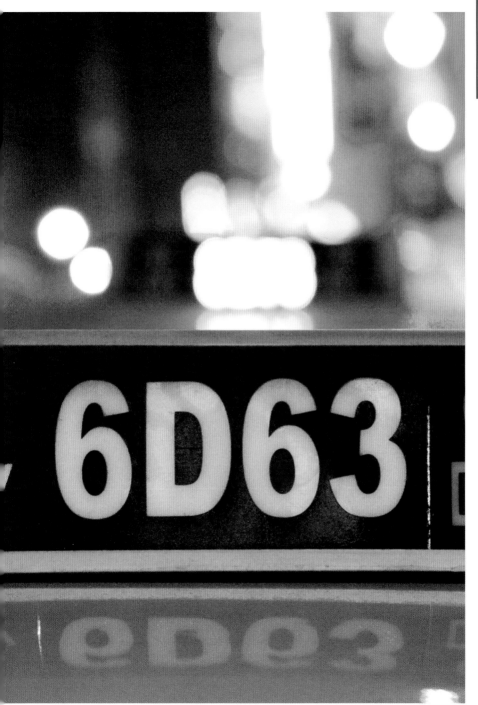

Photo Matt Wittmer

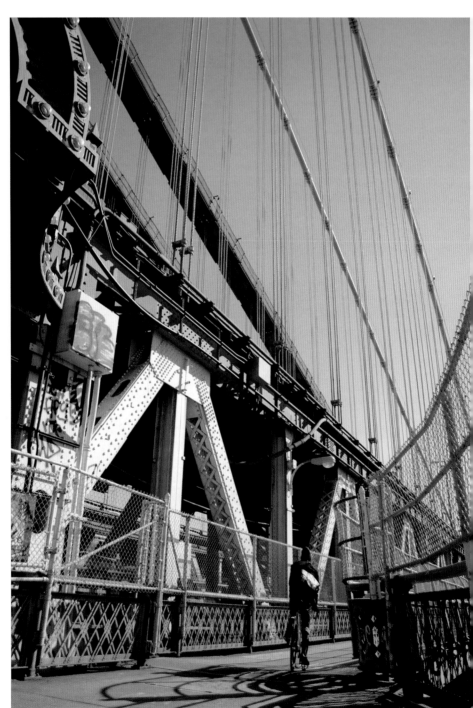

Photo Matt Wittmer

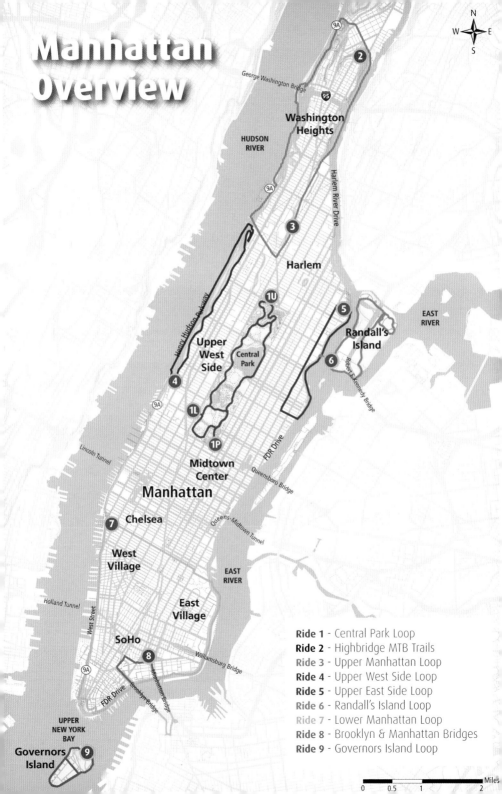

Manhattan Overview

N W-E S

9A

2

George Washington Bridge

95

HUDSON RIVER

Washington Heights

9A

Harlem River Drive

Harlem

3

1U

5

Randall's Island

EAST RIVER

Upper West Side

Central Park

4

Henry Hudson Parkway

Robert F. Kennedy Bridge

6

9A

1L

1P

Midtown Center

FDR Drive

Lincoln Tunnel

Queensboro Bridge

Manhattan

7 **Chelsea**

Queens–Midtown Tunnel

West Village

Holland Tunnel

EAST RIVER

East Village

West Street

SoHo

8

9A

Williamsburg Bridge

FDR Drive

Brooklyn Bridge

UPPER NEW YORK BAY

Governors Island

9

Ride 1 - Central Park Loop
Ride 2 - Highbridge MTB Trails
Ride 3 - Upper Manhattan Loop
Ride 4 - Upper West Side Loop
Ride 5 - Upper East Side Loop
Ride 6 - Randall's Island Loop
Ride 7 - Lower Manhattan Loop
Ride 8 - Brooklyn & Manhattan Bridges
Ride 9 - Governors Island Loop

Miles
0   0.5   1   2

Central Park Loops Ride 1

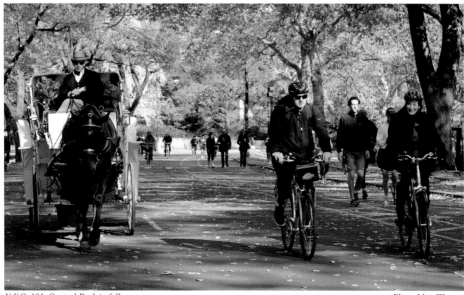

N.Y.C. 101, Central Park in fall. *Photo Matt Wittmer*

At a Glance

Distance Long Loop: 6.7 miles,
Lower Loop: 1.9 miles, **Upper Loop:** 1.4 miles
Total Elevation Long Loop: 560',
Lower Loop: 149', **Upper Loop:** 157'

Terrain
Ring park paths in good condition.

Traffic
Central Park is completely closed to car traffic much of the time—on weekends and official New York City holidays, and from 7pm to 7am weekdays. The park is open to southbound traffic from 7am to 10am and open to northbound traffic from 3pm to 7pm. The northbound section of the park drive from 59th to 72nd is open to traffic from 10am-3pm. Even when the park is completely open to car traffic, there's still a dedicated bike lane. Clueless pedestrians will be your biggest threat.

How to Get There
Located in the middle of Manhattan Island, just about every subway goes there.

Food and Drink
Loeb Boathouse by East 72nd Street is a popular stop, but there are also plenty of food carts along the road and a few cafés in the park as well.

Side Trip
There is no shortage of things to do. From skating to swimming to the Charles Dana Discovery Center at Harlem Meer, to the botanical garden at Fifth Avenue and 100th, SummerStage, and Shakespeare in the Park, there are things to experience year-round in the park.

Where to Bike Rating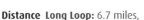

Central Park has extensive auto-free hours. See Traffic above.

About...

Central Park is the crown jewel of the New York City Parks System and arguably the premier urban park in the United States of America. Central Park, which opened in 1859, was inspired by parks in London and Paris. The park drives were built for horse-drawn carriages, and shortly after the bicycle first appeared, it was banned from the park. In more recent times, cyclists have helped spur the resurgent popularity of the park.

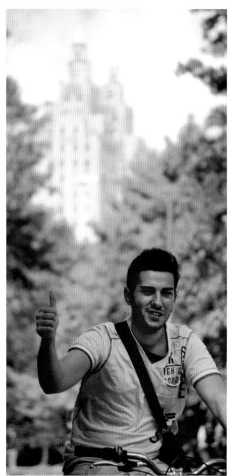

Central Park is designed so well that thousands of people can be in the park at the same time and there's still plenty of room for bike riding. People commuting, out for a little air, exercising, and training for bicycle races and triathlons can all do their thing and rarely get in each other's way. Cyclists first start filtering into the park around 5am, and you can find them riding around until midnight just about every day of the year. That the road is lit makes it a great place to get some nighttime exercise in a very safe environment.

Thumbs up, indeed.   *Photo Matt Wittmer*

The park drive winds through a number of different environments and gives the cyclists plenty to see. It's hard to get bored when you can change your focus from watching people to admiring architecture to checking out the skyline to looking out over fields and lakes or pondering what's going on inside dense forests, all in the space of a few minutes.

If there's a drawback to Central Park, this book is only going to make it worse. The park is incredibly popular. Go for a ride on a summer Saturday afternoon, and it can feel like you're expending more energy dodging people than riding your bike.

Central Park is one ride, but there are four common routes inside it. The first is the Long Loop. For the sake of variety, we have this starting at Grand Army Plaza at the corner of 60th Street and Fifth Avenue. On this loop, you'll encounter the other three loops in the park. The shortest loop is the Upper Loop, which goes around the North Woods and starts at 110th Street and Adam Clayton Powell Boulevard. Next is the Lower Loop that goes around the south end of the park. We started this ride at 67th Street and Central Park West. The final sub-ride is the 5.2 mile loop, which is the ride people do when they want to skip the big hill, which many racers call 110berg. We start this ride at 100th Street and Central Park West.

Ride Log

0.0 Start at Grand Army Plaza and head into the park along the one road you see.

0.3 Join the park drive proper heading north.

0.7 Pass 72nd St transverse. Go straight to do the whole loop, turn left to do the lower loop.

0.8 Pass Loeb Boathouse. There's a bathroom here as well as a cafeteria, a sit-down restaurant, and a bike rental operation.

2.5 Pass the 104th St transverse. If you want to do the 5.2 mile loop and skip the hill, turn left here.

3.1 This is the northern edge of Central Park. We start the Northern Loop here. If you stay on the park road, you'll start to climb the big hill. If you exit the park, you can get on the bike path that will take you to the northern end of Manhattan Island.

3.8 This is the 100th St entrance to the park. We start the 5.2 mile loop here.

4.8 Look to your left and you'll see a building that houses bathrooms. Beyond it is the Delacorte theatre, where Shakespeare in the Park takes place.

5.4 Strawberry Fields is on your right. Coming up on your left is the 72nd St transverse where you'd be coming from if you took the lower loop ride.

5.6 This is the 67th St entrance to the park where we started our Lower Loop ride.

6.0 This is the Seventh Ave exit to the park. You're now at the south end of Central Park and will start heading north.

6.4 You'll see the park road where you started on your right. Make the hard right turn to go back to Grand Army Plaza.

6.7 Finish at Grand Army Plaza.

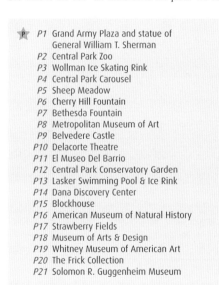

P1 Grand Army Plaza and statue of General William T. Sherman
P2 Central Park Zoo
P3 Wollman Ice Skating Rink
P4 Central Park Carousel
P5 Sheep Meadow
P6 Cherry Hill Fountain
P7 Bethesda Fountain
P8 Metropolitan Museum of Art
P9 Belvedere Castle
P10 Delacorte Theatre
P11 El Museo Del Barrio
P12 Central Park Conservatory Garden
P13 Lasker Swimming Pool & Ice Rink
P14 Dana Discovery Center
P15 Blockhouse
P16 American Museum of Natural History
P17 Strawberry Fields
P18 Museum of Arts & Design
P19 Whitney Museum of American Art
P20 The Frick Collection
P21 Solomon R. Guggenheim Museum

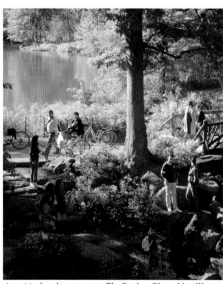

A positively sylvan scene at The Pool.   *Photo Matt Wittmer*

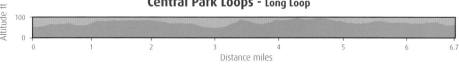

Central Park Loops - Long Loop

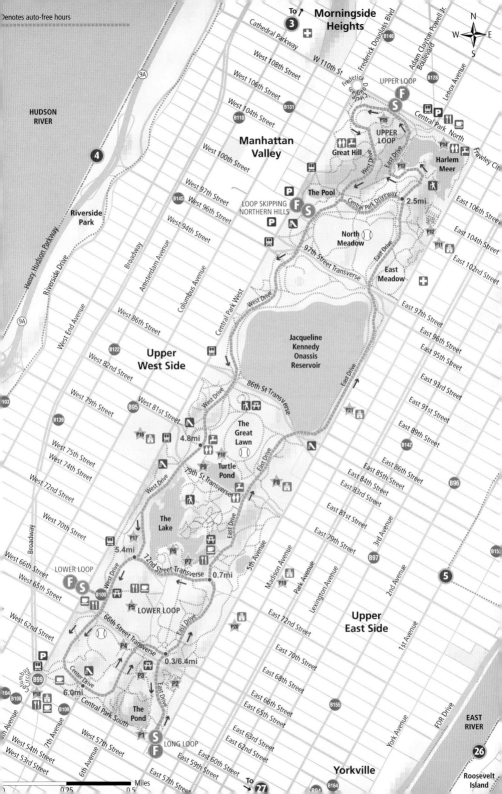

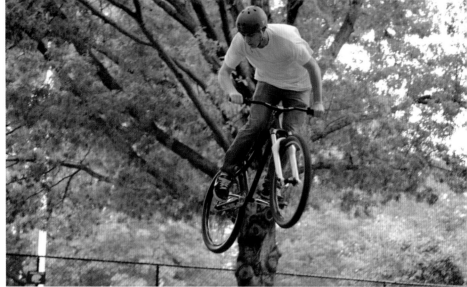

Mile high at Highbridge.   Photo Matt Wittmer

At a Glance

Distance Dirt Jump Loop: 0.2 mile,
MTB Loop One: 0.2 mile, **MTB Loop Two:** 0.7 mile
Total Elevation Dirt Jump Loop: 54',
MTB Loop One: 119', **MTB Loop Two:** 124'

Terrain
Smooth dirt trails.

Traffic
None.

How to Get There
The 1 train stop at Dyckman Street is the closest subway stop, though you'll have to ride up the steep Fort George Hill to get to Highbridge Park or ride to the eastern end of Dyckman and try to climb the trails there—know that these trails are steep and rooty.

Food and Drink
There are no shortage of Latin American restaurants along Nagle Avenue right after you get off the train. The nearest and simplest food is the 24 7 Deli Grocery at the intersection of Fort George Hill and St. Nicholas Avenue.

Side Trip
If you go down the hill and cross the Harlem River Drive, you're just up the greenway from Swindler Cove Park. The park, part of the New York Restoration Project, has salt marshes and a forest. Open seven days a week from 8am-4pm, save holidays.

Links to ❸

Where to Bike Rating

About...

Highbridge is a deceptive park. Considering that it is a few miles long, there's very little room for riding. That's because most of the park is a ridge; a little space before a cliff that falls down to the Harlem River Drive. Still, there is a network of paved and unpaved trails and atop the ridge at the north end are the Highbridge trails.

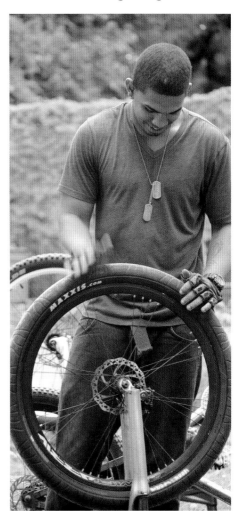

Fat tires make fast friends here off Fort George Avenue. Photo Matt Wittmer

There is an irony to riding trails in Highbridge Park. Just below is the Harlem River Drive, once known as the Harlem Speedway. The Speedway was a popular site for bicycle racing in the heady early days of the sport. Bicycles supplanted horses back then. And cars have supplanted bikes. Now bikes are allowed between the Harlem River Drive and the Harlem River along the greenway and here in the park above.

The trails in Highbridge, few in number, short, and relatively simple, undermine the difficulty of getting them built and the importance of them. The Highbridge mountain bike trails were the first MTB trails to be approved and allowed by the New York City Parks Department.

As written above, riding on these trails is allowed by the Parks Department. The New York City Mountain Bike Association built the trails and maintains them, as they do all the official N.Y.C. MTB trails. If you find you love urban mountain biking, volunteer to help them in their mission.

While the park has beginner, intermediate, and advanced trails and a dirt-jump park, noobs should stick to the beginner's trails at the top of the park. They should also work on balance skills in the dirt jump

park, though only when it is on the empty side of things most of the time. You can go down the hill for the intermediate trails and link up to a small lower loop of beginners trails, including a skills loop, but we found it pretty easy to accidentally end up on an expert trail or the short double black-diamond drop.

Yes, these trails are short, only three miles of trails if you ride every one, but if you want to get a taste of mountain biking or work on your skills, the convenience these trails offer is hard to beat.

Ride Log

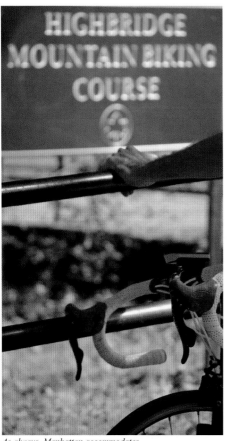

Enter the dirt jump park on Fort George Ave across the street from Javits Athletic field and next to the baseball field.

All three rides start and finish on the edge of the dirt jump park. There is a trail map at the trailhead. The map is quite clear and the trails are marked, at least at the start; it can get confusing in the woods. Know that the trails for expert riders call for full-suspension mountain bikes with several inches of travel. But you'll figure out which these are pretty quick as they have very steep drop-offs. So long as you stay away from pointing your bike down a steep trail, you'll be fine.

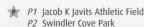

P1 Jacob K Javits Athletic Field
P2 Swindler Cove Park

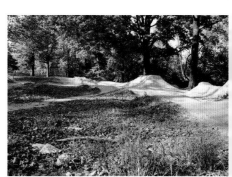

Dirt Jump Park.

As always, Manhattan accommodates.
Photo Matt Wittmer

Highbridge MTB Trails - Loop One

Highbridge MTB Trails - Loop Two

Altitude ft

Distance miles

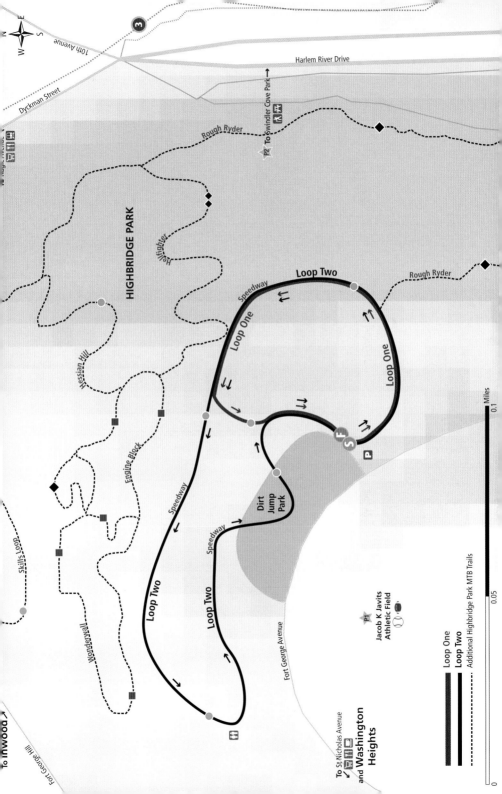

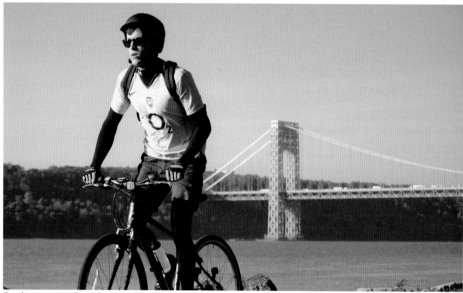

Breaking away on the upper Upper West Side.

Photo Matt Wittmer

At a Glance

Distance 9.4 miles   **Total Elevation** 605′

Terrain

Hilly bike paths and streets. There are stairs to climb and some tricky twists and turns.

Traffic

Varied. Very few people typically on bike paths, to busy on 125th and Dyckman.

How to Get There

The B and C trains stop just underneath the start of this ride, but the ride is easily accessible via the A, D, 1, 2, and 3 trains as well.

Food and Drink

Dyckman Street and 125th Street are fairly busy commercial corridors, so you'll have your choice of fast food joints, pizza places, Chinese food, and even gour-met offerings (Fairway is on the path by 132nd Street and the Hudson River).

Side Trip

If you make a right on Seaman Avenue and take it less than a mile, you'll come to Inwood Hill Park. Great place for picnicking, silent contemplation and hiking, it also has plenty of open grounds, courts and fields.

Links to

Where to Bike Rating

About...

This ride is a study in contrasts. The greenway segments along the Harlem and Hudson rivers are amongst the least utilized greenway paths on Manhattan Island. Riding along Dyckman and 125th shows Manhattan at its most commercial.

The Manhattan Waterfront Greenway is good and getting better all the time. Eventually, this greenway will encompass the entire perimeter of Manhattan Island, but for now, it exists in sections with some on-street linkages. Indeed, we take advantage of the greenway for many rides.

This is probably our favorite greenway loop. Even though the ride takes in some busy roads, the greenway sections are so quiet they more than make up for the car traffic on the street.

We're on this loop a few times a month. Our favorite section is the part along the Harlem River, as we usually have it to ourselves and because it parallels a bit of New York City cycling history, as the Harlem River Drive from north of the exit for the George Washington Bridge to Dyckman is the site of the Harlem Speedway, a venue for bicycle racing in the late 19th and early 20th centuries.

There is a short set of stairs to be climbed at the end of Dyckman, and even though the walking is a bit of a hassle, we like the way it feels as if we're climbing into a treehouse. It's rare that we find another person on the stairs or even on the next segment of path. Occasionally, we'll find a musician practicing with his instrument at one of the better vistas that takes in the Hudson and the Palisades.

The descent to the Hudson is also a blast, as the drop feels like you're on a roller coaster coming off a cliff. Once on the water, the view south to the mouth of the

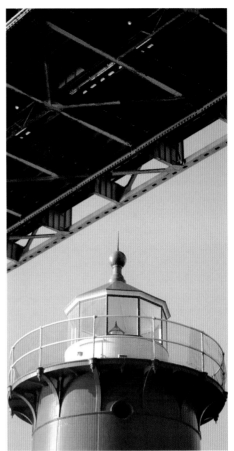

The Little Red Lighthouse beneath the George Washington Bridge. Photo Matt Wittmer

Hudson is usually incredible.

The Hudson River side of the ride, once you get south of the ballfields, can get over-crowded on summer weekends, but with this exception, the path is pretty empty at all times.

And if you want to extend the ride, you can stay on the path down to 96th Street, or further depending on how you're feeling or what kind of time you have. If you want to go longer, you can basically just start doing the reverse of the Riverside Park loop, which is also detailed and take it to 72nd Street, before turning around and heading back north to 125th, and then onto St. Nicholas Park.

Ride Log

0.0 Start where Edgecombe Ave splits from St. Nicholas Ave. Head north. St. Nicholas Park will be on your left.

0.8 Bear right onto St. Nicholas Pl.

1.0 Cross 155th St. There are barriers splitting the bike path from the street. Keep the barriers on your left.

1.3 Slow! To a crawl. You need to make a sharp left across traffic onto a narrow sidewalk that runs alongside an entrance ramp to the Harlem River Dr.

1.6 You're now on the greenway heading north to Dyckman. While the path is narrow, it's almost always empty.

3.2 The path ends. You'll now cross the end of the Harlem River Dr and start riding west on Dyckman St.

3.7 Bear left at light onto Riverside Dr. Fort Tryon Park will be on your left.

4.0 Roll onto the sidewalk to get to the stairs leading to the greenway.

4.1 Dismount bike and walk up gentle steps to greenway. You can roll your bike on the smooth curb on your right or left.

4.1 Start riding south on greenway with Hudson on your right. It's a long, gentle climb.

5.1 If you want to get to Washington Heights or the George Washington Bridge, you can take the bridge over the highway.

5.3 Slow down! You'll be taking a hairpin turn as the

 P1 St. Nicholas Park
P2 The City College of New York
P3 Hamilton Grange National Memorial
P4 Jackie Robinson Park
P5 The Highbridge
P6 Peter Jay Sharp Boathouse
P7 Swindler Cove and Swindler Cove Park
P8 Inwood Plaza
P9 The Cloisters
P10 Fort Washington
P11 Inspiration Point
P12 Little Red Lighthouse
P13 West Harlem Piers Park
P14 The Cotton Club
P15 General Grant National Memorial
P16 Columbia University
P17 Apollo Theatre

road starts to twist and drop precipitously.

5.7 You're down to the Hudson now. If you look to your right, just next to the bridge supports, you'll see the Little Red Lighthouse.

6.8 If you want to leave the park, you can make a left here and start climbing 158th St up to Riverside Dr or Broadway.

7.3 Riverbank State Park is the big structure on your right.

8.0 Turn left onto 125th St. This could be busy, but it's also typically very slow.

8.7 Bear right onto 124th St.

8.8 Turn left onto St. Nicholas Ave.

9.4 Arrive at 135th and St. Nicholas.

Upper Manhattan Loop

Altitude ft / Distance miles

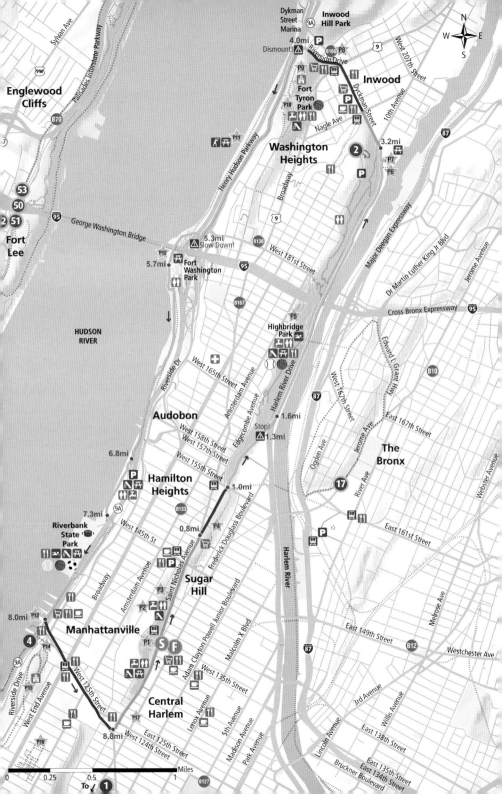

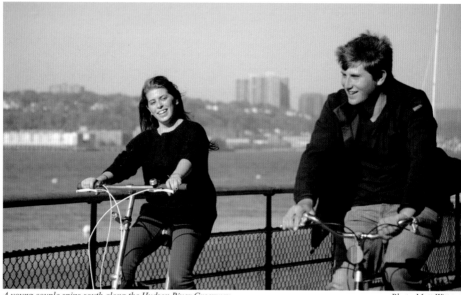

A young couple spins south along the Hudson River Greenway.

Photo Matt Wittmer

At a Glance

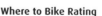

Distance 6.5 miles   **Total Elevation** 372′

Terrain

Flat and rolling bike paths with one big on-street hill.

Traffic

The bike path can get crowded on summer weekends. Riverside Drive is usually lightly trafficked by cars and the occasional bus. The nice thing about Riverside is once you're going south there are only two roads that cross it, 95th and 79th streets.

How to Get There

This loop represents the western edge of both Morningside Heights and the Upper West Side, so for people who live in these neighborhoods, all they have to do is go west. Otherwise, the West Side Greenway takes you there by bike and the 1, 2, and 3 trains get you very close; take them to Broadway and 72nd.

Food and Drink

There's a seasonal café at the 79th Street boat basin, on your trip north. There's a Fairway supermarket just north of the loop at 132nd Street. You can also find a food vendor by the tennis courts at 97th Street. And at 68th Street and the Hudson, there's another seasonal café.

Side Trip

On summer weekends, there are free kayak lessons at 72nd Street and the river. Check out **www.downtownboathouse.org.**

Links to ③

Where to Bike Rating

About...

Riding along the Hudson River is a relaxing experience, and it has gotten easier thanks to the new section of bike path that extends over the river just north of 79th Street. Lots of people just go up and back on the greenway path, but our preference is for loops, so we threw in Riverside Drive, one of the best on-street riding roads on Manhattan.

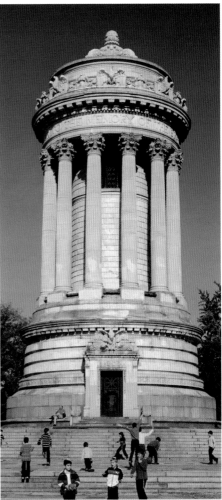

Riverside Park's Soldiers' and Sailors' Memorial.
Photo Matt Wittmer

Riverside Park, despite being in existence since the 19th century, probably only started to match the founding vision of the park within the last 20 years. Even though a train line runs beneath it and a highway through the middle, you can easily forget that you're riding through a major motorized transportation corridor. With the leafy park or the Hudson at your side, the city that never sleeps seems miles away even though it's just out of sight. The path along the river is dead flat and Riverside Drive is rolling.

Circumnavigating the park would be a very easy ride if not for the big hill we threw in at the north end. The Riverside Drive climb to Grant's Tomb is one of the hardest hills on Manhattan Island. Still, we like this hill as a reminder that the city isn't flat and that glacial outcroppings form much of the topography of the upper part of the island. If you have to walk the hill, just roll to the sidewalk and start hoofing it; the tomb is worth it.

We love riding around Grant's Tomb, the final resting place of President and Mrs. Grant, and a popular cycling spot dating back to the 19th century. There's an annual race around the tomb put on by the Columbia University cycling team, and it's a great training spot

for racers as well, easy riding so long as it's not during the morning or evening rush. The tomb itself hosts concerts in the summer. (And for the record, nobody is buried in Grant's Tomb).

Before the city got into building off-street bike paths, Riverside Drive was one of the easiest places to ride in the city. You can take it from 72nd to 165th Street, which is what countless cyclists do when they're fixing to ride over to New Jersey via the George Washington Bridge.

Ride Log

0.0 Start at the Eleanor Roosevelt monument just inside the park at West 72nd St and Riverside Dr. You'll roll onto the sidewalk and around Mrs. Roosevelt. As this is the park entrance for everybody, take it easy. Ride west towards the Hudson River. Start going downhill.

0.2 Bear right on path. Still descending.

0.3 Arrive at Hudson, turn right to go north.

3.1 Turn right. Be careful here, as you'll be crossing an on-ramp to the West Side Dr.

3.2 Turn right onto Riverside Dr. Here's the big hill. Put the bike in its lowest gear.

3.5 Turn right onto Riverside Dr proper. Grant's Tomb is across the street. At your first opportunity, get in the left-hand lane.

3.6 Turn left to make U-turn and start heading south.

5.3 Cross 95th St. If you want, you can bear right and ride into Riverside Park here.

6.2 Cross 79th St. Here, too, you can make a right and go into the park. This time, however, you're riding on the road, and there are both on and off ramps to the west side highway.

6.5 Back at the Roosevelt monument.

P1 Eleanor Roosevelt Monument
P2 79th Street Boat Basin
P3 West Harlem Piers Park
P4 The Cotton Club
P5 General Grant National Memorial
P6 Manhattan School of Music
P7 The Riverside Church
P8 Columbia University
P9 Cathedral of St. John the Divine
P10 Soldiers' and Sailors' Monument

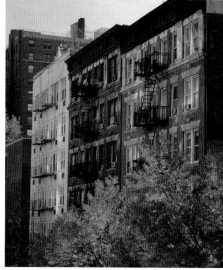

Seasonal glow on the Upper West Side.
Photo Matt Wittmer

Upper West Side Loop

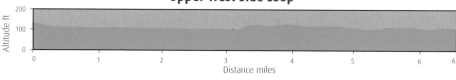

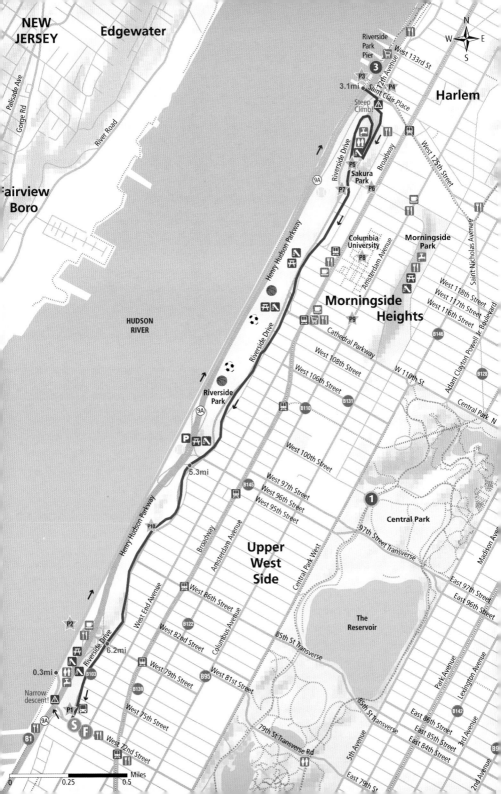

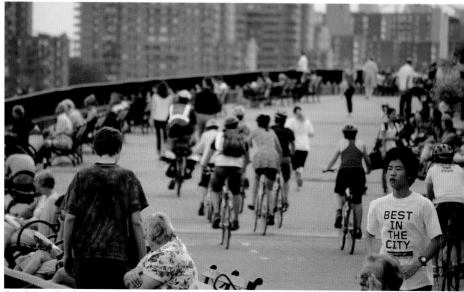

Join the crowd at Carl Schurz Park.

Photo Matt Wittmer

At a Glance

Distance 4.9 miles   **Total Elevation** 126′

Terrain

Flat city streets with bike lanes and some greenway loop. A few stairs to negotiate.

Traffic

Varied. Half the loop, the river half, is free from car traffic. The other half is on city streets, where you'll be riding in a protected bike lane.

How to Get There

You can take the 4, 5, and 6 trains to 125th Street and Lexington Avenue and ride down to 120th on Lex. You can also take Metro-North to the 125th Street-Harlem stop, though you'll need a bike pass for it. Metro-North is on Park. Just ride down to 120th on it.

Food and Drink

There is no shortage of coffee shops, bagel joints, res-taurants, and delicatessens along First Avenue. The culinary star along this avenue is probably Patsy's Pizzeria at 2287 First Avenue, between 117th and 118th streets. You'll probably have to lock your bike outside.

Side Trip

Gracie Mansion, located in Carl Schurz Park. The official residence of the city's mayor since 1942, it is also a historic home, built in the federal style in 1799 at a spot on the shore of the East River overlooking Hell-gate. There are tours on Wednesdays. Call ahead for a reservation; dial 311.

Links to

Where to Bike Rating

About...

This ride displays the contrasts of the Upper East Side, with the high-tone apartments along the East River on one end of the scale, and the developing East Harlem along First Avenue on the other. This loop will serve up opportunities that only New York can. Pleasant riverside stops, a gourmet feast or quick N.Y. bite, and some historical architecture just to round off a perfect day on the bike.

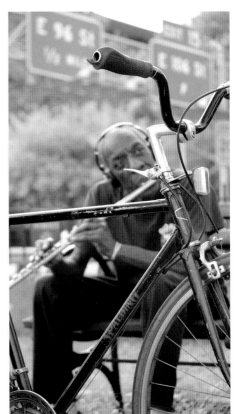

A flutist with his bicycle in East Harlem.
Photo Matt Wittmer

We're looking forward to the day when we can circumnavigate the island entirely on bike paths. The west side is just about done; the east side has a long way to go.

This is a very simple ride. It would be perfect for virgin bike riders, if it weren't for the two-mile stretch along First Avenue, which calls for the usual attention needed for navigating city streets, even with a bike lane to ride in.

This loop starts on the East River, takes you from Randall's Island down as far as you can go without climbing lots of stairs. The river section north of Gracie Mansion is typically empty, and the benches facing the river and the piers, of which you pass two, invite stopping.

Carl Schurz Park, home of Gracie Mansion, is a pleasant little diversion. The park and the site of the mansion itself, was, thanks to its position on the river, a strategically important location for General George Washington. While he did stay there, the building he used was torched by the British when they overran the city. The current mansion was build after the Revolutionary War.

Watching the East River south of Hellgate and north of the 59th Street Bridge is fascinating, as you can see the strong currents that dominate this tidal strait. Even big boats seem to have difficulty fighting the current.

Being a cyclist, the river can hold your attention for only so long. You have to get back in the saddle. Just before you come to a long staircase, you turn right and go down a few steps to East 81st and then you head west before turning north. First Avenue displays many phases of urban planning and how city planners saw the city or didn't. You start with luxury high rises, but then pass old tenement buildings, modern mixed income housing, and classic city housing projects. Which ever way your taste leans, enjoy exploring the contrast and diversity of this area on two wheels.

Ride Log

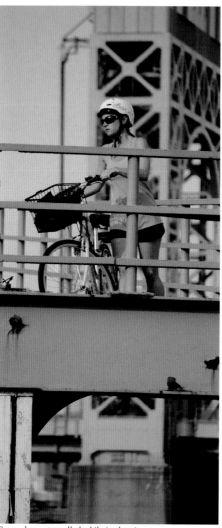

Some choose to walk the bike/pedestrian overpass.
Photo Matt Wittmer

0.0 Start at East 120th St and Paladino Ave. Head for the bike/pedestrian bridge and climb it.

0.2 You're on the greenway. Head south, with the river on your left.

1.1 Pass under bike/pedestrian bridge to Randall's Island

1.9 Enter Carl Schurz Park.

2.6 Turn right out of the park and onto East 81st St.

2.7 Turn right onto First Ave.

4.8 Turn right onto East 120th St.

4.9 End where you began, East 120th and Paladino.

P1 Jefferson Park
P2 Mill Rock Park
P3 Asphalt Green
P4 Gracie Mansion
P5 Carl Schurz Park

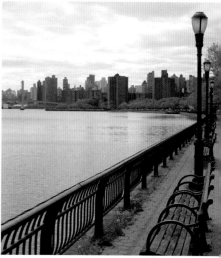

The view downtown

Upper East Side Loop

Altitude ft

100

0

0   1   2   3   4   4.5

Distance miles

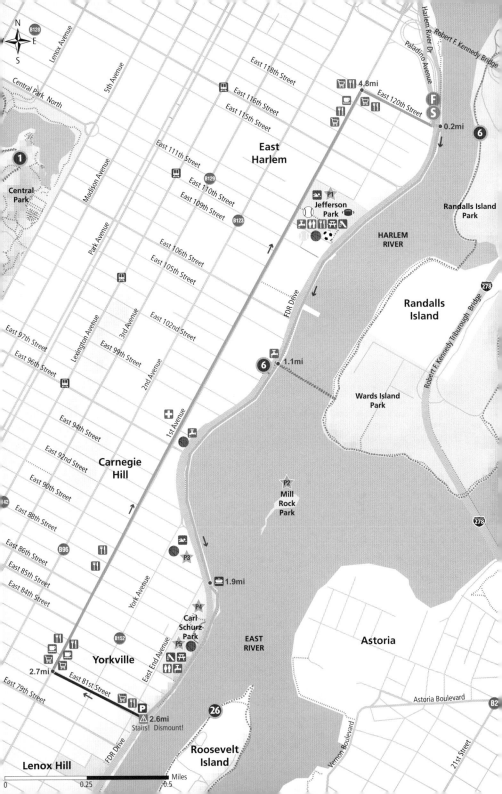

Randall's Island Loop

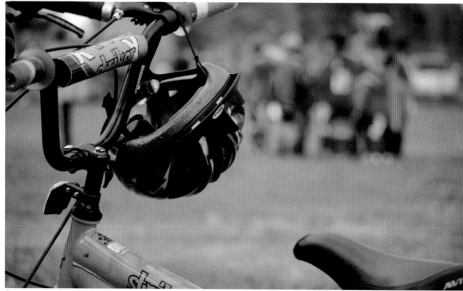

Recreation is this island's new middle name.

Photo Matt Wittmer

At a Glance

Distance 5.4 miles   **Total Elevation** 213'

Terrain

Flat bike paths and access roads. Some pathways may still be under construction.

Traffic

Light. Much of the ride, you'll be on mixed-use paths, sharing space with cyclists and pedestrians. For the rest of the ride, you'll be on access roads where cars are driving pretty slowly.

How to Get There

The ride starts about a block north of the eastern end of East 102nd Street where it stops at the FDR Drive. You can take the 6 train to Lexington Avenue and 103rd Street, exit the subway at 103rd, ride down Lex one block, make a left onto 102nd and go from there. When 102nd turns right to parallel the FDR Drive, get off your bike, lift it over the curb, and ride about one block to the bike/pedestrian bridge over the drive.

Food and Drink

There are food vendor carts typically set up around the island near places the vendors think people congregate. There are also small cafés at both the golf center on the west side of the island and the tennis center on the east. The golf center also has a small beer garden.

Side Trip

The Randall's Island Golf Center has a 36-hole miniature golf course, which is big enough to keep the tee times from backing up.

www.randallsislandgolfcenter.com

Links to 5

Where to Bike Rating

About...

Randall's Island is what happens when a city can't expand; undesirable space eventually becomes desirable. Most people probably know the island for the bridge that uses the island to help join three boroughs. And while the Manhattan Psychiatric Center may dominate the island with a long history, here the playgrounds are what the island is nowadays known for. Luckily, for cyclists, there's plenty of space for us to do our thing without being in the way, or even noticed.

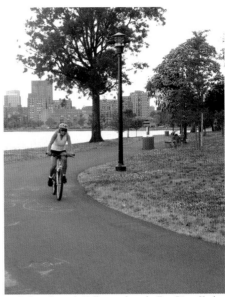

Riding alongside Hellgate, where the East River, Harlem River, and Long Island Sound meet and create viciously strong currents.

Technically, Randall's Island is the northern half of the island, with Ward's Island being the southern half. The two were joined by landfill more than a half-century ago, though there's still an inlet marking the differences on the western side. Baseball fields have long been a part of the scene, but with time doing its thing, the park has recently been upgraded, and there are plenty of soccer fields as well, a tennis center and driving range, and Icahn Stadium, a venue for international-class track and field events. The performance spaces and concert venue are world class with Circque de Soleil also taking residence here.

Despite being underneath busy bridges, Randall's feels pretty quiet most of the time. Lots of water and open space seems to dissipate the hum of automotive traffic and the waters have a calming effect. It's pretty cool to watch the current change at Hellgate on the southern end closest to Astoria, Queens.

The riding here is relatively flat and mostly on bike paths. The only hills of note are the bridges that take you to and from the island. By the time this is published, there will almost certainly be more bike paths on the island than there were at the time of writing. Still, it's a small island, so even if you find yourself

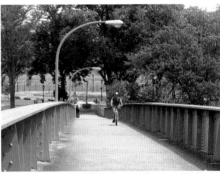

Riding back over the bridge that goes from east 104th street to Randall's Island.

detouring to check them all out, you can't get lost for more than a few minutes.

We've started and finished this route on the 103rd Street pedestrian bridge in Manhattan; Randall's Island is also accessible via the Robert F. Kennedy (formerly Triborough) Bridge from The Bronx, Manhattan, and Queens. There is bike and pedestrian access on all the spans, and there will be a bridge from east 132nd Street in The Bronx dedicated to human-power in the near future.

Ride Log

P1 Hellgate Railroad Viaduct
P2 Icahn Stadium
P3 John McEnroe Tennis Academy
P4 Sportime Randall's Island
P5 Randall's Island Concert Field
P6 Ward's Island Estuary

0.0 Start at the foot of the 103rd St bridge access ramp on the city side of the East River Dr.

0.3 Arrive on Randall's Island. Turn right to follow bike path.

0.9 Hellgate is on your right. Check out the currents. Sometimes it looks like it's going two different ways at the same time.

1.1 The road forks. The bike path is supposed to bear right at the fork, go up the hill, and then follow under the train trestle. That may or may not be completed by the publication of this book. In the meantime, bear left and follow the road.

1.7 The road ends at a T-intersection. This is Triborough Plaza. Turn right.

2.0 Indoor tennis complex is on your right.

2.3 Turn right. You're entering a newly-created area of the park. You're taking a loop road that goes counter-clockwise around the fields.

3.3 Exit the playing fields loop. Go straight.

3.6 The roads start to get confusing. Stay to the right until after you pass under the Manhattan segment of the Robert F. Kennedy (Triborough) Bridge.

4.4 Turn right and ride over wooden bridge.

4.5 Turn right at end of wooden bridge.

5.1 You've finished the loop. Turn right to go back over the bridge to Manhattan.

5.4 Finish at 103rd S and the FDR Dr. You can ride back to 102nd St or go north a little bit and go west on 104th.

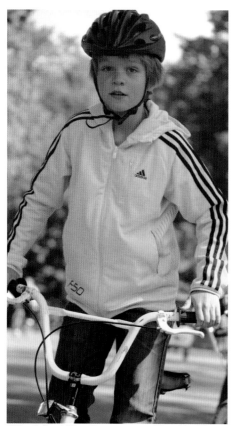

Kids rule Randall's trails.   *Photo Matt Wittmer*

Randall's Island Loop

Altitude ft

Distance miles

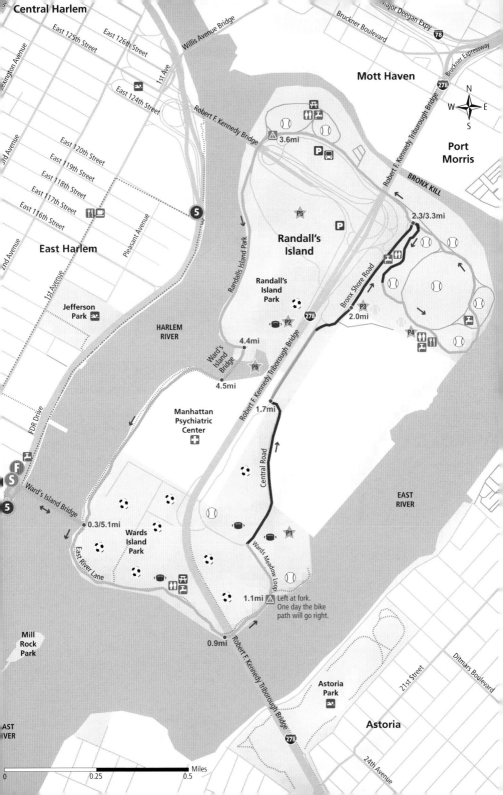

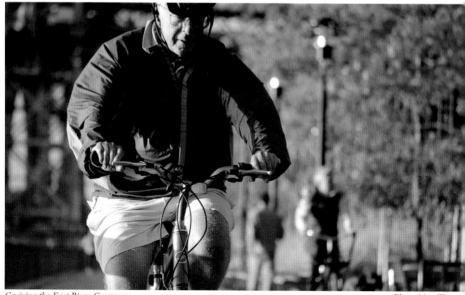

Cruising the East River Greenway.

Photo Matt Wittmer

At a Glance

Distance 9.6 miles   **Total Elevation** 110′

Terrain

Flat streets and bike path.

Traffic

Human-powered traffic for most of the ride, and on the streets traffic is mostly light.

How to Get There

If you're in Manhattan and live north of 21st Street, head south. If you live south of 21st street, head in any direction, you'll eventually link up with this ride. For people who prefer public transit, just about every train line in New York City passes through the lower part of the island. Just take a train and you'll eventually get inside the circle.

Food and Drink

Lower Manhattan's food options are so numerous that we'll simply focus on what's convenient. This loop passes South Street Seaport; the tourist magnet could suck you in. Or, you can find food carts along both the bike paths. Or the carts in front of Battery Park and the Staten Island Ferry terminal. For sit-down, you could stop by Petite Abeille at 20th Street and First Avenue or nosh on a bagel from Ess-a-Bagel at 21st Street and First.

Side Trip

Hudson River Park, which runs from Battery Park to 59th Street along the Hudson, is not only a great playground and a great place to relax, but they have plenty of events, concerts, and films on evenings and weekends all summer long. **www.hudsonriverpark.org.**

Links to

Where to Bike Rating

About...

People love clear sight lines. Maybe it's an evolutionary thing about feeling secure. Riding along the Hudson and East rivers, as this loop does, is calming. And there are plenty of places where you can stop, sit down, lie down, read, or watch the river go by.

The West Side Greenway is the closest thing to a bike highway in New York City. It is said to be the most traveled bike path in the United States. Check it out during the morning and evening rush hours or on summer weekends and you'll agree. You'll probably wonder why the city doesn't widen the path or start turning over streets entirely to bikes.

Both the East and West Side Greenways are great for commuting, sightseeing, and exercise. When it comes to places to go in New York where you can just cruise with your head in the clouds or turned sideways to take in the view over the river, this ride is nearly unparalleled.

There is a marked contrast between the east and west portions of this ride. The east side is both more crowded and less developed. More crowded because of the tourist traps on the East River and because the pathway winds around parking lots and working industrial spaces. And less developed because you can see that the path is a work in progress. Where the path is finished on the east side, it feels immaculate.

In terms of exercise value, fit cyclists who are looking to go hard should probably skip this ride. For them, this loop qualifies as a recovery day. For all other cyclists, this will be good exercise and a decent day's outing.

Riding across the island at 21st Street is much easier than it seems. The only blocks that really have traffic are from Park to Sixth avenues. Both before and after, traffic is pretty light. All the way, you have a marked, on-street bike path.

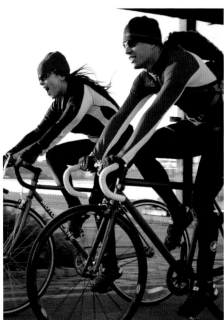

Going fast is fun.　　　　　*Photo Matt Wittmer*

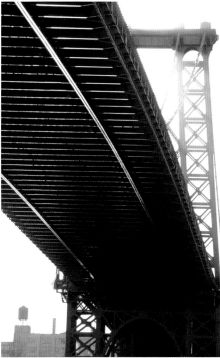

The Manhattan Bridge at dawn.　　　*Photo Matt Wittmer*

Ride Log

P P1 Pier 66 Kayaking
   P2 High Line Park
   P3 Chelsea Market
   P4 The Apple Sculpture
   P5 Pier 40
   P6 Pier 25 Mini Golf
   P7 Governor Nelson A. Rockefeller Park
   P8 National September 11 Memorial
   P9 Battery Place Market
   P10 Castle Clinton
   P11 Battery Park
   P12 New York City Vietnam Veterans
       Memorial Plaza
   P13 South Street Seaport
   P14 Washington Square Park
   P15 Union Square
   P16 Gramercy Park
   P17 Flatiron Building
   P18 Madison Square Park
   P19 Madison Square Garden
   P20 Empire State Building

Who says the city is about conspicuous consumption? These guys rode their bikes to the East River to fish for their food.

0.0 Start at the corner of 10th Ave and 20th St.

0.1 Cross the West Side Hwy. Turn left onto West Side Greenway bike path.

3.3 West Side Greenway ends. You should be able to ride through Battery Park, which is directly in front of you, but the signage can be confusing and the crowds can make riding nearly impossible. Turn left onto Battery Place. Car traffic moves slowly.

3.4 Turn right onto State St with Battery Park remaining on your right.

3.6 State St turns into Water St right in front of the Staten Island Ferry.

3.7 Turn right onto Broad St.

3.8 Turn right onto South St.

3.9 Make U-turn at Whitehall St. You're about to pass the terminal for the Governor's Island Ferry. East Side Greenway bike path starts here.

4.1 The separated bike path begins here, at Old Slip and South St.

5.8 East River Park begins.

6.3 Just after the tennis courts, you'll find some bathrooms tucked away on your right.

7.0 Park ends. Path is pretty narrow for about a block.

7.5 Turn left onto 20th St. There's an on-street bike path and traffic is kind of light.

7.7 Turn right onto First Ave. Get to the left-hand lane immediately, as you'll be making the first left.

7.8 Turn left onto 21st St. There's an on-street bike path on the left side. Take this all the way to 10th Ave.

9.6 End ride at 10th Ave and 21st St.

Lower Manhattan Loop

Altitude ft

Distance miles

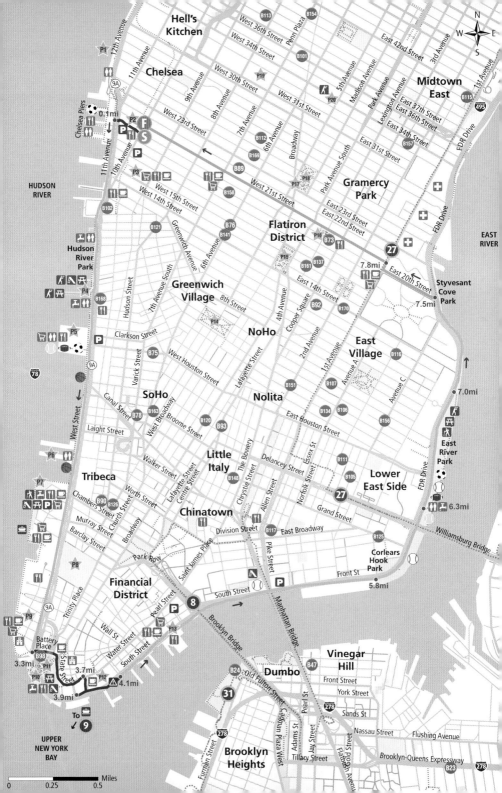

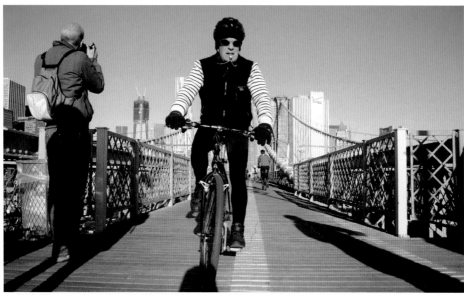

A whistle-blower on the ready on Brooklyn Bridge.   Photo Matt Wittmer

At a Glance

Distance 4.0 miles   **Total Elevation** 199′

Terrain

Hilly streets with some on-road bike paths.

Traffic

Varied. From nearly none to rush hour bustle. The foot traffic can be thick on the Brooklyn Bridge.

How to Get There

Just about every train line passes through Lower Manhattan, and both the East Side and West Side Greenway bike paths have signage leading you to the Brooklyn Bridge. The East Side path also has signage to the Manhattan Bridge.

Food and Drink

Food carts basically line the first few blocks between the Brooklyn Bridge and Worth Street. There is also a permanent food stand/outdoor café just behind the city municipal building at Centre and Reade. Finally, there's Chinatown, which is between Baxter Street and the Manhattan Bridge.

Side Trip

In the middle of Federal Plaza, the green space in front of the court buildings on Centre Street, is a permanent home for Story Corps, an oral history project. Tell your story. You'll need to make a reservation, so be sure to visit **www.storycorps.org**, first.

Links to ⑦ ㉗ ㉛

Where to Bike Rating

About...

Riding over city bridges is one of the many cool things about cycling in New York City. The two most striking water crossings, in my opinion, are the Brooklyn and George Washington bridges, and if you've got a bike and any yen to ride, going over these is an absolute must. The Brooklyn Bridge, riding from the Kings County side, gives you both a great view of the bridge as well as a great view of the canyons of Lower Manhattan.

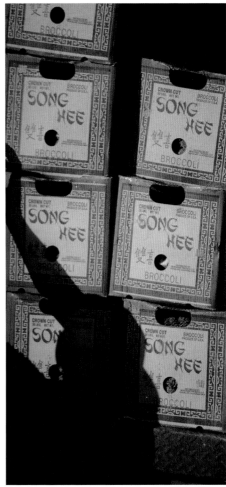

Ever-busy, ever-beguiling Chinatown.   Photo Matt Wittmer

Walking over the Brooklyn Bridge is a popular activity for tourists. There's no reason we should cede this bridge to them. It's our city; let's enjoy all we can of it. It's also a bridge for commuters and exercisers, which is what we cyclists are, too. Still, they might not be ready for us, so we need to ride patiently and politely and forgive the transgresses of the two-footed set. And if you ride it late at night or early in the morning, you'll find out it's for canoodlers, too. Riding over the bridge near sunrise you'll see people stumbling home, or sleeping a night off, or getting that last smooch before returning to their lives. It's as public as a place gets, yet the bridge atmosphere is intimate and personal.

The two bridges are a study in contrasts on many levels. Appearance-wise, they couldn't be more different. The views are equally diverse. Possibly most importantly, the riding conditions are as different as night and day. The Manhattan's path is just for bikes and feels empty. The Brooklyn Bridge is crowded much of the time and you always have to be ready to politely ask pedestrians, tourist gawkers mostly looking for that iconic N.Y.C. image to show their friends, to get out of your way. It is this last reason that many daily cyclists prefer the quietude of the Manhattan over the

chaos of the Brooklyn.

Doing the two bridges in quick succession does prompt a person to ask which style of travel they prefer. We love being able to ride without being disturbed, but the view that the Brooklyn Bridge affords is one we have a hard time passing up.

This ride is essentially two hills. In both cases, the gradient is gentle and the ascent is long. People on single-speed and fixed-gear bikes can do it so long as they're prepared with either a low gear or ready to pedal slowly.

Ride Log

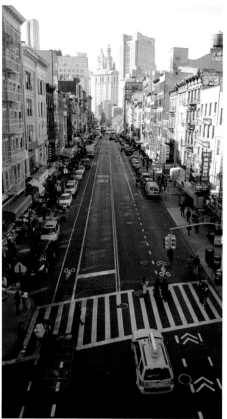

A view down East Broadway off the Manhattan Bridge.
Photo Matt Wittmer

 P1 Korean War Veterans Plaza
P2 Brooklyn War Memorial
P3 PowerHouse Arena
P4 Galapagos Art Space
P5 New York City Hall
P6 Tweed Courthouse
P7 Story Corps Story Booth
P8 United States Court House
P9 US District Court
P10 Chinatown

0.0 Start at the intersection of Canal and Forsyth streets. This is the southern tip of Sara D. Roosevelt Park, where you can find bathrooms. Cross Canal to start the Manhattan Bridge bike path.

1.4 Cross under Manhattan Bridge.

1.4 Exit bike path. Turn left on Jay St. Follow on-street bike path.

1.7 Turn right on Tillary St. Follow on-street bike path.

1.8 Turn right onto Brooklyn Bridge Bike Path. There are two lanes. The right lane is for bicycle traffic. The left for foot traffic.

3.3 Exit the bridge bike path onto Centre St. There's an on-street bike path on the right-hand side.

3.4 Turn right onto Worth St. There's a bike lane as well as signage directing you to the Manhattan Bridge bike path.

3.6 Crossing Baxter, you're entering Chinatown. Across the street is Columbus Park, site of soccer, marathon mahjong, and bathrooms.

3.7 At the intersection of Worth and Park Row, bear left onto Park, then make an immediate right onto East Broadway.

3.9 After passing under the Manhattan Bridge, make a left onto Eldridge St.

4.0 Turn left onto Canal. Finish back at Canal and Forsyth.

Brooklyn & Manhattan Bridges

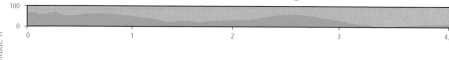

Altitude ft

100

0

0   1   2   3   4.0

Distance miles

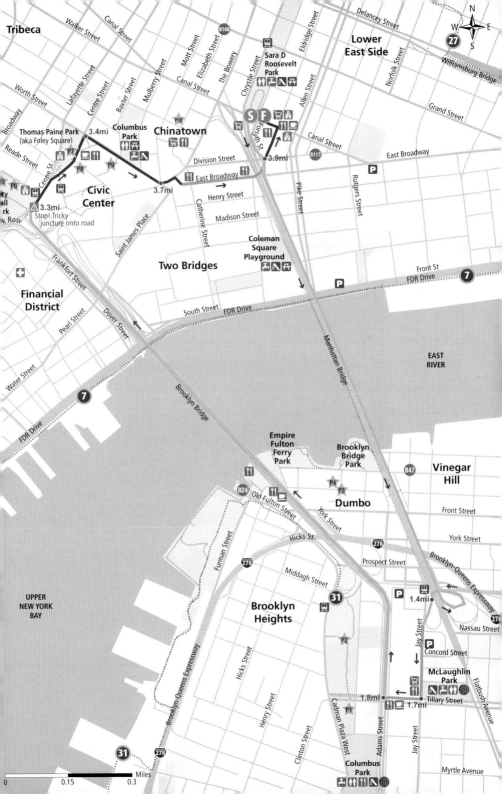

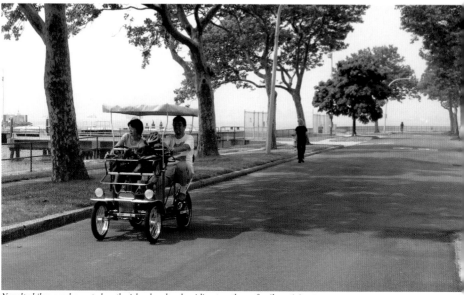

Novelty bikes can be rented on the island and make riding together a family activity.

At a Glance

Distance **Island Perimeter Loop:** 2.1 miles, **Southwest Loop:** 1.4 miles, **Northeast Loop:** 1.5 miles
Total Elevation **Island Perimeter Loop:** 54', **Southwest Loop:** 32', **Northeast Loop:** 56'

Terrain

Flat. Paved roads with a small cobblestone section.

Traffic

Almost entirely foot and bicycle traffic. There are occasional cars and carts on the roads as well as buses that take people (slowly) around the island.

How to Get There

Take the free Governors Island Ferry from downtown Manhattan, 10 South Street. The ferry slip is located just to the northeast of the Staten Island ferry terminal. The ferry runs on Fridays and weekends in the summer. There's a Brooklyn ferry from Pier Six in Brooklyn Bridge Park. It runs on weekends only.

Food and Drink

An outdoor café and beach are just east of the Manhattan ferry landing. There are several food trucks and stands situated throughout the island.

Side Trip

Check out the Sculptors Guild Gallery at 403 Colonels Row toward the middle of the island. There are both indoor and outdoor installations. If that's too much work, there's a beach for sunning, volleyball, and eating right next to the ferry.

Where to Bike Rating

Governors Island is on-road, but almost entirely traffic-free.

About...

The riding on Governors Island is short and easy, and you can easily exhaust all the roads within an hour. While people come here to ride, they also come to make a day trip of the island, so many of the cyclists are here for lunch and a slow afternoon on the water; an escape from the bustle of the city. The car-free roads also make it a great place for kids to ride along with their parents. Bike rentals are available and within easy walk of ferry.

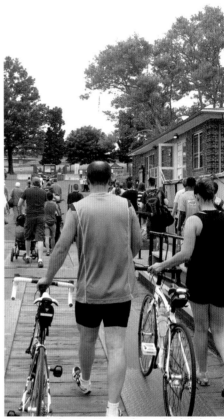

Exiting the ferry. Fort Jay is at the top of the hill, the only hill on the island.

Turning Governors Island into a public park has been a dream of New York City officials for over a century. It's only been in the last few years that the vision has become a reality.

Originally a residence for the Governor of New York Colony, hence the name, the island had been a military installation since the Revolutionary War. First, it housed a fort that helped hold off the British in the Battle of Long Island. Then a second fort was added in anticipation of future wars. It remained a military training ground and military prison, and eventually a Coast Guard base.

Now, it is a summertime destination. The free ferry service helps, as does the private beach that has been built, though this one is mainly for sun and concerts; there's no swimming in the East River (and that's a good thing). But the art gallery, the forts, the classic architecture, not to mention the great views of New York Harbor and the seemingly omnipresent cool breeze are also big draws.

We can attest to the fact that the physical separation as well as the charms of the island have a calming effect. On our first trip, we had a hard time leaving, though we weren't doing anything in particular. The

beach gets boring? Find a hammock on the south end. Tired of that, move on to the art gallery. Want to have lunch, find a food truck and a table and some chairs? Easily done. Work on your tan, sit in the shade under a tree. It's all possible in this beautiful little corner of the city.

The riding is so simple, you don't really need a log. The perimeter loop is just over two miles long, most of the roads are on the northern end of the island, and they're pretty short. The Northeast Loop we have listed is the only one you might want to pay attention to. If you ever get lost, you'll find your bearings, if not a posted map of the island, within a few minutes.

Ride Log

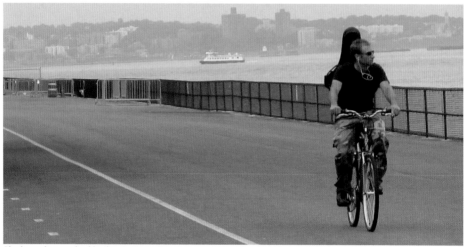

If riding solo is preferable, there's plenty of space for that as well.

Island Perimeter Loop

0.0 Walk bike off ferry up to Kimmel Rd. If you try to ride, you'll be stopped by park officials pretty quickly, as they don't want chaos or crashes by the ferry slip.

0.1 Go left or right. Keep the water on your left or right.

2.1 You're back at Ferry Rd.

Southwest Loop

0.0 Start at the corner of Main St and Craig Rd S.

0.4 Turn left at end of Main onto Craig Rd N.

1.4 End at Main St and Craig Rd S.

Northeast Loop

0.0 Start at the intersection of Kimmel and Clayton roads. Follow Clayton Rd northwest.

0.3 Turn right at Wheeler Ave. Follow Wheeler to Andes Rd.

0.5 Turn right onto Andes Rd. Andes will take you around Fort Jay.

0.7 Andes will turn left at the entrance to Fort Jay.

0.9 Turn right onto Barry Rd. There's a short stretch of cobblestones to traverse.

1.2 Turn left onto Comfort Rd.

1.2 Turn right onto Kimmel Rd.

1.3 Finish at intersection of Kimmel and Clayton.

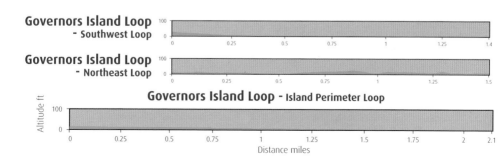

Governors Island Loop - Southwest Loop

Governors Island Loop - Northeast Loop

Governors Island Loop - Island Perimeter Loop

Altitude ft

Distance miles

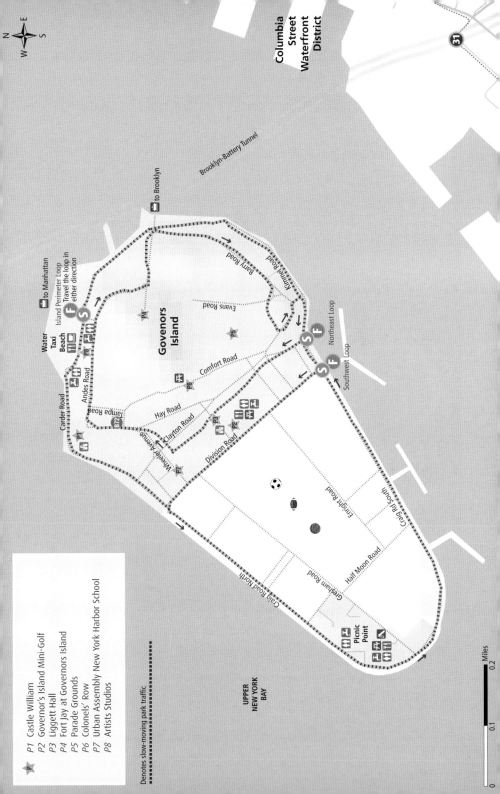

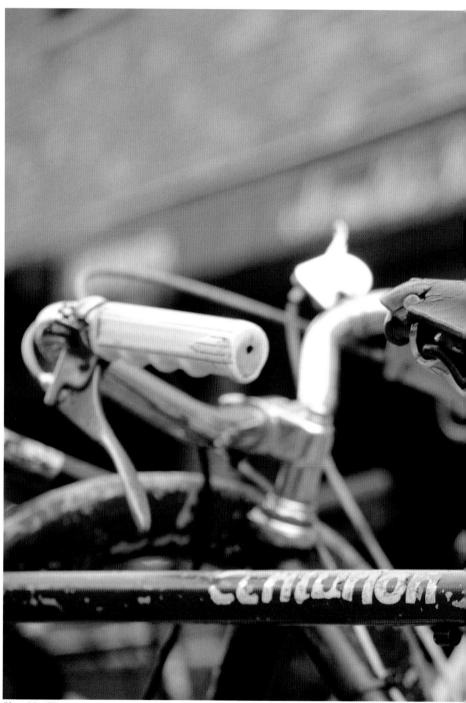

Photo Matt Wittmer

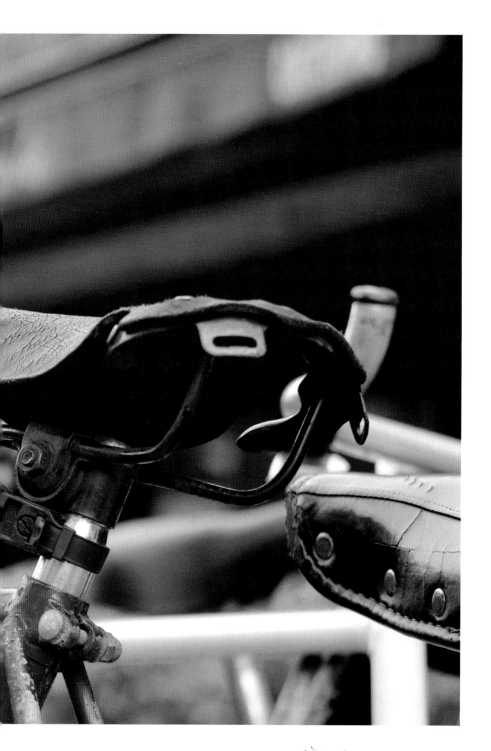

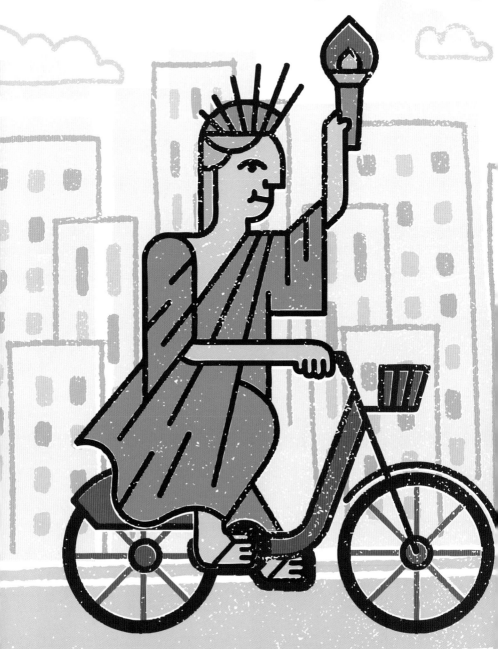

WHERE TO GO BEFORE YOU ROLL

BIKENYC.ORG IS YOUR SOURCE FOR TIPS, EVENTS AND DEALS. POWERED BY NYC BICYCLISTS.

A PROJECT OF 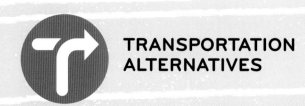 **TRANSPORTATION ALTERNATIVES**

The Bronx

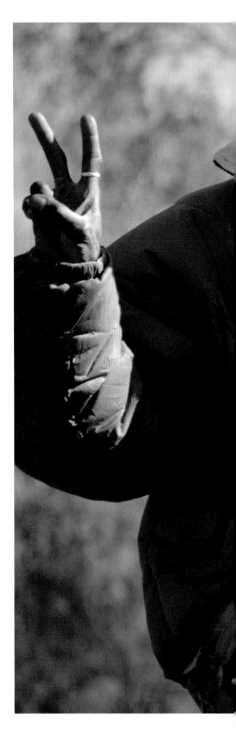

The only borough attached to the United States mainland, The Bronx, to an outsider coming from Manhattan on a bicycle, feels like a giant transition zone to the world beyond the city. It's a simplistic assessment, as Bronx County, with a population of almost 1.4 million, would be the seventh-most populous city in the United States, and a diverse metropolis just about anywhere else. The southern end is urban and industrial, and the parks and streets become ever more verdant as you travel north. It is for this reason that we did most of our rides at the far edges of the borough.

Word has it that The Bronx is the hilliest borough. I've found little proof of this, and only two of the rides, Wave Hill and Yankee Stadium, seemed hilly from the saddle. As with the other boroughs, the natural resistance you'll feel most on the rides here will probably be wind when you're riding along the water.

Many of The Bronx rides overlap, so if you're at all adventurous or seeking more miles, it is easy to combine rides or join them by taking an on-street bike path. Most of the rides either ring or go through parks, so if you're looking for bucolic respite, you'll find no shortage of places to pull over for recreation and relaxation.

Currently, there are plenty of bike lanes running on the north-south avenues, so getting to the northern edge of the borough and the routes we've mapped is fairly easy if you're coming from Queens or Manhattan. At the same time, there are not many lanes running east-west. We're hoping that these start to appear and that more bike lanes appear in the South Bronx. The southern tip seems to have riding potential, as the industrial areas are generally fairly quiet much of the time. And when the new human-power-centric bridge linking The Bronx to Randall's Island is built, we'll realize lots of new places to ride and encourage you to do some exploration in this area as well.

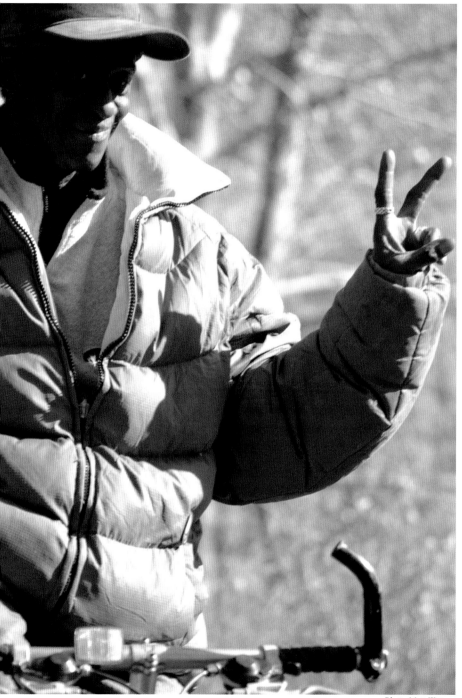

Photo Matt Wittmer

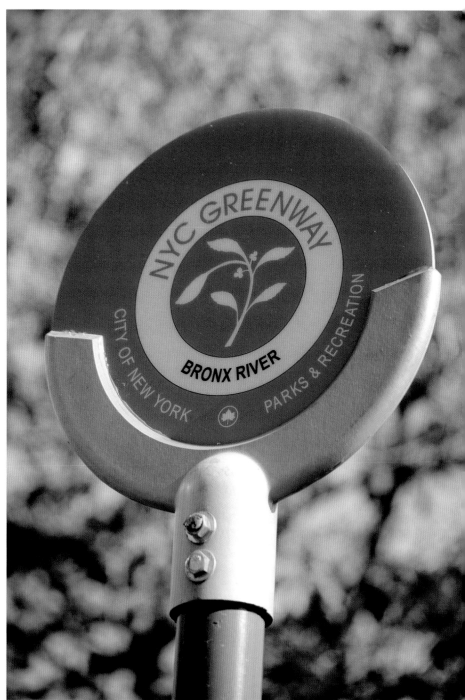

Photo Matt Wittmer

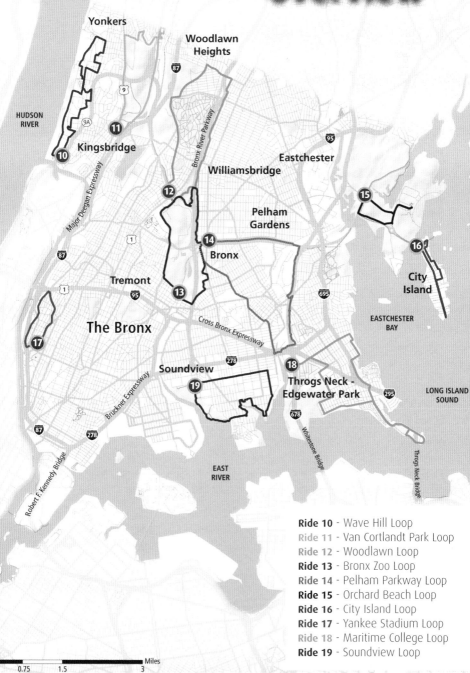

Bronx Overview

Yonkers

Woodlawn Heights

87

9

HUDSON RIVER

9A

11 Kingsbridge

10

Eastchester

95

Williamsbridge

12

Pelham Gardens

14 Bronx

1

Tremont

95

13

15

16 City Island

EASTCHESTER BAY

695

The Bronx

Cross Bronx Expressway

1

17

278

Soundview

19

18 Throgs Neck - Edgewater Park

295

LONG ISLAND SOUND

Bruckner Expressway

87 278

678

Whitestone Bridge

Throgs Neck Bridge

Robert F. Kennedy Bridge

EAST RIVER

Major Deegan Expressway

Bronx River Parkway

Miles
0.75   1.5   3

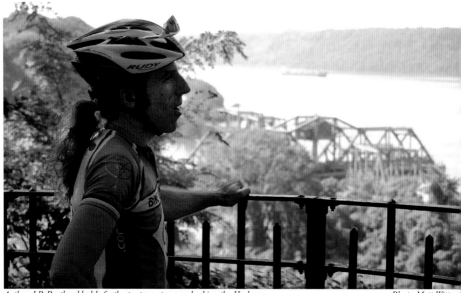

Author J.P. Partland holds forth at a tour stop overlooking the Hudson.

Photo Matt Wittme

At a Glance

Distance 6.5 miles   **Total Elevation** 732'

Terrain
Meandering suburban streets with one steep climb.

Traffic
Mixed. Mostly light, with a few busy sections.

How to Get There
Wave Hill is just across the Harlem River from Manhattan. The Henry Hudson Bridge is one way for cyclists and drivers to get there. The bike path is on the west side of the bridge. People can also take Metro-North to the Spuyten Duyvil stop or the 1 train to 225th Street in The Bronx.

Food and Drink
This ride is mostly residential, though there are som delis and restaurants at the far end of the ride, just a you turn onto Riverdale Avenue.

Side Trip
The Wave Hill estate is a great place to visit. Onc home to Theodore Roosevelt as well as Samuel Clemens (Mark Twain), the estate is now a public garde and cultural center. The views of the Hudson River an the New Jersey Palisades are incredible.
www.wavehill.org

Where to Bike Rating

 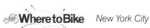

About...

While probably everyone in New York City has gone by Wave Hill, few know of it. It is surrounded by well-used trains, highways, and rivers, and yet few ever stop by. It's in the Riverdale section of The Bronx, which many consider an elite suburb of New York City.

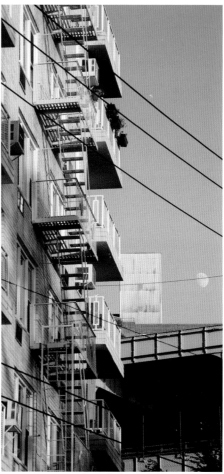

Sunset bathes the heights of Riverdale.
Photo Matt Wittmer

Wave Hill is a quiet spot on the eastern bank of the Hudson River. An oasis of calm in a bustling city. The Riverdale neighborhood that surrounds it has a similar laid back charm. Many of the roads here are narrow, winding, and remarkably traffic-free. If it weren't for the hills, this would be a great ride for beginners.

The Wave Hill Loop is a decidedly suburban ride that starts within sight of Manhattan and under an apartment building. Going north, the ride quickly turns to feeling like a distant locale, more northern Westchester than New York City. Adding to the remote feel are the hills. The first of which is Wave Hill, a stiff climb up from the train tracks. The rest of the ride north to the Yonkers border takes you on narrow suburban streets and past a well-appointed private school, a lush nursing home, and a pretty college.

When you turn right onto Riverdale Avenue, you're confronted with the first and only commercial strip of the ride. Riverdale is also pretty well trafficked, though with the decent width, there is plenty of room for riding. Luckily, you're only on it for a short stretch in the busy section, and then return to it twice more in less-trafficked areas.

On the way south back to the start, the ride turns repeatedly. This was an effort to stay as removed from traffic as possible. You're ducking onto Riverdale Avenue several times just to make connections to quieter, prettier roads. It also lengthens the ride; if you find

yourself running short on time or getting tired, you can just stay on Riverdale longer. Riverdale merges into Henry Hudson Parkway West, which can take you almost the entire way back to the start.

As you're winding south, you pass by several parks, the first of which is when you pass Wave Hill, briefly covering the same road you did on the ride north. A few turns past Wave, and you're at Seton Park. Once through Seton, you're just a minute or so from Henry Hudson Park and then at the finish of the ride. For us, the distance is such that we like doing at least two laps of this loop.

Ride Log

0.0 Start at the intersection of Independence and Palisade avenues. Head west on Palisade.

0.2 Road curves north and descends.

1.4 Road curves right onto West 248th St and starts to climb.

1.6 Turn left onto Independence Ave.

1.7 Pass entry to Wave Hill.

1.9 Turn left onto West 252nd St.

1.9 Road turns right.

2.0 Jog left, then right onto Sycamore Ave.

2.1 Turn left onto West 254th St.

2.2 Turn right onto Palisade Ave.

2.8 Road turns right onto West 261st St.

3.0 Turn right onto Riverdale Ave. Busy street. Also a commercial strip.

3.2 Turn right onto West 259th St.

3.4 Turn left onto Arlington Ave.

3.6 Turn left onto West 256th St.

3.7 Turn right onto Riverdale Ave.

3.8 Turn right onto West 254th St.

4.0 Turn left onto Independence Ave.

4.4 Pass Wave Hill on your right.

4.4 Turn left onto West 249th St.

4.6 Turn right onto Henry Hudson Pkwy West.

4.8 Turn right onto West 247th St.

4.9 Turn left onto Arlington Ave.

5.0 Turn right onto West 246th St.

5.2 Turn left onto Independence Ave.

5.4 Turn right onto West 239th St.

5.5 Turn left onto Hudson Manor Terrace.

5.6 Turn right onto West 236th St.

5.7 Turn left onto Douglas Ave. Douglas turns onto West 235th St.

6.0 Turn right onto Independence Ave.

6.5 Finish at start, Independence and Palisade avenues.

P1 Spuyten Duyvil Shorefront Park
P2 Henry Hudson Memorial Park
P3 Riverdale Park
P4 Wave Hill Environment Center
P5 Cardinal Spellman Retreat House
P6 Hebrew Home at Riverdale
P7 Judaica Museum

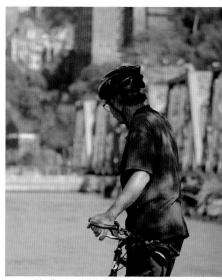

Northernmost Manhattan backed by Spuyten Duyvil, The Bronx. Photo Matt Wittmer

Wave Hill Loop

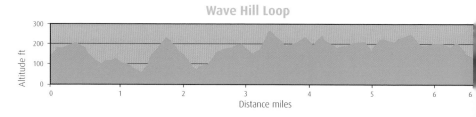

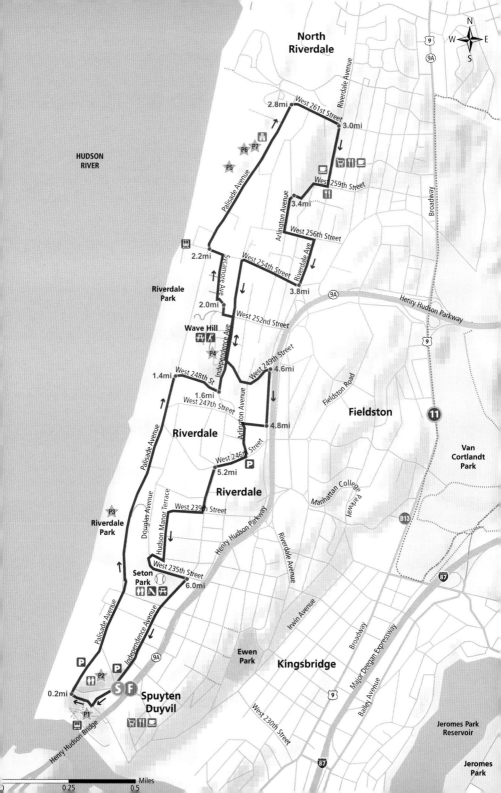

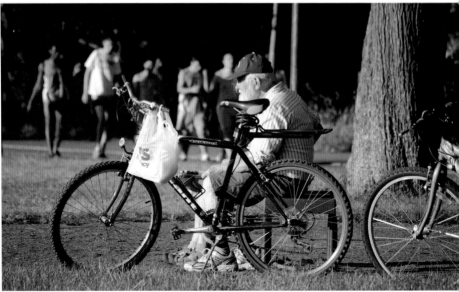

A couple takes a breather at the Van Cortlandt's historic parade grounds.

Photo Matt Wittme

At a Glance

Distance 5.5 miles   **Total Elevation** 358'

Terrain

Rolling terrain through one-way streets and park bike paths. At time of writing there was one section of dirt path due to be sealed.

Traffic

Mixed. Light for the first half, then on park paths for the second.

How to Get There

For city cyclists, Broadway goes right to the park, so it's a fairly simple route through The Bronx. For those who prefer public transit, the 1 train stops at 242nd Street and Broadway.

Food and Drink

Just up the street from the start of the ride, and righ next to the subway stop is a commercial strip across th street from the park. Just north of the stop is Broadwa Joe's Pizza as well as the M&M Deli.

Side Trip

After you've done a loop or two, check out the Va Cortlandt House Museum. It's The Bronx's olde house, an 18th century Georgian fieldstone and bric estate. It's a city and national landmark and has been museum since 1897.

www.vancortlandthouse.org

Where to Bike Rating

About...

Van Cortlandt Park is the fourth-largest city park, comprising 1,146-acres along the Bronx-Yonkers border and containing the city's largest lake. It's a long-time city playground, with the nation's first-ever public golf course, the "parade ground," which is a hugely popular cross-country running venue, and room for baseball, basketball, bocce, fishing, hiking, horseback riding, soccer, swimming, tennis, and, of course, cycling.

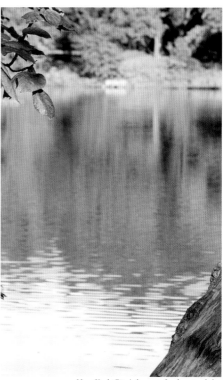

New York City's largest freshwater lake.
Photo Matt Wittmer

Cyclists look at the size of Van Cortlandt, and all the activities that go on within its confines and imagine the park would be perfect for mountain biking and cyclo-ross. The park could be ideal for these kinds of riding, but the time isn't right. For now, we can accept riding around the park and inside it on the designated bike paths.

The ride starts at the southwestern corner of the park just on the street by the wolf statue that greets park visitors. Ride north with the park on your right and the end of the 1 train on your left. You'll immediately see the more traditional urban park facilities: baseball, soccer, basketball, a playground, and the entrance to a swimming pool.

Just after those amenities, you'll pass the Van Cortlandt House Museum and beyond that the Parade Grounds where soccer, baseball, and cross-country running takes place. The park then turns to forest, and will pretty much remain forest until you reach the northern end of the park on the Yonkers border.

Once in Yonkers, you hug the northern edge of the park while meandering through the southern edge of Yonkers; the meanders are due to following the direction of traffic on one-way streets.

Once over the Saw Mill River Parkway, you're looking to get on the bike path. When you hit the South County Trailway, you're turning left to head south. If you turn right, you can take this trailway north, ride it 13 miles to Elmsford, then get on the North County Trailway and take it another 22 miles to the Putnam County line. And then continue on another 12 miles on the Putnam County Trail to Brewster where you can take Metro-North back to New York City. But I digress.

Turn left to get on the path. The path eventually turns to dirt. By the time you're reading these words, it is supposed to be paved, but in case it isn't, know that it could be muddy in or immediately following a rain. This is a pretty section that takes you past Van Cortlandt Lake, and eventually leads back to the southern edge of the park, which is a few hundred feet from the start.

The Bronx

Ride Log

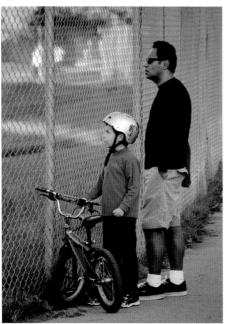

 P1 Van Cortlandt House Museum
P2 Riverdale Riding Club
P3 Sheridan Triangle

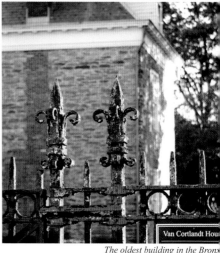

Activities here range from cricket to cross-country running.
Photo Matt Wittmer

The oldest building in the Bronx
Photo Matt Wittmer

0.0 Start at the corner of Broadway and Van Cortlandt Park South. Head north with park on right.

1.8 Turn right onto Caryl Ave.

2.1 Turn left onto Van Cortlandt Park Ave.

2.2 Turn right onto Coyle Place.

2.3 Turn right onto McLean Ave.

2.6 McLean Ave starts turning left.

2.8 McLean Ave forks right.

2.8 Go over Saw Mill River Pkwy.

2.9 Turn left onto Harrison Ave.

3.0 Road turns right onto Lawton St.

3.1 Turn left onto Tibbetts Rd.

3.2 Turn left onto Alan B. Shepard, Junior Place.

3.2 Turn left onto bike path.

3.6 Path turns to dirt.

5.0 Turn left, go under tracks, turn right, continue on path.

5.1 Turn right, go under tracks, turn left.

5.4 At park end. Turn right to finish.

5.5 Ride finishes at Broadway and Van Cortlandt Park South.

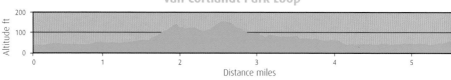

Van Cortlandt Park Loop

Altitude ft

Distance miles

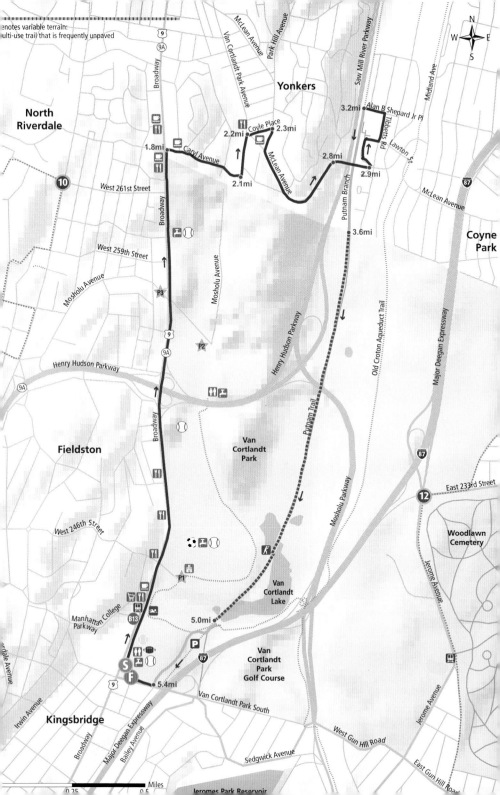

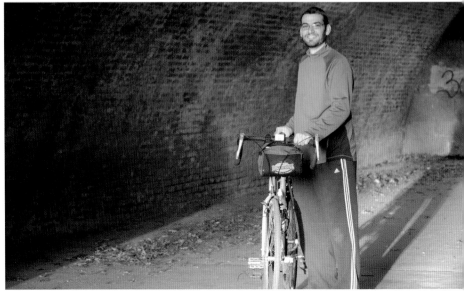

"E" casts a long shadow in a tunnel leading to Williamsbridge Park.

Photo Matt Wittmer

At a Glance

Distance 6.3 miles   **Total Elevation** 392′

Terrain

Predominately flat bike paths, which you will be hopping off and on.

Traffic

As with most of these rides, traffic is mixed. Close to half of the ride is on bike paths, and much of the rest is alongside parks.

How to Get There

Metro-North has a Botanical Garden stop that puts you close to the route. The B, D, and 4 trains all have Bedford Park Boulevard stops that will put you close as well.

Food and Drink

Nicky's Pizza and Ristorante, at 3070 Bainbridge Avenue, just off the route, is known for having huge, tasty, cheap slices. This section of Bainbridge also has a few diners and delis, so whatever your taste runs to, you can probably find it.

Side Trip

The Woodlawn Cemetery was designed in the 19th century as an attractive place to enjoy living, or at least visiting the dead. Woodlawn is considered a "garden cemetery," and is the result of work by both prominent landscapers and architects of its era. While we see anything with a road as a place to ride, a saunter through the grounds, which are open every day, offers beauty and a chance for reflection.

www.thewoodlawncemetery.org

Links to ⓭

Where to Bike Rating

About...

The Woodlawn Cemetery is in the middle of the ride, and as the final resting place for over three hundred thousand individuals, it is pretty huge, but most of it is out of your sight unless you're willing to venture inside the grounds. Even without Woodlawn, there is plenty to see and plenty of parkland to enjoy, even if you're riding on the edge of it most of the time. The ride also takes you to the edge of Van Cortlandt Park and through Bronx Park.

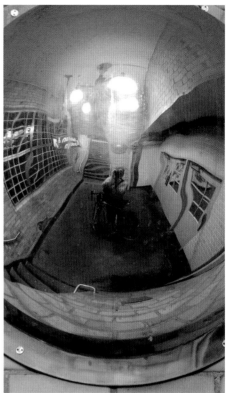

The subway assists cyclists here and throughout the city.
Photo Matt Wittmer

If we can't ride through parks, we like riding next to them. Parkland means long stretches of roadway without driveways and intersections, and this ride takes advantage of this great park feature.

The ride starts on the Mosholu Parkway, which has a nice protected bike path on the eastern side of the roadway. The ride quickly turns off Mosholu to take you to Bainbridge Avenue and the longest park-free stretch of the ride. Once out of the stores, you'll pass the Valentine-Varian house, the second-oldest house in the county, and now a museum. Before you know it, you're riding past Woodlawn and enjoying almost two miles of parkland borders before ending up on McLean Avenue in Yonkers.

McLean is a commercial strip but short and mostly downhill until you cross the Bronx River. Then you take your first right and start heading back.

Bronx Boulevard narrows just where the Bronx Park bike path begins. The park is also fairly narrow here, as is the path, but this section of the park is underutilized so it creates no real problem.

You'll probably have a moment or two of confusion when you cross East 211th Street. As of this writing, the park seems to end, and there is construction mak-

ing it hard to figure out where to go. Ride underneath the overpass, which is Gun Hill Road and continue on your southerly trajectory. You should be on Bronx Boulevard again. The path should resume by Magenta Street, if not sooner.

Shortly after returning to the parkland, you'll find your first right-hand turn, which will take you under the Bronx River Parkway and then over the Bronx River. (Straight, btw, will take you on the Bronx Zoo loop). It's a pretty bridge, an attractive spot, and there are benches for pause and reflection. Soon enough, you'll be coming to a more popular area of the park, with playgrounds and playing fields.

Once through the park, you'll return to a protected bike lane on Kazimiroff Boulevard, which takes you to Mosholu Parkway and its protected bike lane. From here you're pretty much back at the start.

Ride Log

0.0 Start on the Mosholu Pkwy Bike Path at Hull Ave. Head northwest on path.

0.1 Turn right onto Bainbridge Ave. This will take you off bike path.

0.2 Bear left to stay on Bainbridge.

0.5 Pass Valentine-Varian House. It will be on your right.

0.9 Woodlawn Cemetery is now on your right.

1.3 Bainbridge merges into Jerome Ave.

1.8 Turn right onto East 233rd St. Cemetery is on right. Van Cortlandt Park on left.

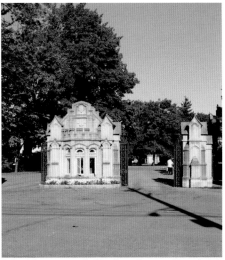

1.9 Turn left onto Van Cortlandt Park East. Get onto on-street bike lane. Park is on left.

2.7 Turn right onto McLean Ave.

3.2 Cross over Bronx River Pkwy.

3.3 Turn right onto Bullard Ave.

3.6 Turn right onto Bronx Blvd.

3.7 Cross East 233rd St.

3.8 After passing highway on-ramp, ride off road onto bike path.

4.9 Bike path ends. Ride back onto Bronx Blvd. Continue heading south.

5.0 After crossing under East Gun Hill Rd, you should be able to get back on bike path.

5.4 Turn right to go under highway overpass. Crossing Bronx Zoo Loop here.

5.5 Go straight over Bronx River.

5.7 Turn right on bike path. Followed by a left. Follow path.

6.0 Turn right onto Mosholu Pkwy. Remain on bike path.

6.3 Finish at Mosholu and Hull.

P1 Valentine-Varian House
P2 Woodlawn Cemetery
P3 New York Botanical Gardens

Behind these gates is the Woodlawn Cemetery. Not only is it a resting place of the famous, but famous architects left their mark on the space as well.

Woodlawn Loop

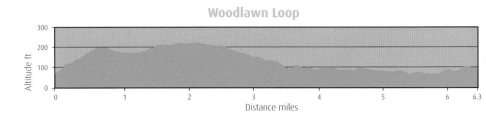

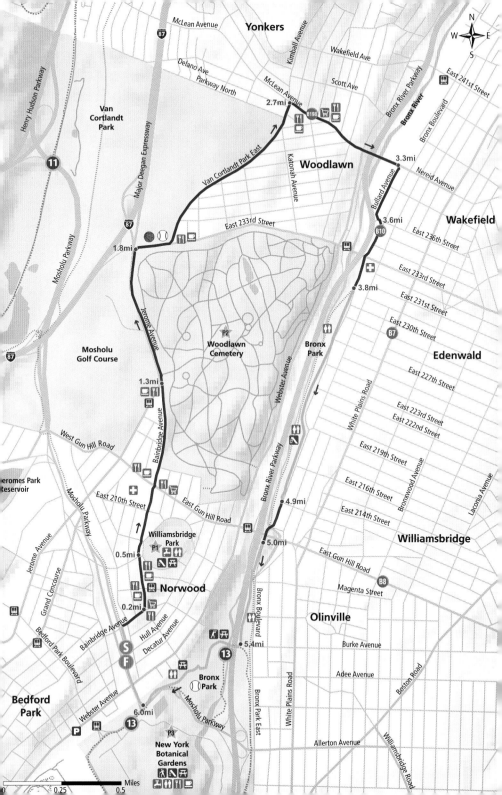

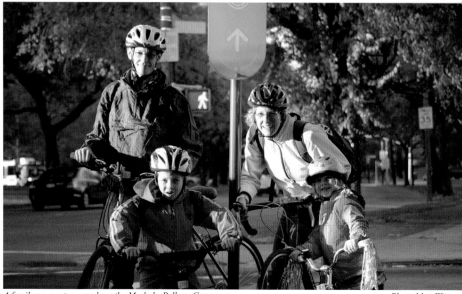

A family pauses to pose along the Mosholu-Pelham Greenway.

Photo Matt Wittmer

At a Glance

Distance 5.9 miles   **Total Elevation** 333′

Terrain

Flat bike paths and streets.

Traffic

Varied. At least a third of this route is on park bike paths, a third is on a busy street, Southern Boulevard, and the rest is on moderately trafficked roads. Most of the streets you're riding on have a park on one side, so very few opportunities for cars to turn into you.

How to Get There

The Bronx Zoo is pretty centrally located in The Bronx. But if you want to take the train, there's a 2 and a 5 stop at East Tremont a few blocks from the ride start.

Food and Drink

If you take Southern Boulevard and turn left on East 187th Street, you're just seven blocks from great Ital-ian fare on Arthur Avenue. There are several bakeries if you just want a snack, and many restaurants if you want a sit-down meal.

Side Trip

The name gives it away. The Bronx Zoo, the jewel of the Wildlife Conservation Society, is the best zoo in the city. There is no shortage of things to see, do, and learn, and even those opposed to zoos will come away the better for having experienced it.

www.bronxzoo.com

Links to 12 14

Where to Bike Rating

About...

The Bronx Zoo takes up a pretty large swath of land in The Bronx. The New York Botanical Garden, which is just across the street, takes up another big patch. This ride takes you around both. Both are sufficiently large that it seemed wisest to break them up into two rides. Beginners might want to do one at a time, while the more experienced should be able to handle both. It's a shame we can't ride inside these places, but maybe it's something we can look forward to in the future.

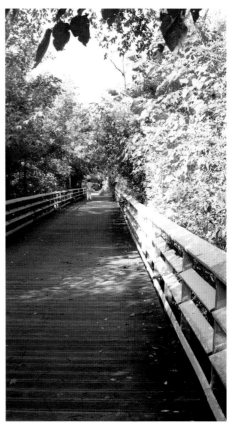
Ride through nature.

Start at the southern entrance to The Bronx Zoo. It's a quiet corner on a lightly trafficked street. The entry is so plain that it's hard to believe much goes on behind the gate.

The start is a contrast to the second road you'll be riding on, Southern Boulevard. Southern is a busy street, and not a terribly pleasant experience. But the road is plenty wide, so drivers should have no problem giving you room. The Southern becomes decidedly more pleasant after crossing Fordham Road, which is only a short distance. Once north of Fordham, it's only a short distance to the Mosholu Parkway Greenway, which is off the street.

The greenway takes you into Bronx Park, and a remarkably remote-feeling stretch of pathway. You'll head north to where the Woodlawn Loop crosses over the Bronx River and under the Bronx River Parkway.

Once under the parkway, you'll start heading south. Bronx Park is narrow here, but the path is lightly-used. If it ever gets busy, you can ride over to Bronx Park East, a quiet road that parallels the park.

Shortly before getting out of the park, you'll pass a skate park where adventurous cyclists, or those with bmx or jump bikes can practice their skills on ramps, half-pipes, and rails. Even if you're uncomfortable with trick riding, you owe it to yourself to see how it's done, and it's usually hosting some kids working their moves.

The path seems to end at Pelham Parkway, but if you go left, you'll see there's an extension that takes you to Boston Road. Follow the path until you reach Boston and then turn right.

This is the old Post road, though because it has just re-started here, it is not too busy. Boston turns into Bronx Park East. Following Boston takes you to the northern entrance to the zoo. From hereon, you'll be hugging the edge of Bronx Park, skirting parkland, elevated train tracks, and quiet edge streets, until you've reached East 180th Street, and then you're just a short ride to the start, which will be your finish.

Ride Log

0.0 Start at the corner of Boston Rd and East 182nd St (aka Bronx Park South).

0.4 Turn right onto Crotona Pkwy.

0.5 Turn right onto Southern Blvd.

1.1 Southern Blvd turns into Dr. Theodore Kazimiroff Blvd.

2.0 Traffic light at Mosholu Pkwy. Cross street and get on bike path that runs along other side of Kazimiroff Blvd.

2.4 Make sharp left into park.

2.9 Turn right to go under highway overpass. Start heading south.

3.3 Cross Allerton Ave.

3.9 Leaving Bronx Park bike path. Cross Bronx River Pkwy on-ramp.

4.0 Turn right onto Boston Rd. Cross Pelham Pkwy.

4.2 Boston Rd turns right. Go Straight onto Bronx

 P1 Bronx Zoo
P2 New York Botanical Gardens
P3 Enid A. Haupt Conservatory
P4 Fordham University
P5 Skate Park
P6 Bronx River Art Center

Park East.

4.5 Turn right onto Unionport Rd.

4.6 Turn left onto Sagamore St.

4.7 Turn right onto White Plains Rd.

4.8 Turn right onto Rhinelander Ave.

4.9 Turn left onto Unionport Rd.

5.1 Turn right onto Morris Park Ave.

5.4 Turn right onto East 180th St.

5.8 Turn right onto Boston Rd.

5.9 Finish at the corner of Boston Rd and East 182nd St.

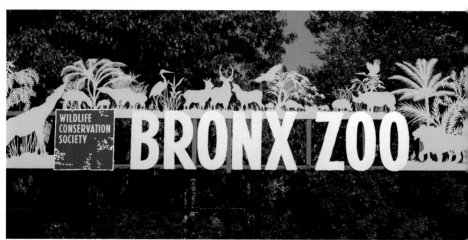

The Bronx Zoo is the largest metropolitan zoo in the United States.　　　*Photo Matt Wittmer*

Bronx Zoo Loop

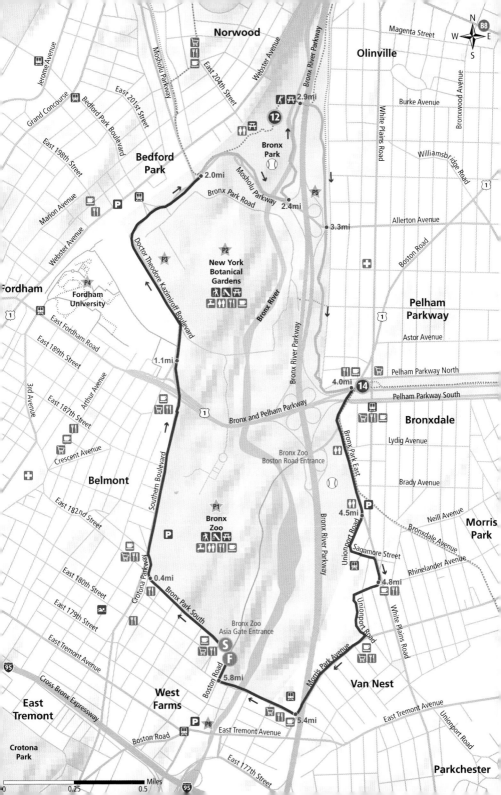

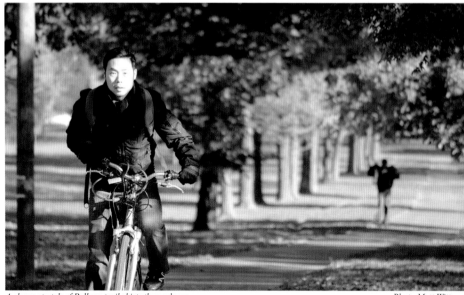

A classy stretch of Pelham trail skirts the parkway.

Photo Matt Wittmer

At a Glance

Distance 7.1 miles   **Total Elevation** 250'

Terrain

Flat bike paths with some major street crossings.

Traffic

Mixed, not just with cars but also with people. Over half of the ride is on separated bike paths, but the other half is on streets that go from being lightly-trafficked to somewhat busy.

How to Get There

You can take the 2 or 5 subway to Pelham Parkway at White Plains Road, which is right at the start of the loop. You can also take Metro-North to the Fordham Station, which is less than a mile west of the ride.

Food and Drink

There's a commercial alley running alongside the elevated tracks on White Plains Road. The Rainbow Diner at 2197 White Plains road is an anchor of the alley.

Side Trip

The New York Botanical Garden is just to the west of the start and finish of the ride. This one bills itself as a "museum of plants, an educational institution, and a scientific research organization." It was founded in 1891 and is considered to be one of the greatest in the world and largest in any city in the United States. Over one million plants! We've been, it's a great place to spend a day appreciating controlled nature.

www.nybg.org

Links to (13)

Where to Bike Rating

About...

Pelham Parkway, a connecting road between Bronx and Pelham Bay Parks, is a road that was probably designed as a pretty route for drivers back when driving was a novelty. There is a central road for through traffic, fields north and south, and access roads for residential and commercial traffic on the far sides of those fields. Bike paths are largely afterthoughts, but they afford easy riding in the midst of heavy traffic.

For all the traffic you'll see on this ride, the start is possibly the most chaotic. It isn't the cars, but the people. Start on the northeast corner of the Boston Road and Pelham Parkway intersection and follow the bike path east. Within a block, you encounter the elevated tracks of the 2 and 5 subway lines and the White Plains Road stop, where people are not only getting on and off the train, but looking for buses going in all directions.

Once you get away from that hectic transportation hub, the bike path becomes pretty quiet, with large expanses of open field on your left. The path lasts for a bit under two miles and you're only interrupted by the occasional cross street.

At the end of the bike path, you make a right across the parkway, a left onto the bike path on the other side of the street, take an overpass above train tracks, then parallel an access ramp to the Hutchinson River Parkway and start to ride parallel to this highway.

Despite the obvious bustle of the highway, the northern stretch of pathway feels pretty far removed from traffic. Then the path takes you off the highway to Herb Rosenblatt Place. Here, you make two lefts, go over the highway, then make a right immediately after the overpass and get back on the bike path. This stretch

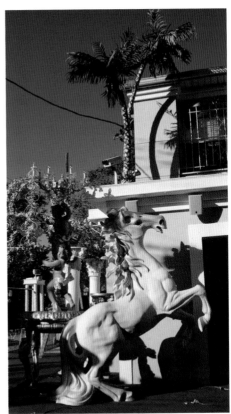

Kudos to all kitsch catchers.   Photo Matt Wittmer

of path tracks much closer to the highway and you'll cross both entrance and exit ramps on your way to the end of the path on Bruckner Boulevard.

Bruckner presents the trickiest part of the ride. You'll come to a light where you'll have to cross the boulevard, then make a right turn onto what seems to be the sidewalk, but is actually the bike path across the bridge and over Westchester Creek.

Once over the bridge, you make a right on Zerega. The ride to Westchester Avenue is pretty easy as the traffic is light. After you make the right on Parker, you'll have another easy stretch until you get to Castle Hill Avenue. Once on Castle Hill, traffic will be moderate but consistent pretty much the rest of the way. You finish up at the start and can then venture north on Boston to get yourself a reward for your efforts.

Ride Log

P1 Westchester Square
P2 Bronx Zoo
P3 New York Botanical Gardens

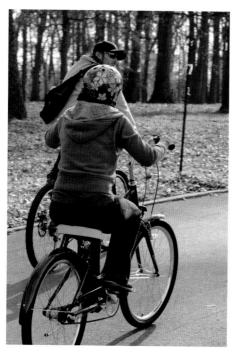

*The Bronx's plentiful green space surprises most everyone.
Photo Matt Wittmer*

0.0 Start at the corner of Boston Rd and Pelham Parkway West. The bike path begins here. Start going east on the path.

1.7 Bike path ends. Cross Pelham Parkway and continue on another bike path.

1.8 Turn right and path will run alongside the Hutchinson River Parkway.

2.8 Bike path ends. Turn left onto Herb Rosenblatt Place.

2.85 Turn left on Westchester Ave.

2.9 Turn right onto bike path.

3.9 Bike path now running alongside Bruckner Blvd.

4.0 Bike path ends.

4.1 Cross Bruckner Blvd. Make right. Ride up on to what appears to be a sidewalk.

4.3 Turn right onto Zerega Ave.

5.0 Turn left onto Westchester Ave.

5.0 Turn right onto Parker St.

5.4 Parker St ends at Castle Hill Ave. Turn right onto Castle Hill.

5.6 East Tremont Ave. Bear left onto Bronxdale Ave.

6.7 Bronxdale ends at Bronx Park East. Bear right onto Bronx Park East.

6.9 Bronx Park turns into Boston Rd.

7.1 Finish at the corner of Boston Rd and Pelham Parkway West.

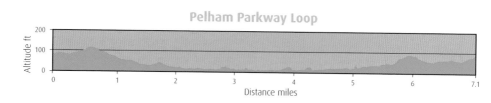

Pelham Parkway Loop

Altitude ft

Distance miles

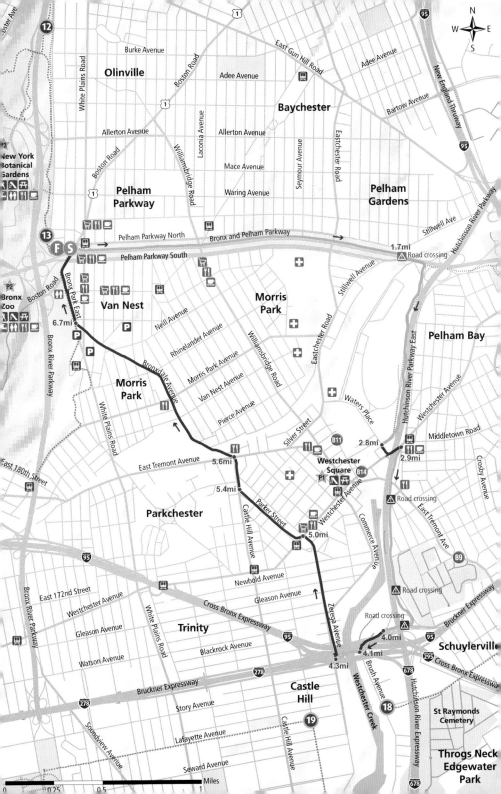

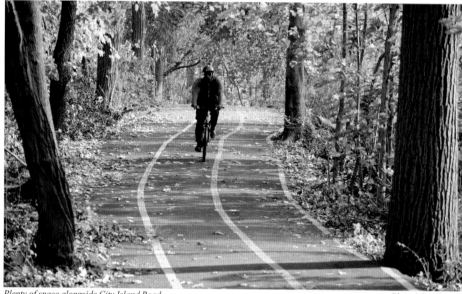

Plenty of space alongside City Island Road.

Photo Matt Wittmer

At a Glance

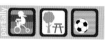

Distance 2.8 miles   **Total Elevation** 112′

Terrain

Flat bike paths and roads.

Traffic

Most of the route is on bike paths, but the first .7 mile is on a one-way street that is likely to have light traffic at its busiest.

How to Get There

Take the 6 train to its Bronx terminus of Pelham Bay Park. Then it's a 2.2 mile ride to the Bartow Pell Circle, almost entirely on bike paths. Alternatively, you can take the BX29 bus from Wilkinson Avenue and Bruckner Boulevard to the intersection of Shore Road and City Island Road.

Food and Drink

In the summertime, you'll find eats at Orchard Beach.

Otherwise, you can stop for a snack at the Turtle Cove Golf and Baseball Center.

Side Trip

Orchard Beach. It's the only beach in The Bronx. Designed as New York's Riviera, it is over a mile long and beautifully designed with a promenade and pavilion, changing areas, playgrounds and more. It's a great hangout in the summer, and for the rest of the year, you get a great view of Pelham Bay, Chimney Sweeps Islands, High Island, Hunter Island, City Island, Hart Island, Kings Point, and Sands Point.
www.nycgovparks.org/parks/orchardbeach

Where to Bike Rating

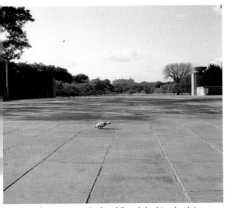

The grand entrance at Orchard Beach looking back into Pelham Bay Park.

About...

Orchard Beach is the best-known facility of Pelham Bay Park, the city's largest park. Much of the park has been left to nature, which is hard to experience, unless you're on foot. What's good about this is it means the few roads and paths that go through the park are generally fairly devoid of traffic most of the time.

The Bronx

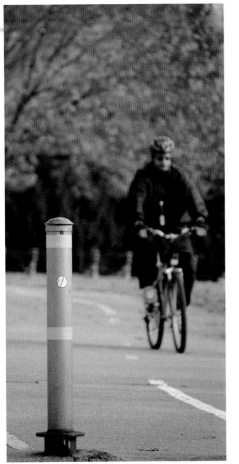

This all-season ride might be prettiest in autumn.
Photo Matt Wittmer

The Orchard Beach Loop starts at the Bartow-Pell Circle. If you stand still for a few minutes, it could be a rural roundabout somewhere upstate. As you start east on Pelham Bay Park Road, the road continues to feel like a ride through the remote woods.

It's only when you get to the parking lot for Orchard Beach that you start to realize you're in a populated area. The lot is huge. And when you see the structures that you're riding to, it becomes clear you're coming to a place designed to draw people in.

Walk up the steps and look out over the promenade, and you'll be impressed. The promenade is majestic, an elegantly sweeping U that faces into Long Island Sound. At the height of a summer heat wave, expect the beach to be crowded. But for much of the year, it feels like a beach town in the off season; peacefully, beautifully underutilized.

Back down the stairs and onto the bike, you retrace your route. When you're back at Pelham Bay Park Road, go straight instead of turning off the path. Shortly thereafter, the path will turn and cross the road. The path will take you by a salt marsh where birds find respite. The marsh empties into Turtle Cove to the south but you continue on a northwest trajectory past the Turtle Cove Golf Center.

Through the woods, and you're at the Shore Road intersection. Cross the road to get to the bike path, turn right on the path, and before you know it, you're back at the circle where you began.

Ride Log

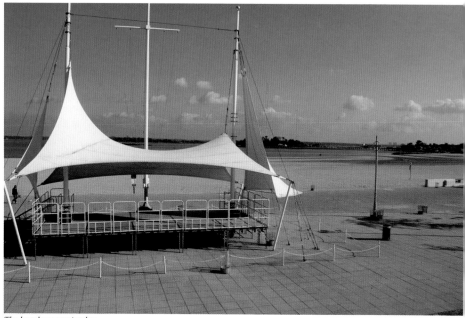

The beach on a quiet day.

0.0 Start at Bartow-Pell Circle at the intersection of Shore Rd and Pelham Bay Park Rd. Head southeast toward Orchard Beach.

0.7 Road ends. Go straight across road. Turn left onto bike path.

0.9 Path bears right.

1.1 Arrive at Orchard Beach. Make U-turn. Follow bike path.

1.4 Bear left to remain on bike path. You are paralleling Park Dr.

1.6 You are passing the spot where you entered the

 P1 Orchard Beach
P2 The Meadow
P3 Salt Marsh
P4 Turtle Cove Golf Center
P5 Bronx Equestrian Center

bike path. Go straight. Remain on path.

1.7 Cross Park Dr. Start following bike path west.

2.1 Pass Turtle Cove Golf and Baseball Center.

2.4 Cross Shore Rd. Make right to go northeast on bike path.

2.8 Finish at Bartow-Pell Circle.

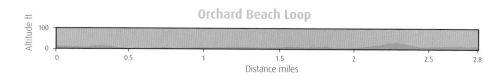

Orchard Beach Loop

Altitude ft

100

0

0   0.5   1   1.5   2   2.5   2.8

Distance miles

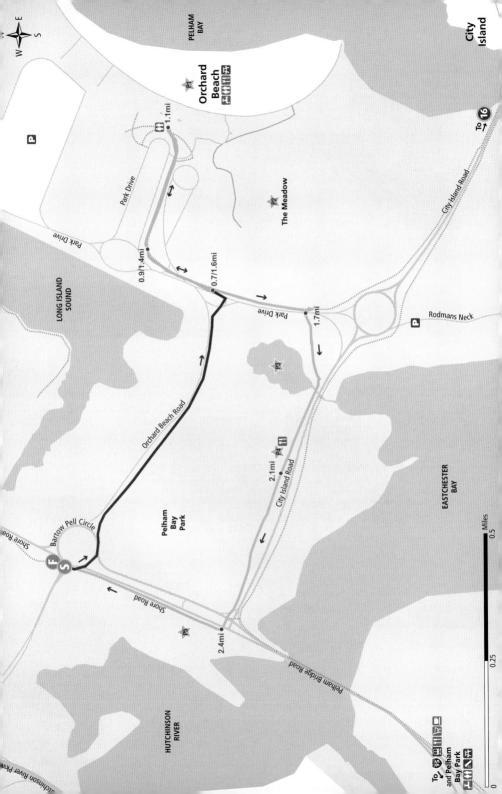

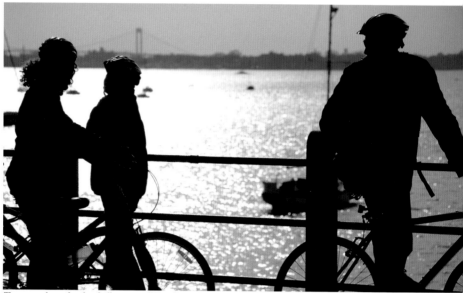

The sun makes a family of silhouettes off Eastchester Bay.

Photo Matt Wittmer

At a Glance

Distance 3.3 miles   **Elevation Gain** 114′

Terrain
Flat suburban streets. Narrow at times, no bike lanes.

Traffic
None to light. It is a very small island.

How to Get There
Take the 6 train to its Bronx terminus of Pelham Bay Park. Then it's a 3.6 mile ride to City Island, almost entirely on bike paths. Alternatively, you can take the BX29 bus from Wilkinson Avenue and Bruckner Boulevard.

Food and Drink
City Island is more about crab shacks and pubs than it is about coffee, but times are changing. City Island Avenue has food venues all the way from the start of the island down to the other end. Check out the Island Café for a quiet break.

Side Trip
If you have the time check out The City Island Historical Society's Nautical Museum. It's on the route at Fordham and King. Open on weekends, it details the history of this isle of seafarers and farmers. Make an appointment before visiting.
www.cityislandmuseum.org

Where to Bike Rating

About...

City Island's name is derived from New City Island. It was given the name because the island's owners had a dream of building a city to rival that on Manhattan Island. Only it came to be populated by farmers, oystermen, and commercial shipbuilders. By 1896, residents were calling it City Island, and they voted to join with New York City, as a metropolis was growing off the coast of America. Today, it's largely residential, with four yacht clubs, and is mostly known for its seafood.

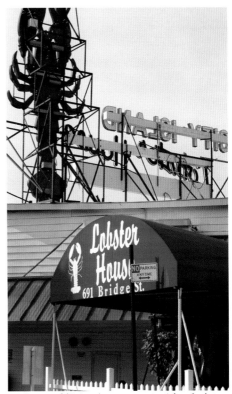

Just one of this jaunt's numerous potential seafood stops. Photo Matt Wittmer

Ride over the City Island Bridge and you'll be heading down City Island Avenue, the backbone of both the island and this ride. You're taking it all the way down, and it runs in a straight line down to the water.

If you want a little adventure, feel free to check out any of the streets on your right. Many of them dead end at the water, so you'll be coming back, but you can make a right on Tier and take it to Hawkins, then go back to City Island, make a right, continue south until Caroll, make a right there, take it to William, then left on William, left on Centre, and back to City Island, and then continue down.

Many say that the island feels like a quaint New England fishing village. They are mistaken. It feels like a quaint New York City fishing village. Many of the older houses have a covered deck atop the roof that is right for looking out over the water. Many of these homes look like they've been brined by the weather. It feels largely untouched by the times, though, like many places that have earned the "quaint" label, there are antique shops, hip coffee joints, and what appears to be a growing art scene. This isn't so much a criticism, but a wonder at how places grow and change and get colonized in similar ways everywhere.

When you reach the end of City Island Avenue, turn around and start heading back. You're on it until Fordham Street, which you'll know by both the stoplight and the signage directing you to City Island Museum. Take a right, then your first left just by the museum. Start following King Avenue north.

From here until you reach the end, you're basically paralleling City Island Avenue on either Minnieford Avenue (the island was called Minneford or a variation thereof in the 18th century) until you reach Terrace Street, the northernmost road on the island. Turn left and follow it back to City Island Avenue and you'll be exactly where you started.

Now that you've seen the entire island, you have, if you've got the appetite, no shortage of seafood restaurants to choose from. If it's a Sunday or Wednesday, stop by the island's museum.

The Bronx

Ride Log

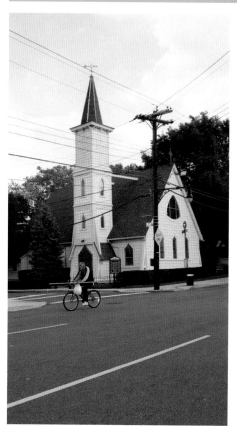

Riding is easy on the island.

 P1 Focal Point Gallery
P2 Starving Artist Cafe and Gallery
P3 City Island Theatre Group
P4 The Sailmaker Marina
P5 City Island Nautical Museum
P6 Pelham Cemetery

0.0 Start across the street from triangle on City Island side of City Island Bridge. Go southeast on City Island Ave.

1.3 End of City Island Ave. Long Island Sound is straight ahead. Make a U-turn and start heading back up City Island.

2.0 Turn right onto Fordham St.

2.2 Turn left onto King Ave.

2.4 Turn left onto Ditmars St. Make immediate right onto King Ave.

2.6 Turn left onto Beach St.

2.7 Turn right onto Minnieford Ave.

2.9 Turn right onto Sutherland St, then a near immediate left onto King Ave.

3.0 Turn left onto Terrace St.

3.1 Terrace becomes Minnieford.

3.2 Right onto Bridge St.

3.25 Bear left onto City Island Ave.

3.3 Go right around triangle.

3.3 Finish at City Island Ave at foot of City Island Bridge.

City Island Loop

Altitude ft

100

0

0   1   2   3   3.3

Distance miles

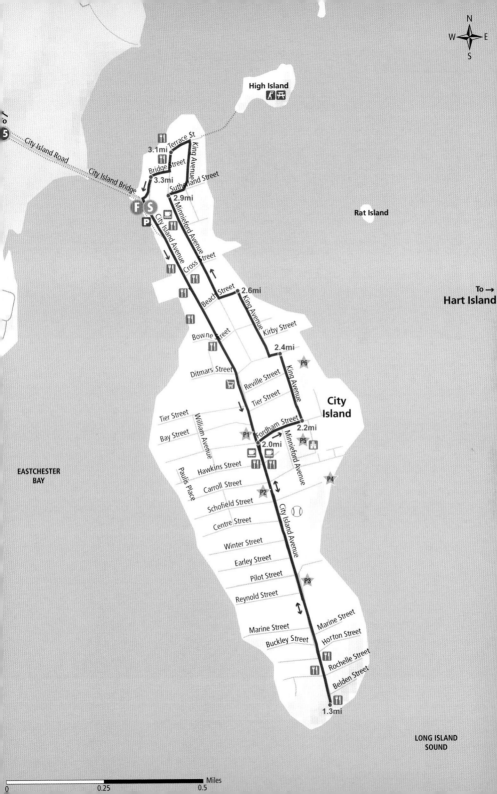

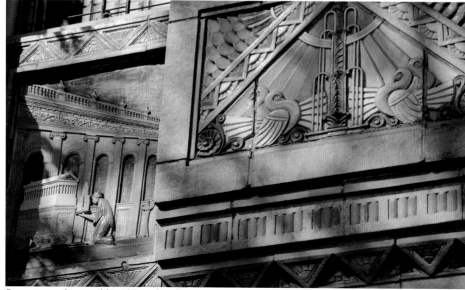

Be sure to sample some of this ride's art deco décor.

Photo Matt Wittmer

At a Glance

Distance 2.5 miles **Elevation Gain** 188'

Terrain

Hilly urban streets, some with bike lanes.

Traffic

Mixed. Light to busy. Could get crowded by the start and finish both immediately preceding and following games.

How to Get There

The ride starts and finishes next to Yankee Stadium, so finding directions is easy. It's at the southern end of Jerome Avenue, which runs through The Bronx. It's just past the Macombs Dam Bridge, which joins The Bronx to Manhattan. If you want to take the train, the 4, B, and D subway lines go to 161st Street and Metro-North stops at East 153rd Street.

Food and Drink

On the other side of Yankee Stadium, there are bars along River Avenue and if you take 161st east from River Avenue, you have a commercial strip with coffee shops, diners, pizza places, and fast food. Coffee, yes, bakeries, yes, ecologically-grown coffee and artisanal bread, probably not.

Side Trip

Two words. Yankee Stadium. The Bronx Bombers are in season from the start of April to the end of September; into November if they make the World Series. If you're going to combine a ride and a game, bring a good lock.

www.yankees.com

Where to Bike Rating

About...

Yankee Stadium was once The House That Ruth Built. Now, it's The House That Giuliani and Steinbrenner Built. But you know about that. This ride rings the Highbridge neighborhood. Highbridge, because it isn't upscale, has a number of underutilized streets and lots of great architecture, particularly art deco exteriors. And the topography not only yields hills, but vistas and great cliffside parks.

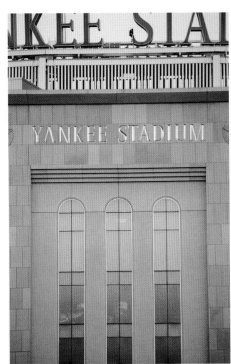

A slice of the new Yankee Stadium.   Photo Matt Wittmer

Yogi Berra, the silver-tongued Hall of Fame catcher who played in pinstripes said, "it's so crowded, nobody goes there." That's why it's been years since we've been to a Yankees game. But we do ride around Highbridge, and this loop is pretty interesting urban riding, and pretty easy to navigate.

Start across the street from Yankee Stadium. You're heading southwest toward the Major Deegan Expressway. Turn right onto Martin Luther King, Junior Boulevard. Start climbing. This road climbs gradually and then flattens out onto a ridge overlooking Manhattan. You'll be on here for over a mile.

When the road ends, you're turning right and heading downhill on Edward L. Grant Highway. This road goes southeast and you're going to lose altitude much faster than you gained it. While Grant is busy, there is a protected bike lane all the way down to Jerome Avenue.

Once on Jerome, you're almost done. Within a block you'll start passing John Mullaly Park, a wonderful oasis of green in this hyper-urban landscape. The park is on your left. Make sure to look right and check out the Art Deco buildings and the staircases leading up the cliff.

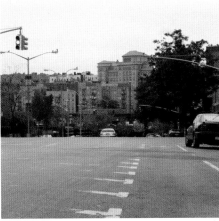

Edward L. Grant Highway, with a bike path on the right.

Once you're in front of Yankee Stadium, just another block and you're done. The route is so easy, so short, go for another loop before calling it quits. You'll see much more the second time around.

The Bronx

Ride Log

0.0 Start at the intersection of Jerome Ave and Macombs Dam Bridge across from Yankee Stadium. Bear right to follow Jerome heading south west.

0.2 Jerome turns right and takes you onto Dr. Martin Luther King, Junior Blvd (also called University Ave). Start climbing.

0.5 Bear right at fork to stay on MLK Blvd.

1.4 Bear right to stay on MLK Blvd.

1.4 Turn right onto Edward L. Grant Hwy.

 P1 Yankee Stadium
P2 John Mullaly Recreation Center
P3 Mullaly Skate Park
P4 Highbridge-Woodycrest Center
P5 Bronx Community Center and pool

2.0 Turn right onto Jerome Ave.

2.5 Finish at the intersection of Jerome Ave and Macomb's Dam Bridge.

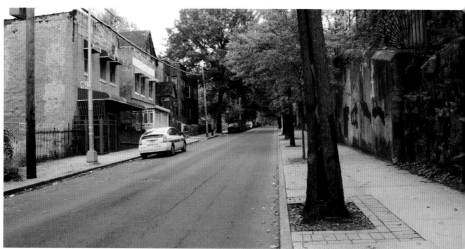

The long climb of MLK Boulevard.

Yankee Stadium Loop

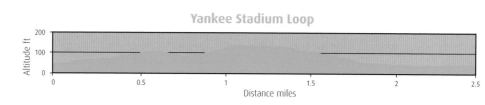

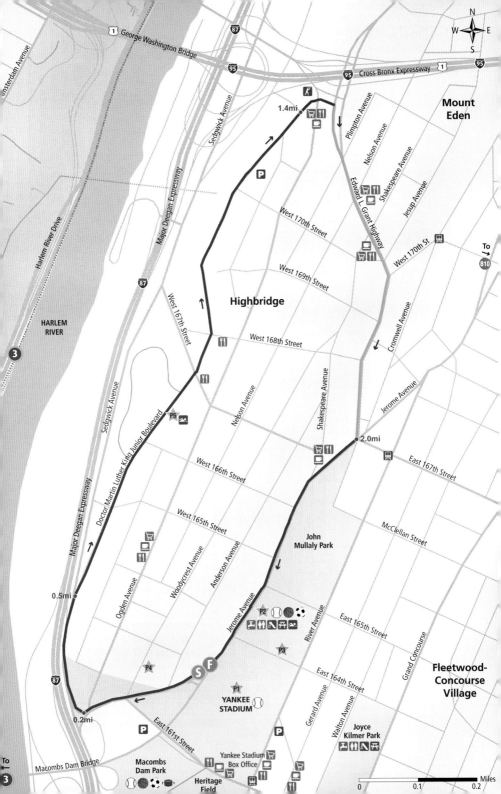

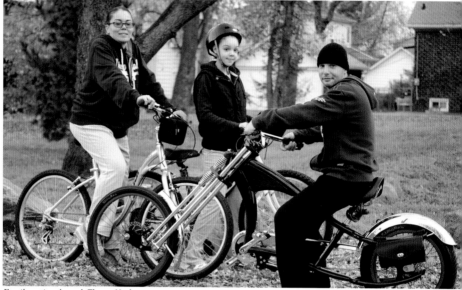

Family outing through Throgs Neck.

Photo Matt Wittmer

At a Glance

Distance 8.2 miles   **Elevation Gain** 277'

Terrain

Flat, mostly well-maintained roads meandering through mostly suburban areas.

Traffic

The start and finish are a bit busy. The rest is very light. By the time you're reading these words, there is probably a bike path being constructed in Ferry Point Park that could result in much of this ride being completely free of traffic.

How to Get There

The 6 train stops at Zerega Avenue, which is actually on the Pelham Parkway Loop. Ride backwards on that loop south on Zerega, then east on the Bruckner bridge, then right on Brush. It's about a mile in all.

Food and Drink

About .8 of a mile after the ride starts, you'll cross East Tremont Avenue, which is the commercial hub of the area. There are two pizza places as well as cafés and delis within a few hundred meters of the intersection. Also, right before (or after) you encounter SUNY Maritime, there's The Harbour Inn, at 50 Pennyfield Avenue.

Side Trip

The Maritime Industry Museum at Fort Schuyler gives you both a historic fort and a history of seafaring, starting with the ancient Phoenicians and detailing the maritime industry of the Americas in the 18th and 19th centuries.

www.sunymaritime.edu

Where to Bike Rating

About...

To many, Throgs Neck is just a bridge. To cyclists, it's a frustrating one, as there's no bike path over it. But Throgs Neck is also a community on Eastchester Bay. And the bridge passes over SUNY's Maritime College, which sits on a peninsula at the southeastern edge of The Bronx and houses a historic fort as well as an institute of higher learning.

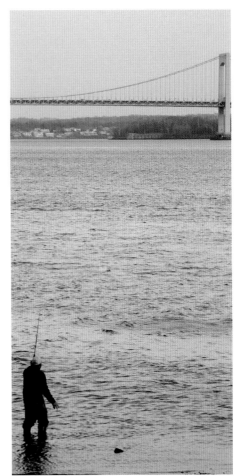

A fisherman casts from Old Ferry Point.
Photo Matt Wittmer

The Bronx

This ride starts on the edge of a gritty industrial area. Don't be fooled by the start, most of the ride is peaceful and on the water. This is also one of many rides that should be even better by the time you're reading these words as there are planned bike paths through Ferry Point Park, which is directly south of where this ride begins at the intersection of Ferry and Brush.

You're heading in a straight line for East Chester Bay. If you want to tarry, you can stop for a snack on East Tremont Avenue. When Lafayette ends, you're just about on the water. Make a right to follow the water's edge south.

When you can't go south any more because the land ends, you make a right onto Schley Avenue and follow it to its end, where it runs into the Throgs Neck Expressway. Parallel the expressway south until you come to your first intersection. Make a right and go under the highway. You're on this road until its end. Make a left at the guard station and you're on college property.

You're now going to follow the road so the water is on your left. This will take you under the Throgs Neck Bridge and to Fort Schuyler, which is at the very tip of the peninsula. On your left, is a tiny spit of land, a pe-

ninsula off the peninsula, a spot that's great for setting down in the grass or at a picnic table.

The first street that actually goes somewhere is Schurz Avenue. In time, you should be able to take this road into Ferry Point Park and almost all the way back to the start, but for now, there's no route through, so turn right just before the road ends onto Hosmer, and then follow the edge of the park, so it's on your right until you get to St. Raymond's Cemetery. Then, follow the edge of the cemetery until you're at the Cross Bronx Expressway Extension, where you'll make a left and ride it until you get to Lafayette, where the ride ends.

Ride Log

0.0 Start at the intersection of Brush and Lafayette avenues. Head east, up the hill.

0.6 Cross Balcolm. The ride will finish here.

0.8 Cross East Tremont Ave. To the right is the commercial strip of the area.

1.3 Lafayette ends. Turn right on Dean Ave.

1.4 Dean ends. Right on Philip Ave.

1.5 Left on Clarence Ave.

1.8 Clarence ends. Right on Schley Ave.

2.0 Schley ends. Left on Throgs Neck Expressway access road.

2.6 Right onto Prentiss Ave.

2.7 Bear left onto Pennyfield Ave.

3.5 Bear left into Maritime College property, then, at water, bear right onto Erben Ave.

4.2 Follow road around Fort Schuyler.

4.3 The road is now Shephard Ave.

4.6 Right onto Crownshield St.

4.7 Left onto Erben Ave. Retrace your ride out of college property.

5.1 Leave college property. Start riding up Pennyfield Ave.

5.6 Left onto Schurz Ave.

6.6 Right onto Hosmer Ave.

6.8 Hosmer ends. Right onto Miles Ave.

7.2 Left onto Balcolm Ave.

7.6 Balcolm ends. Right onto Randall Ave.

7.8 Left onto Cross Bronx Expressway Extension (not a highway).

8.2 Finish at Lafayette Ave and Cross Bronx Expressway Extension.

 P1 Saint Raymonds Cemetery
P2 Fort Schuyler—Maritime Industry Museum
P3 State University of New York Maritime College
P4 Schuyler Hill Performing Arts and Cultural Center

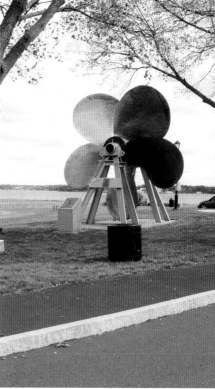

A giant screw standing outside Fort Schuyler

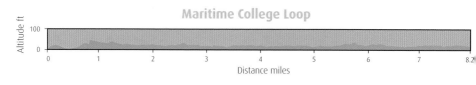

Maritime College Loop

Altitude ft

Distance miles

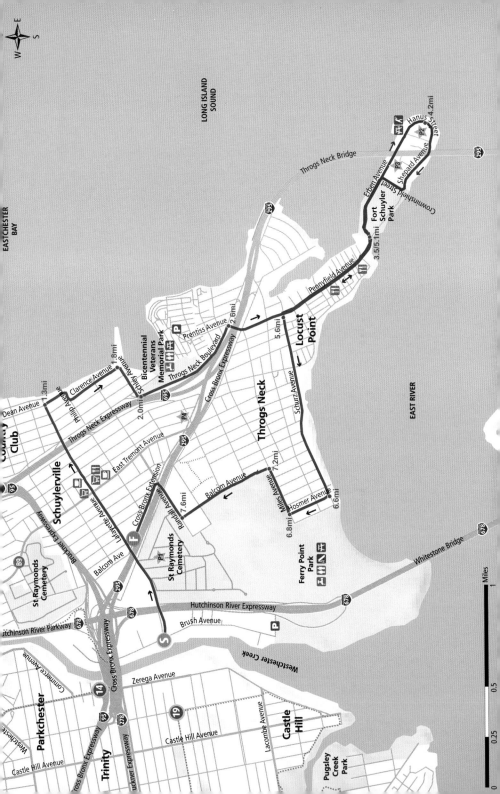

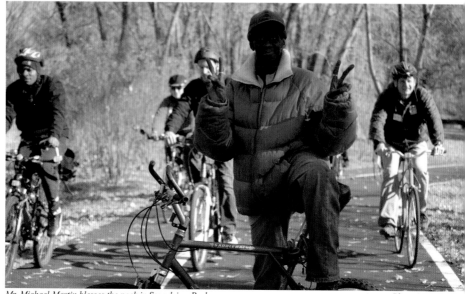

Mr. Michael Martin blesses the pack in Soundview Park.

Photo Matt Wittmer

At a Glance

Distance 5.0 miles   **Elevation Gain** 158′

Terrain

Flat bike paths with plenty of spots to stop and relax.

Traffic

From light to none. Much of the ride is on bike paths and the rest of the ride is on lightly-trafficked roads with bike lane markings.

How to Get There

The 6 train stop at Morrison Avenue is about a mile north of the start. Just ride south down Morrison.

Food and Drink

There are two commercial alleys on the ride. The first, Lafayette Avenue, you'll ride through at the start. The second, Soundview Avenue, you'll cross shortly after leaving Pugsley Creek Park.

Side Trip

Pugsley Creek Park is in the middle of the ride. It is home to freshwater wetlands of the East River that support diverse wildlife, including osprey. The park is largely untouched and mostly undiscovered. And if you plunk yourself down on some benches overlooking the water, it will only be a short matter of time before nature will come to life right in front of you.

www.nycgovparks.org/parks/pugsleycreekpark/highlights

Where to Bike Rating

About...

Reputations can be deceiving. Little good has been said about Soundview. That's thanks to a reputation for drugs and crime back in the 70s, 80s, and 90s, and because few people who live in The Bronx actually see the place, as the only street most know in the area is the Bruckner Expressway. It's a pity, as the streets are quiet, there is lots of waterfront, and the parks are totally underutilized. Both Pugsley Creek and Soundview have been largely left to nature, which makes their paths quiet and peaceful.

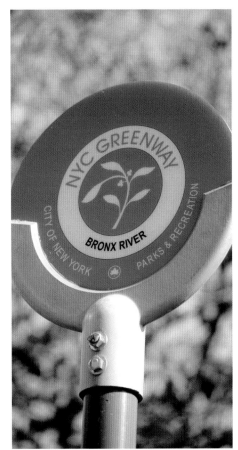

Signs like these help lead the way.   Photo Matt Wittmer

The ride starts at the intersection of Lafayette and Morrison avenues, with two large apartment towers behind you and a stub of Soundview Park on your left. You're going to ride through the park and take Lafayette just about to the end. This is the same Lafayette that is on the Maritime College Loop, only you can't go directly there from here, as Westchester Creek is in your way.

In the first half-mile, you'll come across one of two commercial areas on the ride. One is on Lafayette straddling Soundview Avenue. This is as busy as Lafayette gets.

About a mile and a half in, you'll come to Havemeyer. You'll turn right here and follow it until you're at the very southern end of the road. The road will have become Zerega Avenue on the way. Parkland will be straight ahead. Turn right and keep the water on your left.

On Howe Street, the bike path in Pugsley Creek Park begins. Follow the path. You'll be in trees, riding on the edge of coastal freshwater wetlands. If you need a spot for quiet reflection, there are several in the park.

When you exit the Pugsley Creek Park Bike Path, you should be riding west straight onto O'Brien Avenue. This will quickly pass the second commercial area on the loop, Soundview Avenue.

O'Brien also takes you into Soundview Park. Once in the park, follow the path. On your left, between the path and the water, are a number of spots where benches are facing south and looking out over the East River where the Bronx River joins the East.

The path turns from going west to going northwest where the Bronx River pours into the East River. The water is still on your left as you head north. You'll finish by riding through a stand of trees with open fields on both sides.

You finish up where you start, at Lafayette and Morrison. At only five miles, go for a second lap before stopping off for a bite.

Ride Log

 P1 Bronx YMCA
P2 Puglsey Creek Park untouched freshwater wetlands
P3 Woodrow Wilson Triangle

0.0 Start at the intersection of Lafayette and Morrison avenues. Head east on path through Soundview Park.

0.1 Cross Metcalf Ave and start riding east on street.

1.4 Turn right onto Havemeyer Ave.

1.9 Havemeyer ends at Zerega Ave. Turn right on Zerega.

2.2 Zerega ends at Castle Hill. Turn left onto Castle Hill.

2.3 Castle Hill ends. Turn right on Hart St.

2.4 Turn right onto Howe Ave. Bike path is on left.

2.5 Path turns left onto Olmstead Ave. Follow path.

2.6 Path turns left onto Norton Ave. Follow path.

2.6 Path turns right onto Screvin Ave. Follow path. You're in Pugsley Creek Park. Stay in park continuing on path.

2.8 Path turns left at Lacombe Ave. Follow path.

3.5 Leave Pugsley Creek Park. Ride straight onto O'Brien Ave.

3.8 Enter Soundview Park on bike path. Keep the water on your left.

4.3 Turn right. Continue to follow bike path.

5.0 Finish at the intersection of Lafayette and Morrison avenues.

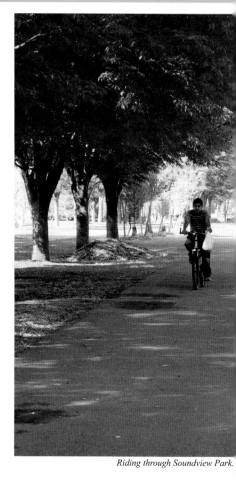

Riding through Soundview Park.

Soundview Loop

Altitude ft

Distance miles

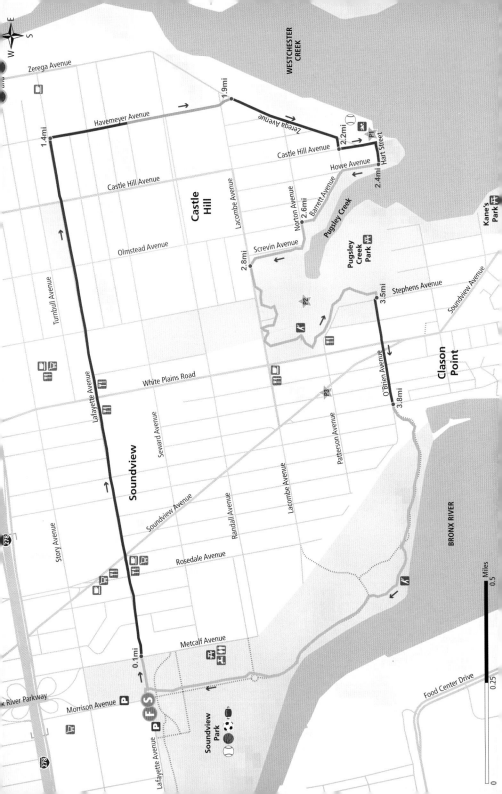

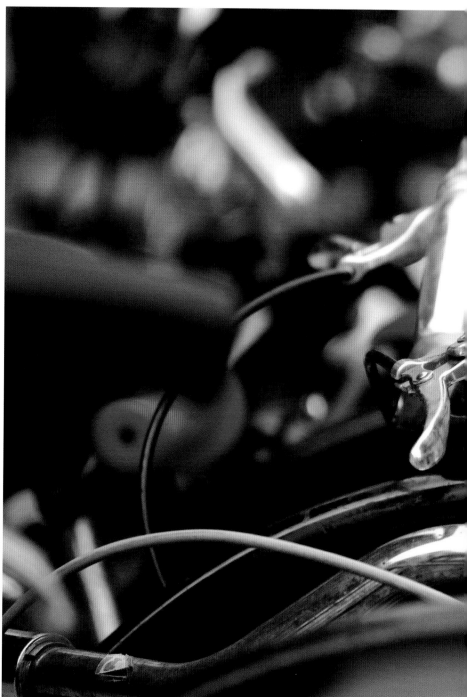

Photo Matt Wittmer

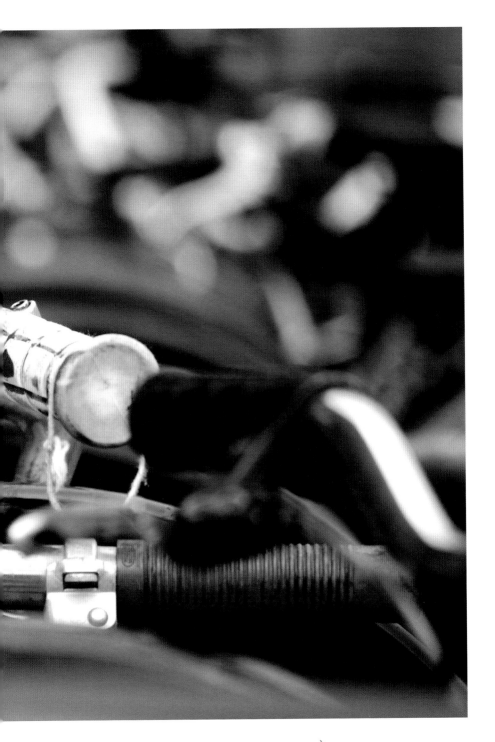

Queens

I've been riding through Queens for years. However, starting in Manhattan and crossing the Queensboro Bridge, it was hard to get beyond the idea that the borough is choked with cars driving too fast. One of my regular destinations in the county was the Kissena Velodrome, for Wednesday night races. To get there, I first tried riding along Queens Boulevard, a ride that was no fun at rush hour thanks to aggressive drivers and a bit scary after dark as the empty road and regular lights seemed to invite excessive speeding.

I then tried Northern Boulevard, which was much better, but still unpleasant. The best part of Northern was that I only had to be on it for a few miles before moving over to the 34th Avenue bike lane.

Now, thanks to the efforts of the Department of Transportation, there is a marked route that takes you from the Queensboro to the 34th Avenue bike lane while avoiding busy streets. It's delightful. Sunnyside Gardens feels like a hidden gem of the city.

Riding around Queens, I found several more places upon which to bestow that designation. My current favorite is the Vanderbilt Motor Parkway. It's hard to believe the road began as a private highway—one that bootleggers used—but that's part of the fun. I only wish the city and state had salvaged more of the road, as it originally went 45 miles out to Lake Ronkonkoma. It would have been a great greenway, if only people thought that way when it was taken over by New York State in 1938.

Looking at a Queens map, it seems that the largest greenspaces are cemeteries. At one time, cemeteries were open to the public for not only communing with the dead, but also as spaces for strolling and reflection. While riding around cemetery grounds might not be appropriate, the roads encircling these final resting places should be ripe for riding. We're hoping that the city sees value in creating bike lanes and paths here, as well as in other places in Queens. It's a big borough, and it needs more places to for riding.

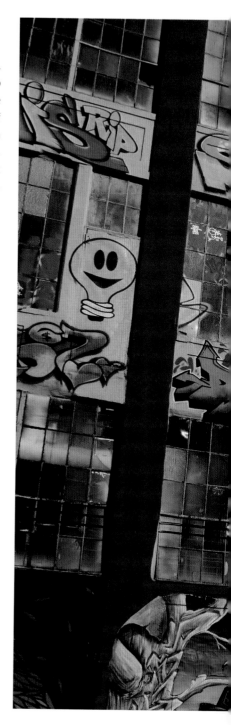

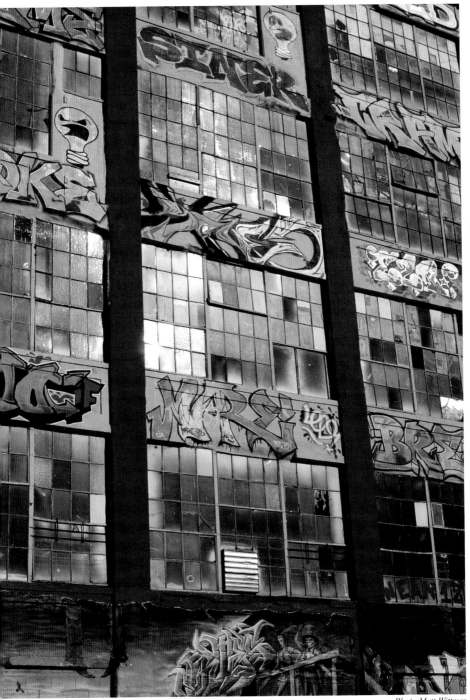

Photo Matt Wittmer

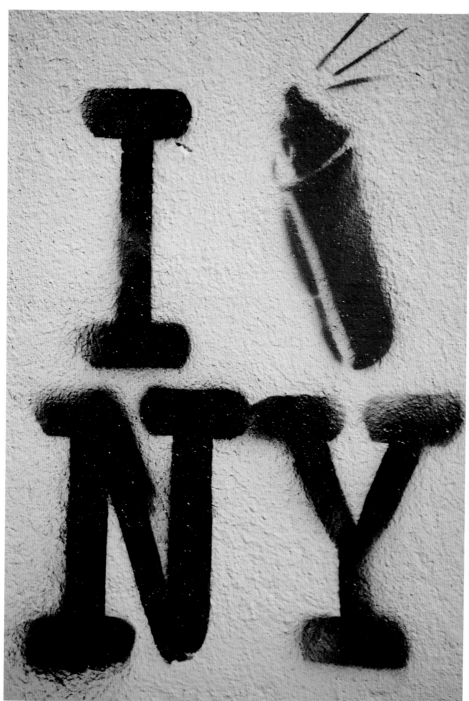

Photo Matt Wittmer

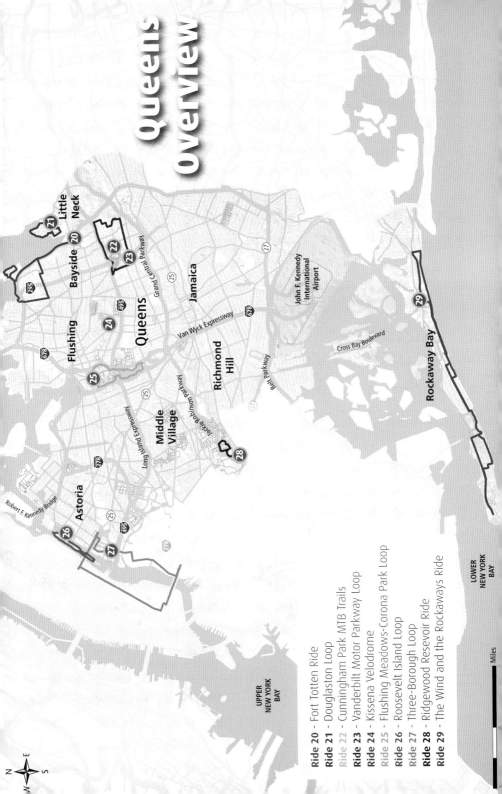

Queens Overview

Little Neck

Bayside

Flushing

Queens

Jamaica

Grand Central Parkway

Van Wyck Expressway

John F. Kennedy International Airport

Cross Bay Boulevard

Richmond Hill

Belt Parkway

Rockaway Bay

Jackie Robinson Parkway

Middle Village

Long Island Expressway

Astoria

Robert F. Kennedy Bridge

UPPER NEW YORK BAY

LOWER NEW YORK BAY

N E S W

Miles

Ride 20 - Fort Totten Ride
Ride 21 - Douglaston Loop
Ride 22 - Cunningham Park MTB Trails
Ride 23 - Vanderbilt Motor Parkway Loop
Ride 24 - Kissena Velodrome
Ride 25 - Flushing Meadows-Corona Park Loop
Ride 26 - Roosevelt Island Loop
Ride 27 - Three-Borough Loop
Ride 28 - Ridgewood Resevoir Ride
Ride 29 - The Wind and the Rockaways Ride

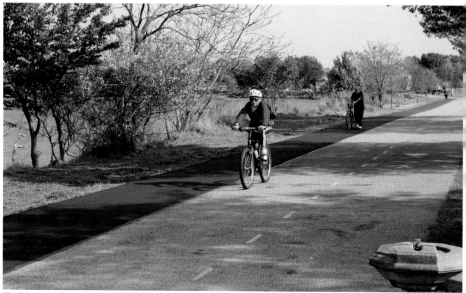

The bike path along the bay is great for both riding and walking bicycles.

At a Glance

Distance 8.7 miles   **Total Elevation** 427′

Terrain

Flat bike paths and roads.

Traffic

None for most of the ride. Light for the rest.

How to Get There

The easiest public transit option is to take the Long Island Rail Road to Bayside, Queens and ride a mile or so to the ride start.

Food and Drink

You'll pass through a commercial alley on Utopia Parkway that highlights the diversity of Queens. Greek, Chinese, pizza, bagels, and a deli are all available in a two-block length of road.

Side Trip

Go for the ride's namesake: Fort Totten. It is a decommissioned fort that was an army installation from the mid-19th century to the 1970s. The old fort is still there, and you can join in the speculation as to whether or not there's a tunnel leading to Fort Schuyler across the Sound. Even if there isn't, there are cool tunnels under the fortifications that are worth checking out.

www.nycgovparks.org/parks/forttotten

Where to Bike Rating

About...

Many people are familiar with Little Neck Bay from driving on the Cross Island Parkway. It's much prettier when you have an opportunity to actually see the bay, rather than sideways glances stolen while navigating highway traffic. Fort Totten is a great, hidden park of the city. Besides the history and architecture, there are plenty of places to plop down and enjoy sitting in a green field with a great view of Long Island Sound.

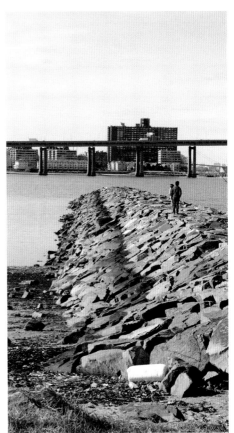

Exploring the jetty at Little Bay Park.
Photo Matt Wittmer

We wish that fewer bike paths were placed on the side of highways. You'll spend over three miles on this path alongside the Cross Island Parkway. This is one of the many times you'll curse Robert Moses when riding around New York. But the good thing is that the city has been pretty good about squeezing in paths alongside parks and waterfront. Both Little Neck Bay and the Long Island Sound are better appreciated from the saddle of a bicycle than from the seat of a car.

The first two and a half miles of this ride are alongside the Cross Island Parkway. If you look left, you see speeding cars. If you look right, you'll see the bay. It's a powerful contrast and appropriate that you can ride in between, using a vehicle, but benefiting from the calming effect of a large body of water.

Fort Totten, while a city park, is also home to an army outpost, and training centers for both the city's finest (NYPD) and bravest (FDNY). The riding is so peaceful, you'll be inspired to explore every road on the island. We turned wrong at some point and got chewed out by a policeman for being in their training grounds. Even after that, we were inspired to do laps around the peninsula.

Leaving Totten, and heading north to the Throgs

Neck Bridge, you get a great view of the bridge as well as a sighting of the SUNY Maritime College, the southeastern edge of the mainland, and part of The Maritime Loop (aka Ride 18).

Once off the bike path, you encounter Utopia Parkway, a misnomer on both counts, but a great name and a pleasant on-street bike path. The traffic is light and slow.

After a mile on Utopia, you're halfway through the suburban sojourn section of the ride. Just a few more roads and a few more turns, most of which are over on-street bike paths. Once you hit 28th Avenue, it's smooth sailing back to the bike path and onto the finish of the ride, back where you started on the edge of Alley Pond Park.

Ride 20 - Fort Totten Ride

Ride Log

0.0 Start at the intersection of Northern Pkwy and the Cross Island Pkwy. The bike path begins on the northeast corner, on the edge of Alley Pond Park. Ride north.

1.3 Bear right to avoid the overpass. On the return leg of the trip, you'll come down the overpass and ride south back to the start.

2.4 Turn right onto 212th St. This leads you into Fort Totten.

2.5 If you're short on time, you can turn left and follow the bike path north. As the route is configured, you're going into the fort for a lap of the grounds, then coming back out and then going north.

2.6 Go straight onto Bayside St.

2.7 Turn right onto Abbot Rd.

2.8 Turn left onto Sylvestar Ave.

2.9 Turn right onto Ordinance Rd.

3.0 Turn right onto Shore Rd.

3.5 Shore Rd turns into Sergeant Beers Ave.

3.6 Turn right onto Murray Ave.

3.8 Bear left onto Totten Ave.

4.0 Crossing over where we started. Follow Bayside out of fort.

4.1 Turn right onto bike path.

4.7 Ride under Throgs Neck Bridge.

4.8 Bike path ends. Turn right onto Utopia Pkwy. Utopia has on-street bike path.

5.6 Entering small commercial strip alongside Utopia. A good place to stop for a bite.

6.0 Turn left onto 26th Ave.

6.4 Cross over Clearview Expressway.

6.8 Turn right onto 212th St.

6.9 Turn left onto 28th Ave.

7.4 Twenty-Eighth ends. Turn right to get on bike path and go over Cross Island Pkwy.

7.6 Rejoin bike path. Head south to finish ride.

8.7 Finish at start; Northern Pkwy and Cross Island Pkwy.

 P1 Bayside Marina
P2 Fort Totten
P3 Start of Officer's Row
P4 Officer's Club, historic building
P5 Bayside Historical Society
P6 Fort Totten Gatehouse
P7 Start of a restaurant alley

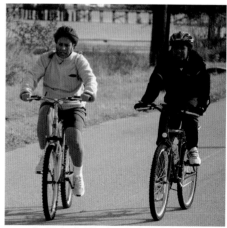

Joe Michael's Mile along Little Neck Bay is wide, flat and scenic.
Photo Matt Wittmer

Fort Totten Ride

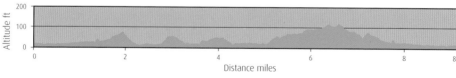

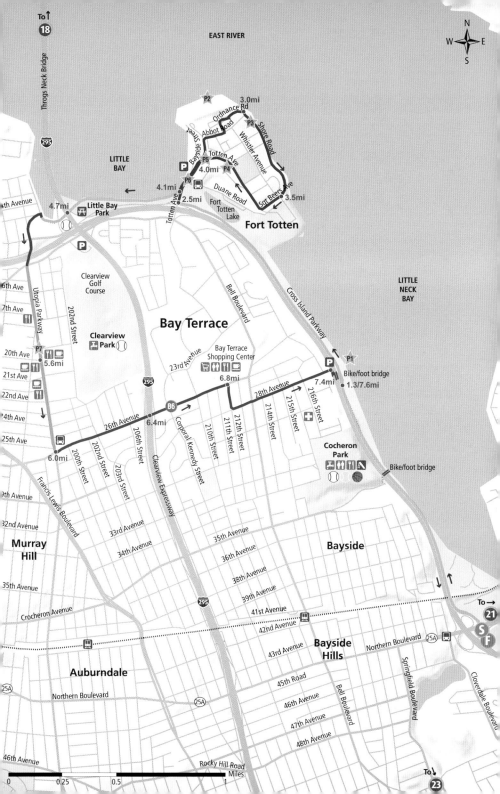

EAST RIVER

To ↑ **18**

N
W ✦ E
S

Throgs Neck Bridge

I-295

P2
3.0mi
Ordnance Rd
Abbot Road
P3
Bayside Street
Whistler Avenue
Shore Road
P5
Totten Ave
4.0mi P4
P6
4.1mi
2.5mi
Duane Road
Sgt Beers Ave
3.5mi
Fort Totten Lake
Fort Totten

LITTLE BAY

←

4.7mi
Little Bay Park

LITTLE NECK BAY

6th Ave
7th Ave

Utopia Parkway
202nd Street

P

Clearview Golf Course

Clearview Park

Bay Terrace

Bell Boulevard
Cross Island Parkway

P1
Bike/foot bridge
1.3/7.6mi

20th Ave
P7
5.6mi

21st Ave
22nd Ave
4th Ave

23rd Avenue
Bay Terrace Shopping Center
6.8mi
28th Avenue
7.4mi
P

25th Ave
26th Avenue
6.4mi
B6

200th Street
202nd Street
203rd Street
206th Street
Clearview Expressway
Corporal Kennedy Street
210th Street
211th Street
212th Street
214th Street
215th Street
216th Street

6.0mi

Cocheron Park

Bike/foot bridge

Francis Lewis Boulevard

9th Avenue
32nd Avenue
33rd Avenue
34th Avenue

Murray Hill

35th Avenue
36th Avenue
38th Avenue
39th Avenue

Bayside

35th Avenue
Crocheron Avenue
41st Avenue
42nd Avenue
43rd Avenue

Bayside Hills

Northern Boulevard
25A

To →
21
S
F

Auburndale
Northern Boulevard
25A

45th Road
46th Avenue
47th Avenue
48th Avenue

Bell Boulevard
Springfield Boulevard
Cloverdale Boulevard

46th Avenue
Rocky Hill Road
25A

To ↓
23

0   0.25   0.5   1
Miles

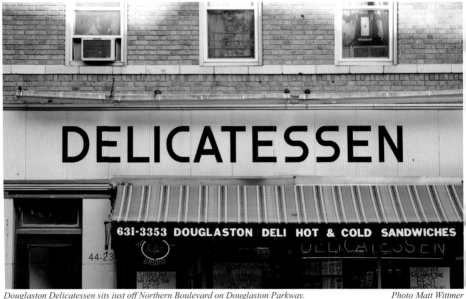

Douglaston Delicatessen sits just off Northern Boulevard on Douglaston Parkway.　　Photo Matt Wittmer

At a Glance

Distance 2.9 miles　　**Total Elevation** 263′

Terrain

Flat, with one steep hill at the start.

Traffic

Light.

How to Get There

Take the Long Island Rail Road to the Douglaston stop. When you get off the train and go to the north side of the tracks, you're across the street from the ride start.

Food and Drink

The Douglaston Market is right next to where the ride starts. It's a pizza place, a deli, a local market in one. Tables are set outside in warm weather months.

Side Trip

Alley Pond Park, just a little west down Northern Boulevard, is one of the many under-appreciated parks in the city. Alley Pond is situated on a glacial moraine, has freshwater and saltwater wetlands, and even old-growth woodlands, including the oldest living organism in the city, The Queens Giant, a tulip tree alleged to be over 400 years old (and the tallest tree in the city as well). The Alley Pond Environmental Center is where you should begin.

www.nycgovparks.org/parks/alleypondpark

Where to Bike Rating

About...

Douglaston is a leafy suburb in the city similar to The Bronx's Riverdale in how it is largely single-family houses and cut off from the rest of the city by water and highway. It's another peninsula with roads designed to discourage fast driving. When the area was settled by non-Natives, the land was laid out with large lots to encourage homeowners to lay out their own extensive gardens.

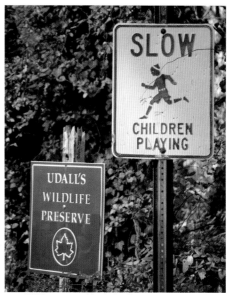

UWP is managed by the NYC Department of Parks and Recreation.   *Photo Matt Wittmer*

Anytime you can find a ride where through-streets are limited by parks, highways, or bodies of water, it's a safe bet that the riding is pretty peaceful. Douglaston being on a peninsula that is cut off from the rest of civilization first by rail road tracks (LIRR) and then by a major thoroughfare (Northern Boulevard, has two layers of protection from traffic). And this makes it a great place to go for a ride. Pity it is so small.

The ride starts at the Douglaston train station. Considering Douglaston is a bedroom community, the station and environs should be busy. They aren't. The

downtown area is tiny and you exit it immediately.

Willow Drive, the second road you're on, is a pretty steep hill, but take it steady and you'll get over the top before you know it. This hill is the reason this ride is only a two-bike ride rather than a one. What goes up must come down; in this case, almost immediately. The payoff isn't huge, but it's a rush and a time to freewheel a bit to recover from your hump up Willow.

Once you're on Douglas Road, you can just about ride on autopilot. Water is on your right, and that also means no streets coming from your right. Douglas wraps around the peninsula and turns into Shore Road and it takes nearly two miles from the moment you turn onto Douglas to hit another turn. You'll pass fields, then water on your right and pretty homes on your left.

And even once you've turned onto West Drive, you're pretty much following the edge of the peninsula and do so right until the end, back at the beginning, in front of the Douglaston train station. Since it ended so quickly, we strongly recommend doing at least another loop or exploring the other roads on the peninsula. Now that you have the perimeter down, it will be nearly impossible to get lost.

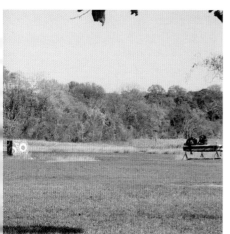

A little art with your park? Udall's Cove Park is a saltwater marsh, and a fine place to sit on the grass.

Queens

Ride Log

0.0 Start at 235th St and 41st Ave across the street from the Douglaston train station. Start heading northwest.

0.1 The first intersection is Douglaston Pkwy. Turn right to start up Willow Dr, the hill of the loop.

0.3 Turn right onto 39th Ave.

0.4 Thiry-Ninth Ave turns into Douglas Rd and then 38th Dr as you exit a big, sweeping turn.

0.5 Turn right onto Circle Rd.

0.6 Turn right onto 38th Rd.

0.7 Road turns left and becomes Douglas Rd.

 P1 Douglaston Pier

1.5 Road turns left and becomes Shore Rd.

2.2 Road turns left and becomes 36th Ave.

2.3 Turn right onto West Dr.

2.4 Turn right onto Bay St.

2.5 Turn left onto 233rd St.

2.8 Turn left onto 41st Ave.

2.9 Finish at 235th and 41st.

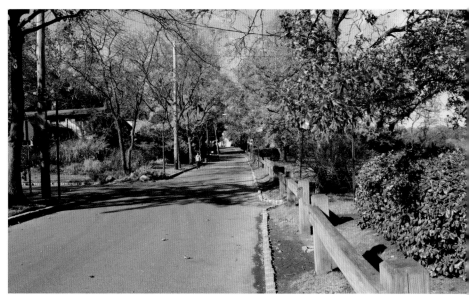

Another busy day on Douglas Road.

Douglaston Loop

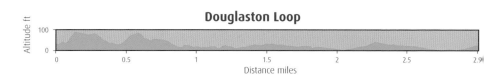

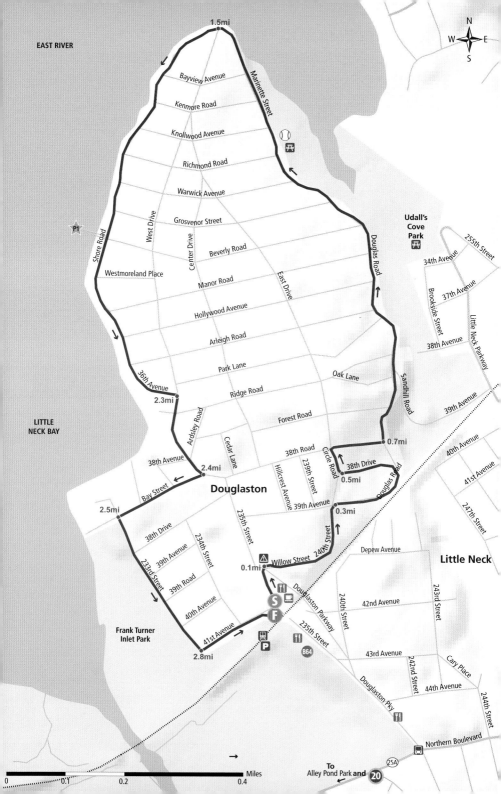

EAST RIVER

N
W E
S

1.5mi

Bayview Avenue

Marinette Street

Kenmore Road

Knollwood Avenue

Richmond Road

Warwick Avenue

West Drive

Grosvenor Street

Center Drive

Beverly Road

Udall's
Cove
Park

255th Street

34th Avenue

37th Avenue

Brookside Street

Little Neck Parkway

P1

Shore Road

Westmoreland Place

Manor Road

East Drive

Douglas Road

38th Avenue

39th Avenue

Hollywood Avenue

Arleigh Road

Park Lane

Oak Lane

Sandhill Road

LITTLE
NECK BAY

36th Avenue

2.3mi

Ardsley Road

Ridge Road

Forest Road

0.7mi

40th Avenue

41st Avenue

247th Street

38th Avenue

Cedar Lane

38th Road

Circle Road

38th Drive

0.5mi

Douglas Road

2.4mi

Bay Street

Douglaston

Hillcrest Avenue

239th Street

39th Avenue

0.3mi

40th Avenue

43rd Avenue

Little Neck

2.5mi

38th Drive

39th Avenue

39th Road

233rd Street

234th Street

235th Street

Willow Street

0.1mi

240th Street

Depew Avenue

42nd Avenue

243rd Street

240th Street

241st Avenue

S
F

Douglaston Parkway

235th Street

42nd Avenue

Frank Turner
Inlet Park

40th Avenue

41st Avenue

P

B64

43rd Avenue

Cary Place

242nd Street

44th Avenue

242nd Street

244th Street

2.8mi

Douglaston Pky

Northern Boulevard

0   0.1   0.2   0.4
Miles

To
Alley Pond Park and 20

25A

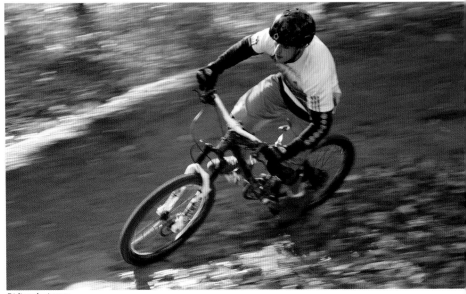

Riding the jumps.

At a Glance

Distance   Perimeter Loop: 2.1 miles
Trails in total: 6.5 miles
Elevation Gain 185′

Terrain

Off-road dirt trail with lots of roots and some rocks.

Traffic

No car traffic. Cyclists and hikers will be more or less present, depending on the weather.

How to Get There

Three trains stop close enough to this ride. The closest is the F Train stop at 179th Street and Hillside Avenue. It's a short spin up Midland Parkway. If you take the 7 Train to its Flushing terminus, you can ride the Brooklyn-Queens Greenway most of the way there, which is a five-mile ride. Or, you can take the Long Island Rail Road to Bayside, Queens, and ride about two miles to the park.

Food and Drink

There's nothing in the park, but there is food aplenty in Bayside and Flushing (great Chinese, said to be the best in the city), and there's a commercial strip at the intersection of 73rd Avenue and Bell Boulevard.

Side Trip

The dirt jump park in the middle of Cunningham is, if you're good enough, a great way to polish your skills and have some thrills. If you're new to mountain biking, it's the perfect place to observe skilled mountain bikers do their thing. Stop, observe, ask questions. Skilled riders are usually happy to share their knowledge.

Links to

Where to Bike Rating

Cunningham's signage is omnipresent and easy-to-follow. Photo Matt Wittmer

About...

This is the first place we legally pedaled off-road in New York City. The trails have been official for less than a decade, but they're already well-known, probably because New Yorkers who ride cherish trails close to home. There's a pretty cool dirt-jump park in the middle of Cunningham. Of the three parks that allow mountain biking in the city, this one has the best trail network, the best signage, the most looked-after trails, and probably the most bike traffic as well.

Cunningham, along with Highbridge in Manhattan and Wolfe's Pond on Staten Island, contain the only sanctioned mountain bike trails in the city. The trails in these three parks are allowed by the Parks Department. The New York City Mountain Bike Association, which was formed to help in the building of the Highbridge trails built the trails here and maintains them, as they do all the official NYCMTB trails. If you find you love urban mountain biking, volunteer to help them in their mission.

While the park has beginner, intermediate, and advanced trails and a dirt jump park, noobs should stick to the beginner's trails that ring the park. The route laid out on the map follows those trails. As you feel your skill and confidence increasing, follow the signs off the beginner loop to the harder trails.

The park is small, so it's impossible to get lost for more than a few minutes. The beginner trails are easy enough that a skilled cyclist can ride them on a road bike, which should mean anyone with knobby tires should be able to handle getting dirty in Cunningham. Cyclocrossers are also known to take their rides into these woods for training.

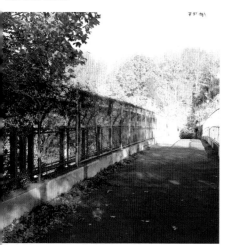

The bridge connecting both halves of the park.

Queens

Ride Log

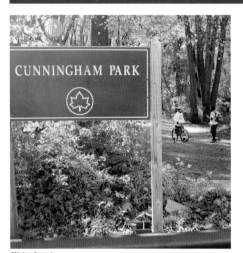

We're here!

0.0 Start at trailhead. It sits at the intersection of 67th Ave and 210th St.

206ft Bear left to start on the perimeter loop.

0.6 Trail crossing. Very wide track. Turn left.

0.7 Ride bridge over Clearview Expressway.

0.8 Bear left to continue on beginner trail.

0.9 Come to clearing. Dirt Jump Park is straight. Follow trail to the left.

1.3 Finish trans-Clearview loop. Turn left to go back over bridge to eastern half of park.

1.5 Bear left to continue on perimeter loop.

2.1 Finish back by trailhead.

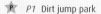 *P1* Dirt jump park

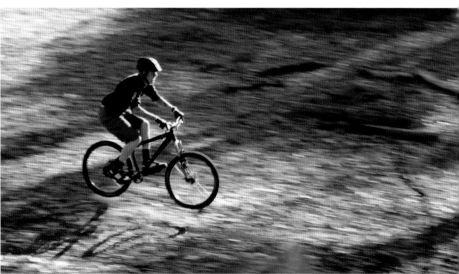

Let's go!

Cunningham Park MTB Trails

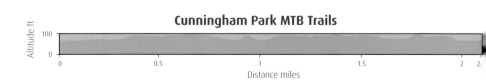

Altitude ft

Distance miles

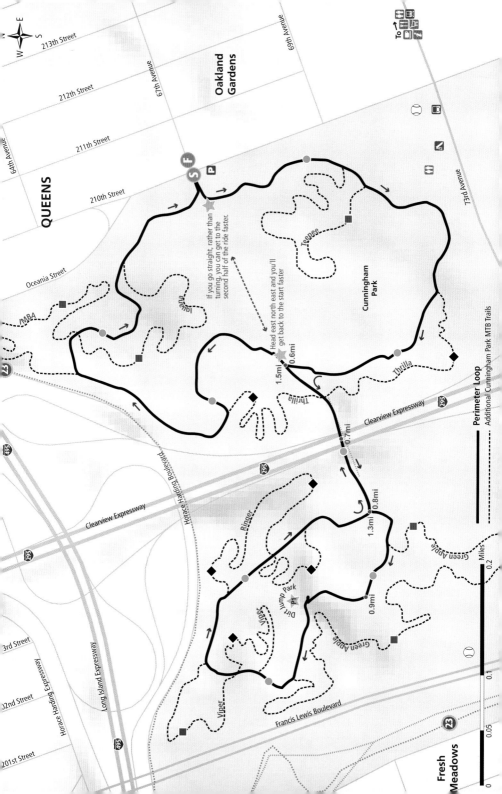

QUEENS

Oakland
Gardens

Cunningham Park

Fresh
Meadows

213th Street
212th Street
211th Street
210th Street

69th Avenue
67th Avenue

64th Avenue

Oceania Street

3rd Street
02nd Street
201st Street

Horace Harding Expressway
Long Island Expressway
Clearview Expressway
Horace Harding Boulevard

Clearview Expressway

73rd Avenue

Francis Lewis Boulevard

If you go straight, rather than
turning, you can get to the
second half of the ride faster.

Head east north east and you'll
get back to the start faster.

1.5mi
0.6mi

0.7mi

0.8mi

1.3mi

0.9mi

Teepee
Thrilla
Thrilla
Ringer
Viper
Viper
Green Apple
Green Apple
Dirt Jump Park
MBA
Iguana

Perimeter Loop

Additional Cunningham Park MTB Trails

Miles
0   0.05   0.1   0.2

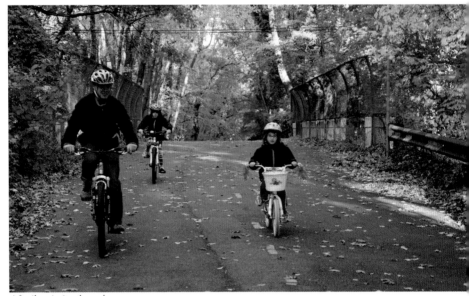

A family enjoying the parkway.

At a Glance

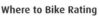

Distance 5.8 miles   **Total Elevation** 404'

Terrain

Lightly rolling, a few hills punctuated by lots of flat roads and a few gentle descents.

Traffic

Dramatic mix. From riding on a highway frontage road that can be jammed with cars on occasion to a bike path that can be completely empty, save you.

How to Get There

This ride goes around Cunningham Park's mountain bike trails (Ride 22), so getting here is largely the same. There are three train stops close enough to ride from easily. The closest is the F Train stop at 179th Street and Hillside Avenue. It's a short spin up Midland Parkway. If you take the 7 Train to its Flushing terminus, you can ride the Brooklyn-Queens Greenway most of the way there, which is a five-mile ride. Or, you can take the Long Island Rail Road to Bayside, Queens, and ride about two miles to the park.

Food and Drink

As we wrote about the eats near Cunningham Park's mountain bike trails, there's nothing in the park. But there is food aplenty in Bayside and Flushing (great Chinese said to be the best in the city), and there's a commercial strip at the intersection of 73rd Avenue and Bell Boulevard.

Side Trip

Just two miles from the southeastern edge of the ride is Queens Farm Museum. The farm has been in operation since 1697. It is both a working farm, and a site that explains the city's agrarian past. Open every day from 10am to 5pm. **www.queensfarm.org**

Links to (22)

Where to Bike Rating

About...

This ride is an interesting study in contrasts – of both successful and unsuccessful visions of uninterrupted highway driving. While we're cyclists first, and New York is a human-powered and public-transit town, cars and the amenities created for driving, are still a big part of life. The parkway this loop is named for was the first purpose-built private highway in the country. It was a high-speed toll road, with bridges making it possible for drivers to avoid slowing, and banked turns to allow high speeds. It was sold to the state 20 years after opening; public highways bankrupted it.

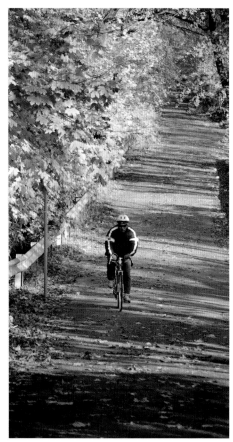

Cyclists are a fixture of the VMP's colorful history.
Photo Matt Wittmer

We don't start many rides on the edge of parking lots, but here, it makes sense. The Vanderbilt Motor Parkway Loop takes you right by this small lot, and the lot itself is in a quiet spot and even has benches where we start.

At the beginning, the ride threads around several large, wide-open playing fields. In good weather, expect to find lots of people meandering and making their way to the fields. After you ride over the first of many bridges path traffic will thin out and you'll get a fun sensation. That's riding through woods in what is clearly the middle of a heavily-trafficked area. You've got a clear path ahead, are surrounded by nature, but you'll still sense car traffic just beyond your vision.

The traffic will become explicit when you ride out of the park and onto the Horace Harding Expressway. You'll be paralleling the Long Island Expressway. The nice thing is that while most of what you see there is cars stuck in bumper-to-bumper traffic, you'll be rolling along unimpeded. Keep your head up and ears perked as drivers frustrated by traffic can end up on the same road with you and can get touchy. All the same, there are enough lights that they won't be tempted to speed.

Once you climb up a hill and get to a point that the highway is beneath you, the road will feel quieter and more manageable, and once you're used to this sensation, you're at the turn. Go right, have Alley Pond Park on your left and start threading suburban streets en route to entering the park.

The highlight is the Vanderbilt Motor Parkway. Here, too, you're in the middle of the woods, a green oasis in very densely-packed suburbia. You feel like you're sneaking through people's back yards, and you can have fun imagining that you're rum-running; lore has it that bootleggers used to utilize this road to elude cops during prohibition. Sixty mph on this road, in early cars, must have been frightening.

Ride Log

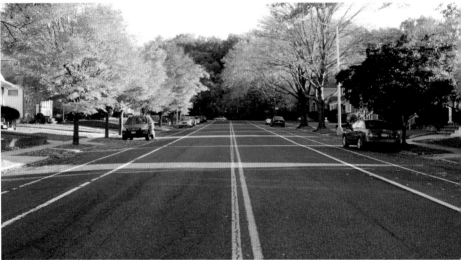

Quiet suburban streets comprise most of the connecting roads.

0.0 Start in parking lot by corner of 73rd Ave and Hollis Hills Terrace. Go west under Clearview Expressway.

0.2 Turn left. You're following the bike path to the end of the park.

0.3 Turn right.

0.4 Take bridge over Francis Lewis Blvd.

0.5 Follow path north. Parallel 199th St, but stay in park.

0.6 Take bridge over 73rd Ave. Turn right.

1.1 Turn left.

1.2 Park ends. Make sharp right onto Horace Harding Expressway South.

3.1 Turn right onto 233rd St. Alley Pond Park is on your left.

3.4 Turn right onto 67th Ave.

3.5 Turn left onto 230th St.

3.7 Turn right onto 69th Ave.

3.8 Turn left onto Cloverdale Blvd.

3.9 Enter Alley Pond Park. Follow bike path.

4.0 Bear left to stay on path.

4.2 Path snakes a bit.

4.3 Exit park. Turn left onto Cloverdale Blvd.

4.4 Enter park. Turn right onto Vanderbilt Motor Pkwy.

5.7 Turn right with path.

5.8 Finish at the start. The parking lot is here.

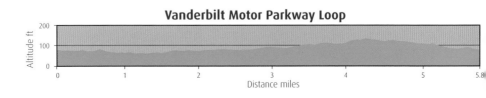

Vanderbilt Motor Parkway Loop

Altitude ft

200
100
0

Distance miles
0   1   2   3   4   5   5.8

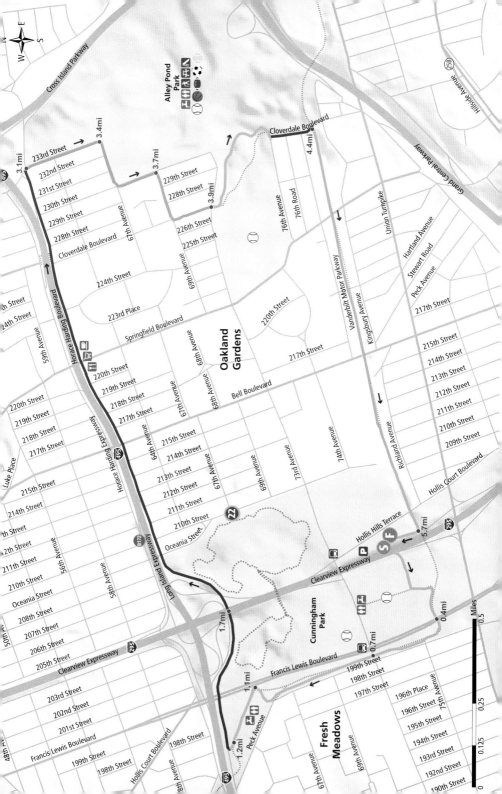

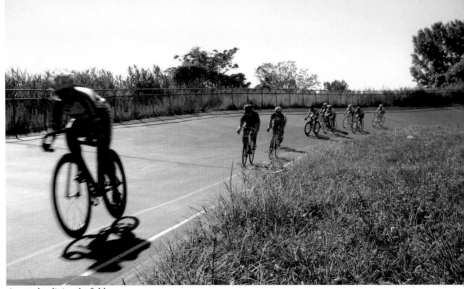

An attack splitting the field.

At a Glance

Distance 0.3 mile   **Elevation Gain** 0′

Terrain
Banked track (aka velodrome).

Traffic
Light. Bicycles only.

How to Get There
Take the 7 Train to its Flushing terminus. Then ride about a mile on Kissena Boulevard. When you get to the park, turn left on Booth Memorial Avenue. The track entrance is the first left. You can also take the F Train to Parsons Boulevard, and ride Parsons until it veers into Kissena, then make a right on Booth. The track is .2 mile after the driveway entrance.

Food and Drink
Downtown Flushing is known for its great Chinese food. It's also an immigrant haven, with lots of ethnic fare; there's also no shortage of Indian, Italian or Korean food.

Side Trip
Take in some track racing. Admission is free, the races are great to watch, and the velodrome is in a pretty setting. Borrow a bike and try racing for yourself.
www.kissena.info/track

Where to Bike Rating

About...

The Kissena Velodrome is one of three outdoor bike tracks in the northeastern United States. It was built in 1962 for the 1964 Olympic Trials, and re-built in 2003 when the city was making a bid for the 2012 Olympic Games. It's a 400-meter banked oval, paved with asphalt, and protected by fencing. New York had a great track racing history; a race was even named for Madison Square Garden. By the time this track was built, all the old velodromes were gone.

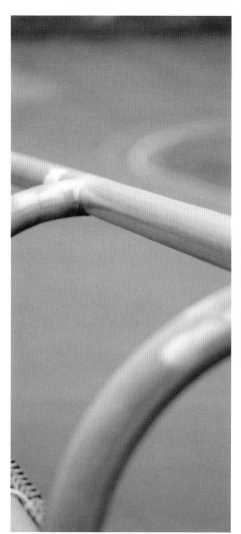

New York City's only velodrome sits ready and waiting. Photo Matt Wittmer

Don't feel bad if you've never heard of the Kissena Velodrome. Many people who live near Kissena Park, for which the velodrome is named, haven't either. But now that you've heard of it, you owe it to yourself to try it out.

The track is open and free to the public. You can ride on it with any bike any time the park is open, the track surface is dry and there isn't racing going on, which is most of the time. The track was designed long, with gentle banks so that just about anyone with a minimum of bike-handling skills can ride it at just about any speed. If you're riding slow, stay high, if fast, you can ride low. Four hundred meters goes by pretty fast, but if you want an uninterrupted ride or a place where you can measure your effort without distraction, the track can be fun.

Track racing is done with "track bikes," fixed-gear bicyles that seem to have no brakes. Since the single cog is fixed to the rear wheel (hence the name), when you pedal the bike moves, when you slow down your pedaling, the bike slows. And if you want to slow down fast, you put your gloved hand on a tire to scrub off more speed.

Go fast, turn left. The motto of track racers doesn't give credit to the exciting and tactically complex world that is mass-start track racing. Races are traditionally held Wednesday evenings from late April to Labor Day. People like racing track because the races are short and intense, the workout great, and despite all the technological advances in the last 20 years, you can still be competitive on an inexpensive bike built with technology that is over 40 years old. And the bike can double as your hipster commuter rig when you want to bust out the flannel.

Ride Log

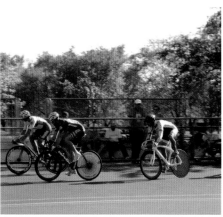

This isn't your regular ride log: From the parking lo approach the track, open the low gate and, with you bike, cross the track at the start/finish line. Watch fo other riders from the left. Ride as many laps as you like When finished, slow and exit the track. Be respectful o other riders by hand signaling before you exit.

Looking around in a match sprint.

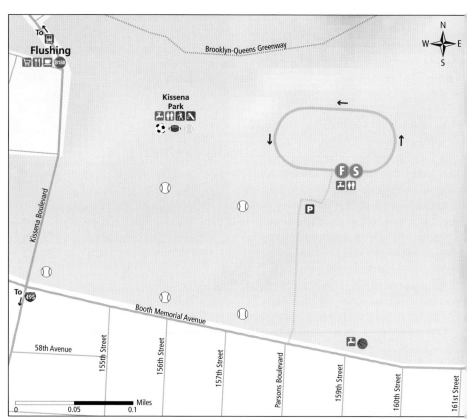

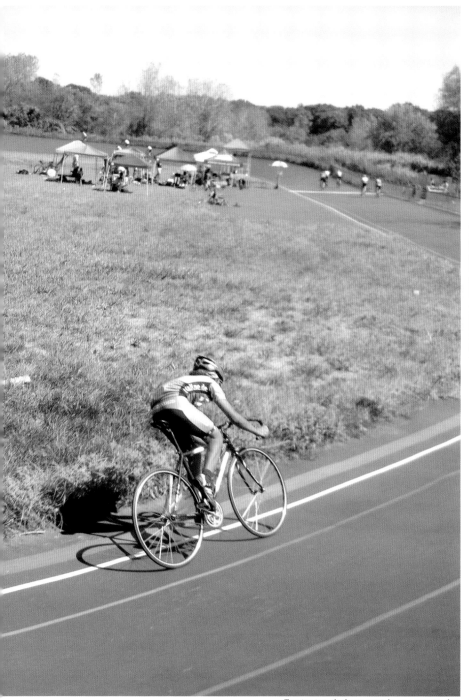

Turning into the home straight on a practice lap.

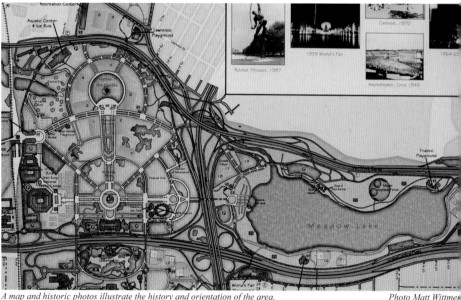

A map and historic photos illustrate the history and orientation of the area.   Photo Matt Wittmer

At a Glance

Distance 4.9 miles   **Elevation Gain** 62′

Terrain

Flat roads and bike path.

Traffic

Light to none. About half the ride is on park access roads, and the rest are on bike paths. Expect it to be crowded on warm weekends, empty on cold or wet days.

How to Get There

There's a Long Island Rail Road stop inside the park! But it's only used when either the Mets are playing or the United States Open tennis tournament is in session. Otherwise, the 7 Train stops at Shea Stadium/Willets Point regardless of who is playing and when.

Food and Drink

During the warmer months of the year, there are food carts set up by both the tennis center and the mini-golf center, and you will also find carts scattered throughout the park. The tennis center usually has something set up in the winter as well. For more of a sit-down meal, you're less than a mile away from the international dining experience known as downtown Flushing.

Side Trip

The Queens Museum of Art is not only the start and finish of the ride, but a great cultural institution. Probably best known for The Panorama, a scale model of the entire city, it is much more. While it has diverse collections, it is very hands-on in its approach to what it exhibits and definitely has New York City as its main focus.

www.queensmuseum.org

Where to Bike Rating

About...

The city's second-largest park, with the most usable space, Flushing Meadows has everything: swimming pools, skating rinks, playgrounds, ball fields, courts, barbecuing, fishing, a zoo, a marina, skate parks, and cycling. This ash dump was transformed into a park for the 1939 World's Fair, was the temporary site of the United Nations (now the Queens Museum), was the site of the 1964 World's Fair, and is designed as a playground for the people. It's easy to go for a ride and make a day of it.

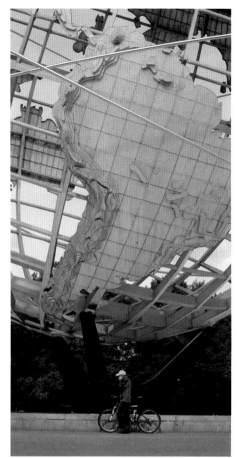

Walking and talking in front of the iconic Unisphere.
Photo Matt Wittmer

There are many ways into the park. We start this ride by the Billie Jean King Tennis Center because it's just past the two train platforms you will be exiting if you take the train here.

The ride goes around the building counter-clockwise and heads for the Perimeter Road, which you'll turn right to join and start riding around the park clockwise. On this ride, you'll get a good look at just about everything the park has to offer.

After passing the aquatic center, you'll scan right and view the manicured walkways that focus the eye's attention on the Unisphere, the 12-story high stainless steel globe that was built for the 1964 World's Fair. Originally, the walkways helped take World's Fair visitors from the Unisphere to various pavilions. This formal design is a contrast to the more natural design of the southern part of the park, which you'll see after making a left turn and heading for Meadow Lake.

Meadow Lake, at 93 acres, is the city's largest lake. It's also man made, and great for boating. When riding clockwise around the lake, you'll see the various playgrounds that are contained in the park. You'll pedal past cricket fields, a marina for rental boats, a field for flying model airplanes, baseball fields, a grilling sec-tion, and even playgrounds for kids.

When you ride over the Meadow Lake Bridge back to the northern half of the park, you'll come across more ruins from the two World's Fairs. Some have been dismantled, some have been utilized as great skate parks, and some have been formally re-purposed into theatres and museums.

After passing through the ruins of the World fairs, you're almost to the Queens Museum of Art, and almost finished with the ride. Our preference is to do another lap, stopping at the Unisphere to reflect, then grabbing a hot dog from a cart, before stopping in to check out the exhibitions.

Ride Log

0.0 Start in front of Billie Jean King Tennis Center.

0.1 Turn right onto Perimeter Rd (aka Meridian, aka Flushing Meadows Park).

0.3 Cross over Flushing Creek. Turn left. This is Meadow Lake Promenade, but you'll just see directions to the bike path.

1.4 At traffic circle, continue going south. After circle, there will be a bridge over the edge of the lake.

1.5 Turn right off road onto bike path.

2.3 Still on path, go over bridge at south end of lake. Bear right to stay on path after bridge.

3.4 Join up with road. Continue straight.

3.5 Go around circle to get to foot of Amphitheatre Bridge.

3.6 Start up Amphitheatre Bridge.

3.7 End bridge. Make a gradual 180-degree turn to the

 P1 Louis Armstrong Stadium
P2 Billie Jean King National Tennis Center
P3 Arthur Ashe Stadium
P4 Skate Ramps
P5 Queens Theatre in the Park
P6 Queens Museum of Art
P7 Queens Zoo
P8 New York Hall of Science

left.

3.8 Turn right onto Perimeter Rd. This will take you back to the start.

4.2 Queens Museum of Art is on the right.

4.5 Turn right. Remain on Perimeter.

4.8 Turn right off of Perimeter to get back to start.

4.9 Finish where you started.

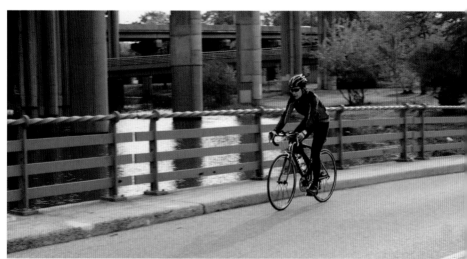

The riding is pleasant, even under the shadow of highways.

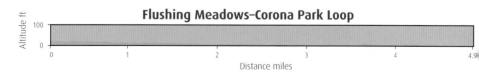

Flushing Meadows–Corona Park Loop

Altitude ft

100

0

0   1   2   3   4   4.9

Distance miles

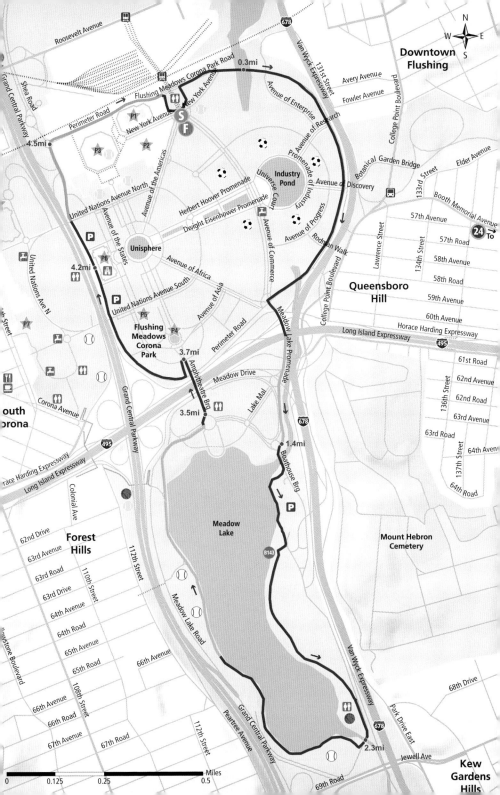

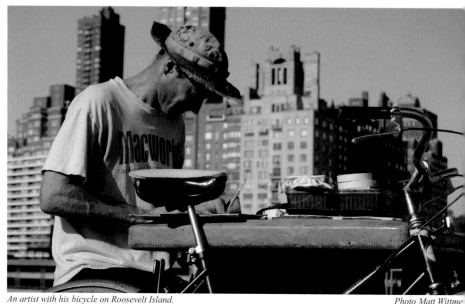

An artist with his bicycle on Roosevelt Island.

Photo Matt Wittme

At a Glance

Distance 3.5 miles   **Elevation Gain** 173'

Terrain

Flat roads and bike paths.

Traffic

Light. The bike paths will have some pedestrians strolling along, some cyclists stroking along, and the greatest danger will be a kid or a dog off-leash. The roads are lightly-trafficked; figure most are residents and know what to expect.

How to Get There

You can ride from Long Island City, Queens over the Roosevelt Island Bridge, aka 36th Avenue. You can also take the F Train. And the Roosevelt Island Tramway, which departs from 59th Street and Second Avenue allows bicycles.

Food and Drink

Ride along Main Street to find your food. There are both delis and sit down restaurants. Locals like Riverwalk Bar and Grill, which is also located next to Nono's Foccaceria and Fuji East.

Side Trip

The ruins of Roosevelt Island, namely the Smallpox Hospital and Stecker Laboratory are amazing. And largely off limits to the public. Still, the Roosevelt Island Historical Society can point you to the Octagon, the Lighthouse, and the Blackwell House, and the Chapel of the Good Shepherd.

www.rihs.us

Links to

Where to Bike Rating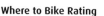

About...

Roosevelt Island is an island off an island, and even though it's considered part of Manhattan, the only bridge to it is from Queens. This onetime home to hogs, then hospitals, is now a small town of roughly 10,000. Since there is nowhere to drive here, there are few roads, and fewer reasons for cars to speed. The views on the south, west, and north sides of the island are excellent. The main street is both modern and quaint at the same time.

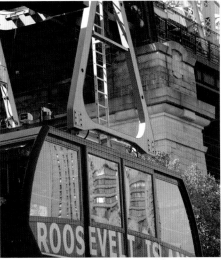

Bikes are welcome on the tram to and from Manhattan.
Photo Matt Wittmer

Queens

This loop starts in East Road, just south of the Roosevelt Island Bridge. There aren't many street names, but the great thing is that on an island two miles long and fifteen-hundredths of a mile wide, with the southern end closed to the public, getting lost is very hard. And even if you do get lost, you'll find your way back very easily.

Just to the east of East Road, between the road and the water is the bike path. Start going south, which means the water will be on your left, and keep going south until you can go south no longer. At the time of writing, the path finished up on East Road, and you follow that to South Point Park, where there's a fence keeping you from going any further. In the near future, there will be a bike path all the way along the water until this point, or even, perhaps, into the park, where you'll be able to check out the ruins.

For now, you'll have to turn right onto Road 3, and travel west to the west side of the island. Much as with the bike path on the east side, the west side path is between W Road and the water, though we found riding on W Road much easier.

Take W north, going under the Queensboro Bridge, past the F Train stop, until you get to the fork for Main Street, where you go left to get onto West Road, and West Road becomes a bike path.

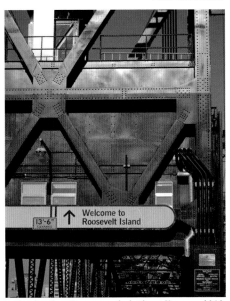

If cycling from Queens, use the bridge at Vernon and 36th.
Photo Matt Wittmer

Take this path all the way to the north end of the island. At the north end, you'll be at the lighthouse of Lighthouse Park, and you ride around that and start down the bike path on the eastern edge of the island and follow it all the way back to the start.

Ride Log

0.0 Start at East Rd (aka E Rd) just south of the Roosevelt Island Bridge (aka 36th Ave).

0.3 Bear right off the bike path while still heading south.

0.4 Bear left to join up with East Rd.

0.6 Go around traffic circle and turn left to follow East Rd.

1.0 Road turns right. Turn right onto Rd 3.

1.1 Turn right onto West Rd (aka W Rd).

1.5 Pass F Train stop.

1.6 Bear left to stay on West Rd.

2.8 Arrive at north end of island. Bear right to start heading south. Follow water.

2.9 East Rd begins. Just keep the water on your left.

3.5 Finish at East Rd just south of the Roosevelt Island Bridge.

P1 Chapel of the Good Shepherd
P2 Blackwell House
P3 Roosevelt Island Lighthouse
P4 The Octagon

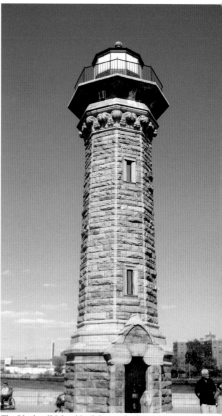

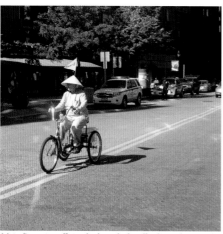

Main Street is sufficiently devoid of traffic that riding a trike down the middle of the road isn't an issue.

The Blackwell Island Lighthouse, built in 1872, stands at the northern edge of the island.

Roosevelt Island Loop

Altitude ft

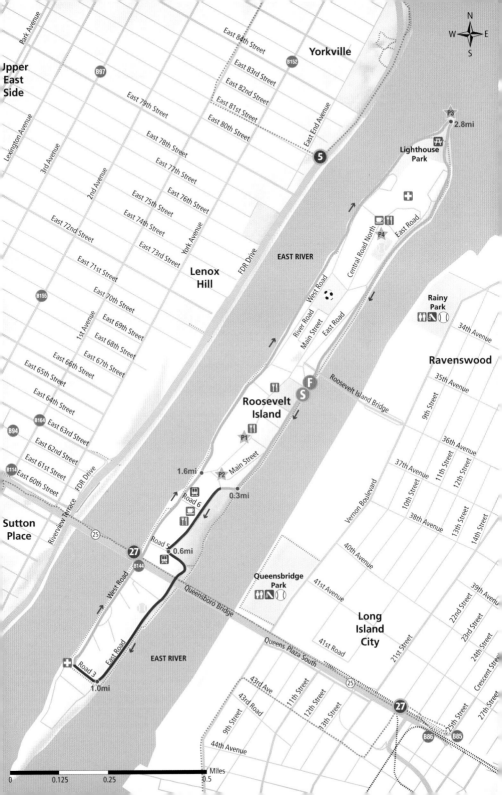

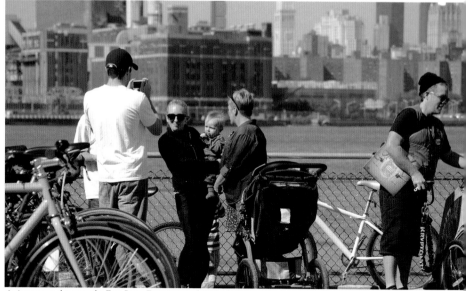

A picturesque day near the East River Ferry terminal in North Williamsburg.

Photo Matt Wittmer

At a Glance

Distance 10.8 miles   **Elevation Gain** 344'

Terrain

Flat, save the three bridges you'll be riding over. The Pulaski Bridge is a pretty small hill, while the Williamsburg and Queensboro bridges are a little on the long side.

Traffic

Varied. Almost the entire route is over bike paths, but they vary from a simple striped lane to protected lanes.

How to Get There

The ride starts on the Queens side of the Pulaski Bridge. The closest subway stop is the Hunters Point Avenue 7 Train stop. It's also a LIRR stop. But you can also quickly ride from the E, F, G, M, N, Q, and R trains, all of which stop in Long Island City by the Queensboro Bridge.

Food and Drink

Oy, you're passing through several excellent foodie alleys on this ride. The ride goes through great restaurant streets in Long Island City, Greenpoint, and the Lower East Side; it's hard to choose. Our preference is the Lower East Side, but there are good eats by the ride start/finish. Literally next door to the start is Manetta's Ristorante, pizza and Italian fare. Just about across the street is Sweetleaf Coffee and Tea for something lighter.

Side Trip

Building 92 at the Brooklyn Navy Yard. It's a bit off the route in Brooklyn, but it's a historic building with art exhibitions in a converted industrial space. The building itself is from 1857, and the area is decommissioned naval property that they're finding new uses for. **www.bldg92.com**

Links to

Where to Bike Rating

About...

This ride is in Queens for less than a third of its duration, but it's a great central location, and the ride demonstrates how easy it is to get around the city. Superb views are also to be had from two big bridges, the Williamsburg and the Queensboro. And the third bridge has some pretty good views as well.

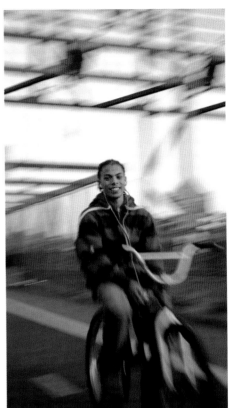

Getting good buzz on the Williamsburg Bridge.
Photo Matt Wittmer

Queens

There's an old joke that you're not a New Yorker until you mourn the loss of something "that used to be right there." Of course, the city is changing every day; even tourists can get in on the act.

While researching this book, we did this ride a few times, and even while riding this route, we saw major changes. The First Avenue bike lane was being created, the Queens side entry to the Queensboro Bridge bike path was being built, among other things. No telling how it will look by the time this book is published.

But in the greater scheme of things, there is lots of loss on display, the greatest of which is the decay of industrial New York. Both the Queens and Brooklyn segments ride through old industrial zones, where lots of stuff was made. Much of the Brooklyn section passes by industrial buildings that are either fallow or have been converted to post-industrial uses. The ride passes the Brooklyn Navy Yard, which had American defense shipbuilding operations from the close of the Revolutionary War until 1966. At one time, the yard employed 10,000 workers. Now, it rises again, but with many fewer workers, and less heavy machinery.

Drivers, no doubt, will be mourning the loss of driving lanes, but those lanes in all three boroughs will make your riding easier and driving safer. You will experience a diversity of on-street bike paths in the city. From the sharrows-type to the protected lane. All the same, the riding in Brooklyn is amongst the most pleasant of the ride, as the balance between bikes and cars seems to shift heavily toward bikes.

Once on the Williamsburg Bridge, you get to survey industrial Brooklyn, and the Navy Yard, survey the East River and the way Midtown rises like a mountain from the plains of old tenements of the Lower East Side. The first mile or so takes you through what was once considered immigrant havens, and what was assumed to be breeding grounds for criminals. Now, it's been largely gentrified, though most of the tenement buildings remain.

First Avenue takes you through the rest of the East Village, and you get to experience various iterations of slum clearance developments en route to midtown, and then back to the Queensboro, which deposits you back where you began.

Ride Log

P1 Williamsburg Art & Historical Center
P2 ABC No Rio Performance Space
P3 Performance Space 122
P4 Theater for the New City
P5 United Nations Headquarters
P6 Union Square
P7 Gramercy Park
P8 Flatiron Building & Madison Square Park
P9 Empire State Building
P10 Rockefeller Center
P11 New York Public Library & Bryant Park
P12 Radio City Music Hall
P13 Broadway Theatre
P14 MoMA (Museum of Modern Art)
P15 Times Square
P16 Grand Central Terminal
P17 Chrysler Building

0.0 Start at the corner of Vernon Blvd (aka 25A) and Hunters Point Ave. Ride onto sidewalk, which takes you to the Pulaski Bridge bike path on the southbound side of bridge.

0.5 Bike path ends. Merge onto McGuinness Blvd.

0.6 Turn right onto Freeman St.

0.9 Turn left onto Franklin St.

1.3 Road forks; stay right on Franklin.

1.6 Franklin becomes Kent Ave.

2.5 Turn left onto South Fifth St.

2.9 Turn right, a full 180°, to get onto Williamsburg Bridge bike path.

4.3 Turn right onto Clinton St.

4.4 Turn left onto Rivington St.

4.7 Turn right onto Allen St.

4.9 Cross Houston. Allen becomes First Ave.

6.9 Just before 41st, bear left to avoid entering the tunnel under 42nd St.

7.1 Pass United Nations on right.

7.3 Tunnel comes up and rejoins First Ave.

7.8 Turn left to ride onto Queensboro Bridge bike path.

9.3 Bike path ends. Make 180° and follow bike path.

9.4 Turn left onto 22nd St.

9.6 Turn right onto 43rd Ave.

10.0 Turn left onto Vernon Blvd.

10.7 Turn left onto Hunters Point Ave.

10.8 Finish at start, the corner of Vernon and Hunters Point.

Rolling to the vanishing point on the Queensboro Bridge.
Photo Matt Wittmer

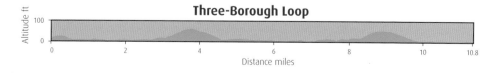

Three-Borough Loop

Altitude ft

Distance miles

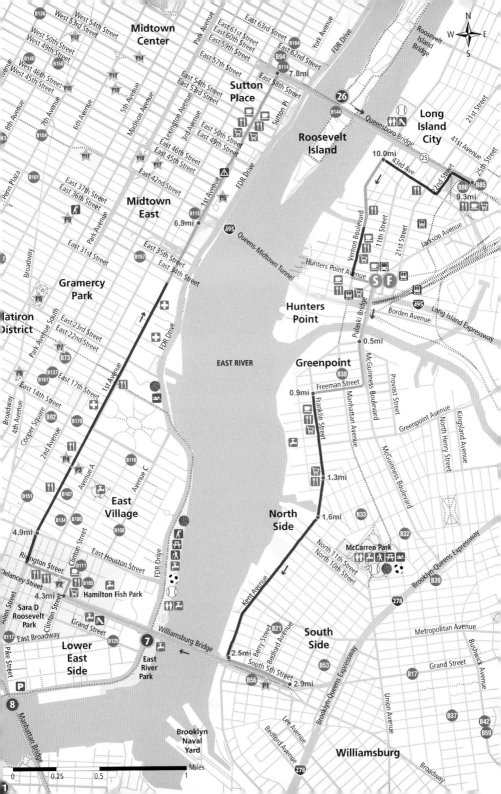

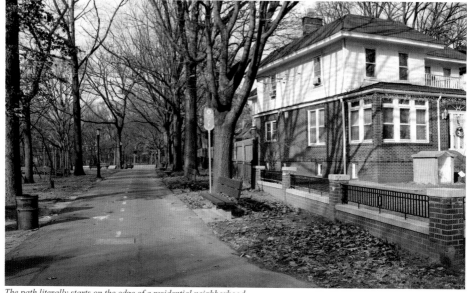

The path literally starts on the edge of a residential neighborhood.

At a Glance

Distance 2.2 miles   **Elevation Gain** 83′

Terrain

Flat bike paths, with one hill leading up to reservoir.

Traffic

The ride is entirely on bike paths, so just about all traffic will be the human-powered kind. You will cross one street, Vermont Place, right before reaching and immediately after leaving the reservoir loop.

How to Get There

Take the A or C to Liberty Avenue. Or take the J or Z to Van Siclen Avenue and L Train to East New York will all get you close. There's an on-street bike path on Liberty. Go east on Liberty, then north on Vermont and you'll get to the start quickly. The LIRR East New York stop is also nearby.

Food and Drink

You can find basic eats by the subway stops. Atlantic Avenue, which is between Van Siclen and Liberty avenues, is a veritable eating alley.

Side Trip

Across the Jackie Robinson Parkway is The Evergreens Cemetery. It's a 225-acre ground designed by landscape architect Andrew Jackson Downing in the 1850s as a burial site and retreat. You'll have to leave your bikes at the entry and walk the grounds. Call ahead to see when there are tours.

www.theevergreenscemetery.com

Where to Bike Rating

About...

The Ridgewood Reservoir is part of Highland Park, which, when you see the street that this ride starts on, feels as suburban as its name. The park straddles the Brooklyn/Queens border, but the reservoir, which was decommissioned in 1990, is in Queens. It sits atop the Harbor Hill Moraine, and is now the home of a reappearing forest, wetlands, even a bog, all of which makes it a good place for experiencing ecological diversity in the city.

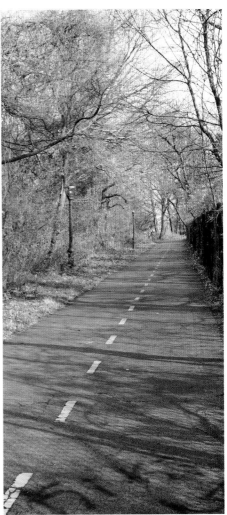

Much of the ride feels secluded and private.

The Ridgewood Reservoir is a great spot for a leisurely spin in a great slow ride. Good for beginners. Good for kids. Good for people who want an out-of-the-way place for experiencing nature in the middle of the big city. If you're riding in from a train, we took the subway, the ride to the ride, from our starting point, is almost as long as the ride itself.

But in that, there is beauty. Getting off the A Train, you'll find an industrial environment, and when you turn the corner onto Highland Boulevard, you'll find yourself thrust into a sleepy suburbia, with large detached homes and comfortable front yards.

The route itself is similarly relaxed. After riding by the playground at the start, you'll be pedaling around woods and through fields en route to the reservoir.

Once you cross the street and climb the short rise up the reservoir, you're suddenly riding a ring above what feels like an arboretum, with the only sense of civilization being the hum of the Jackie Robinson Parkway nearby. But even it feels much farther away than it actually is.

The reservoir, having been decommissioned over 20 years ago, seems to be given to natural decay, with the basins filling in. This is a great thing, as the reservoir is part of an avian migration route, which explains how 127 species of birds were observed during a count in 2007. There are benches along the eastern edge; you can look into the reservoir or out over Brooklyn.

While you can head back to the start of the ride after one short 1.2 mile loop of the reservoir, we'd go around a few more times, stopping now and again to check out both the returning fauna, flora, and wildlife, but also the great views, as on a clear day, you can see all the way past the Rockaways to the Atlantic.

Ride 28 - Ridgewood Reservoir Ride

Ride Log

0.0 Start at the southwest corner of Highland Park. Ride into the park.

0.1 Bear right to stay on path.

0.2 Turn left to stay on path.

0.5 Turn left. Prepare to cross Vermont Place.

0.5 Cross Vermont and ride up hill to Ridgewood Reservoir. Turn left. Ride clockwise around reservoir.

0.7 Path turns right.

1.0 Path turns right.

1.2 Path turns right.

1.3 Path bears right.

 P1 Carmelite Monastery
P2 North Brooklyn YMCA

1.4 Path bears left.

1.5 Path turns right.

1.6 Path turns right.

1.7 Path turns left. Now you are retracing the earlier portion of the ride. Ride downhill and cross Vermont Place.

1.7 Turn right. Follow path back.

2.1 Turn right to stay on path.

2.2 Finish at the southwest corner of Highland Park.

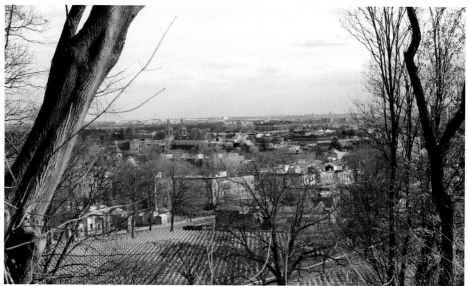

Looking out over Brooklyn and Queens, with the Atlantic in the distance.

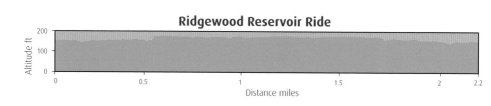

Ridgewood Reservoir Ride

Altitude ft / Distance miles

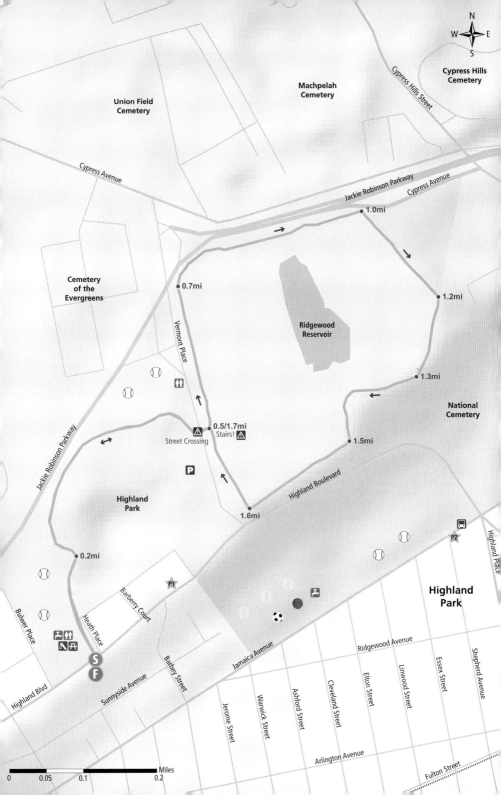

The Wind and the Rockaways Ride

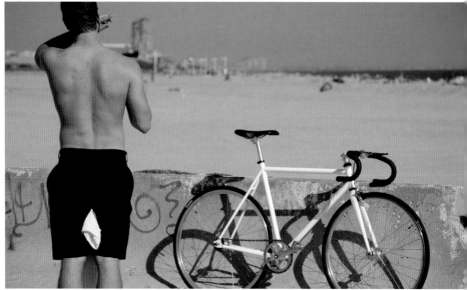

Why not roll to Rockaway?

Photo Matt Wittmer

At a Glance

Distance 20.3 miles **Elevation Gain** 136′

Terrain

Flat.

Traffic

A bit of everything. Much of the ride takes place on bike and multi-use paths, so foot and bike traffic will be what you're dodging. Some of the roads, particularly those out to Breezy Point, are lightly trafficked, and a few, mainly Rockaway Beach Boulevard from 125th to 116th streets, could be on the busy side. Access to the boardwalk is limited from 5-10am during summer.

How to Get There

Take the A Train. Duke Ellington was referring to Harlem with the song, but it applies here. The ride starts at the stop at Beach 67th Street. But since the A sometimes makes a right at the fork and finishes at Beach 116th Street, you can take the train there and join up with the ride half a block from this stop as well.

Food and Drink

Beach 116th Street, which the ride goes through, is the commercial center of the island. Ice cream, pizza, sandwiches, beach food galore. Jacob Riis Park's snack bar opens around Memorial Day and stays open through the summer. There are also vendors, and even a few restaurants along the boardwalk in the summer season.

Side Trip

You can do some quality bike meandering and get a locally crowd-sourced tour of The Rockaways with Rock Spot. Search, text and discover. Visit **www.rockspot-nyc.org** for full details.

Links to

Where to Bike Rating

About...

The Rockaways are different. Scuba divers and surfers take the A Train there. As do pigeons. This shore community on the edge of the city offers New Yorkers the ocean, and it's only a train ride away. The beach is one long strip running the length of the Rockaways, and is managed in parts by the Parks Department and the National Park Service. For cyclists, its more than just a beach, but both part of the city and a community that seems far, far away.

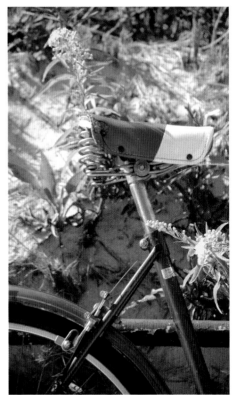

It's a world apart out here.   *Photo Matt Wittmer*

Taking the elevated train to the Rockaways gives you the feeling that the area is pretty urban. Once you get to the beach, it's easy to forget that initial observation. The beach is broad, the waves noisy, and the breeze is either refreshing or bracing, depending on the time of year. Without cars for companions, and with a long open space in front of you, the feeling of speed changes, you're going nowhere, which is fine, unless you're in a hurry.

When you first get off the boardwalk, you're deposited in a lush suburban setting, which even gives you an ample on-street bike lane all the way down to Jacob Riis Park. Once in the park, you're back on the beach, and the bathhouse and promenade are reminders of when the area was developed.

Riding through Fort Tilden, you'll feel like you're not in the city at all, but in a remote shore community. Tilden gives way to Breezy Point, a co-op community that, to the chagrin of cyclists, doesn't allow beach access from most of Rockaway Point Boulevard.

Coming back, there's a second way through Fort Tilden, and both the maritime forest and sand dunes make this decommissioned defense post an interesting spot for a stop.

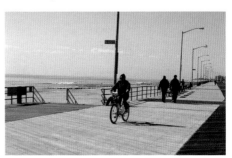

Riding the boardwalk.

Once you're back in Jacob Riis Park, you're largely re-tracing your route out, but now that you're looking east rather than west, you're witnessing a whole new landscape.

Before returning to the beach a final time, you'll ride through Beach 116th Street, the commercial center of beachdom, and the obligatory beach treats.

Queens

Ride Log

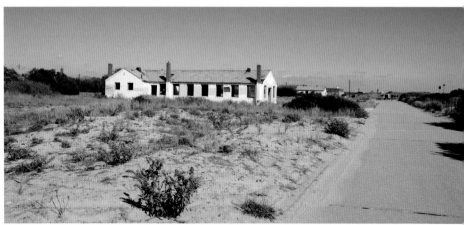

Ruins at Fort Tilden.

0.0 Start at the intersection of Beach 67th St and Rockaway Freeway. Ride south. Turn left onto Rockaway Beach Blvd.

1.7 Turn right onto Beach 34th St. Take to end.

2.0 Turn right onto boardwalk.

5.5 Boardwalk ends. Turn left onto Ocean Promenade.

6.4 Ocean Promenade ends. Turn right onto Beach 126th St.

6.5 Turn left onto Rockaway Blvd.

7.6 Entering Jacob Riis Park.

7.7 Turn left to get onto bike path.

7.8 Turn left on path towards beach.

7.9 Turn right to follow bike path.

8.8 Turn right and head away from beach.

9.1 Turn left onto Rockaway Point Blvd.

11.9 Make U-turn at Breezy Point Park.

13.3 Turn right at Beach 193rd St.

 P1 Rockaway Museum
P2 Rockaway Artists
P3 Fort Tilden

13.5 Turn left.

13.6 Turn right.

13.8 Turn left.

14.9 Turn right.

15.0 Turn left.

15.9 Turn left away from beach.

16.0 Turn right onto Rockaway Beach Blvd.

17.7 Turn right onto Beach 116th St.

17.8 Turn left onto Beach Promenade

18.1 Start on Shorefront Pkwy.

20.0 Turn left onto Beach 69th St.

20.2 Turn right onto sidewalk under the elevated A Train tracks.

20.3 Finish at Beach 67th St.

The Wind and the Rockaways Ride

Altitude ft

100

0

0   3   6   9   12   15   18   20.3

Distance miles

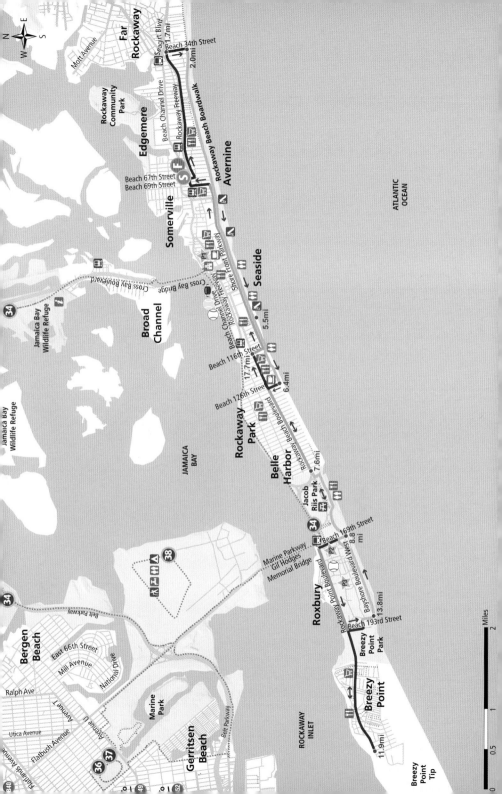

Brooklyn

Brooklyn is the old country in so many ways. Not only does it seem to have been the first stop for millions of immigrants, and millions of immigrants still seem to land there first, but much of the borough's past can still be seen.

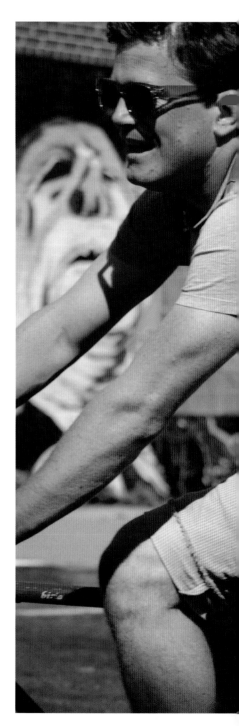

Whether it's the artfully-decaying Red Hook, the gentrifying Crown Heights, the abandoned-seeming Floyd Bennett Field, or any number of places, there's a comfortable, well-worn vibe. And despite the incredible population density, and very few parks of any great size, there are plenty of quiet streets for easy riding.

The Brooklyn waterfront, whether on the East River, or all the ocean bays (Upper New York, Lower New York, Gravesend, Dead Horse, and Jamaica) seem to be where it's easiest to find good riding. But western Brooklyn, from Greenpoint down past Prospect Park, seems to be where bike culture is most alive. Maybe it's the want of the residents, maybe it's the streets, maybe it's the city's efforts to make riding better. Whatever the causes, cycling is woven into the life of these places.

The bridges of Brooklyn are the biggest hills of the borough, and they're a must for any city resident or tourist. At the same time, keep in mind that most bridges are pretty popular with everyone. The one named for the borough is often swarming with people. Do it for the thrill and the views, but know the Manhattan Bridge has a bigger, less-trafficked bike lane.

While the bridges are something everyone should ride because people know the city for bridges – with 759 of them linking this archipelago together, they are something to know – Prospect Park is a place that people flock to. It's worthy of many visits. While you're at it, check out the bike lane on Prospect Park West. It has been a flashpoint for many disputes about what constitutes improving or destroying an urban area, but as time passes, I expect those arguments will seem small and silly and the lane will merely be another good place for cyclists to ride.

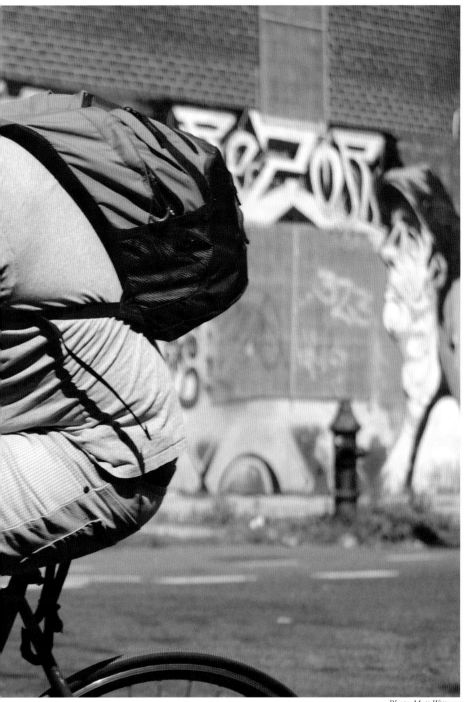

Photo Matt Wittmer

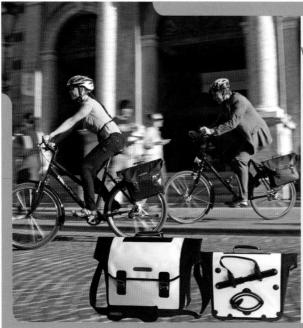
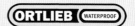
MR. C'S CYCLES
serving cyclists since 1982

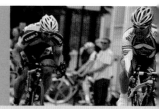

Since opening their doors in 1982, Mr C's Cycles has pursued the goal of providing an unparalleled level of excellent quality customer service. Taking the time to go the extra mile to learn about each individual's needs has earned Mr C's the well deserved respect of the cycling community.

Come visit Mr C's Sunset Park showroom and experience it for yourself!

- **Rental Bikes Available!**

- **Join our store rides every weekend! 3 different ride lengths to suit all riders.**

- **Brooklyn's biggest selection of bike brands including Trek, Specialized, Cannondale, Schwinn, Bianchi, Raleigh, Fuji, GT, Breezer and more!**

4622 7th Avenue
Brooklyn, NY 11220
T 718 438 7283 | F 718 438 0360

Mon	Wed	Thurs	Fri	Sat	Sun
10am-7pm	10am-7pm	10am-7pm	10am-7pm	10am-6pm	10am-5pm

www.mrccycles.com

You can find us on facebook and Twitter!

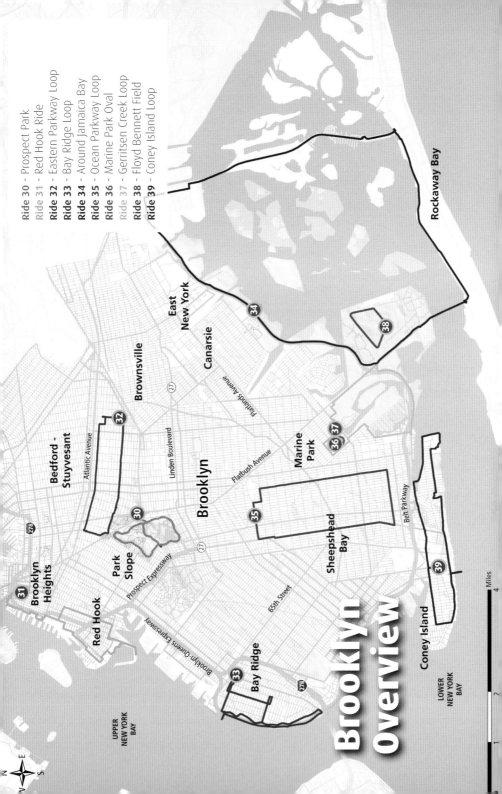

Brooklyn Overview

Ride 30 - Prospect Park
Ride 31 - Red Hook Ride
Ride 32 - Eastern Parkway Loop
Ride 33 - Bay Ridge Loop
Ride 34 - Around Jamaica Bay
Ride 35 - Ocean Parkway Loop
Ride 36 - Marine Park Oval
Ride 37 - Gerritsen Creek Loop
Ride 38 - Floyd Bennett Field
Ride 39 - Coney Island Loop

Brooklyn Heights
Bedford - Stuyvesant
Brownsville
East New York
Canarsie
Red Hook
Park Slope
Brooklyn
Marine Park
Sheepshead Bay
Bay Ridge
Coney Island

UPPER NEW YORK BAY
LOWER NEW YORK BAY
Rockaway Bay

Atlantic Avenue
Linden Boulevard
Flatlands Avenue
Flatbush Avenue
Prospect Expressway
Brooklyn-Queens Expressway
65th Street
Belt Parkway

Miles
0   2   4

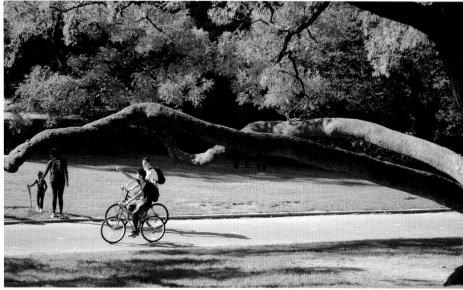

Brooklyn's original oasis of exercise since 1867. Photo Matt Wittmer

At a Glance

Distance **Perimeter Loop:** 3.4 miles, **Southern Loop:** 2.1 miles, **Northern Loop:** 2.9 miles
Elevation Gain **Perimeter Loop:** 185′,
Southern Loop: 78′, **Northern Loop:** 181′

Terrain

Rolling. One hill, a few rises. Good pavement.

Traffic

Light to moderate. Extensive car-free hours. Weekends and holidays, the park is closed to car traffic. Weekdays, the West Drive is open to car traffic 5pm-7pm, and the East Drive is open to cars 7am-9am.

How to Get There

Most roads in Brooklyn lead to Prospect, and many of those have on-street bike paths. You can also take the 2, 3, B, F, Q, and S trains; all stop at Prospect.

Food and Drink

Connecticut Muffin, 206 Prospect Park West, is just across the Bartel-Pritchard circle from the end of the West Drive. There's a Saturday Farmers' Market at the Grand Army Plaza entrance and a second at the Bartel-Pritchard Circle, Wednesdays May through October. In the park, you can find food vendors and a few cafés and bars, though most are seasonal and have limited hours.

Side Trip

Just across Flatbush is the Brooklyn Botanic Garden. To get there you'll have to take Empire Boulevard one block before turning left onto Washington. Open Tuesday through Sunday, it has 13 gardens and five buildings all on an idyllic campus. Find out more at **www.bbg.org**.

Links to **32**

Where to Bike Rating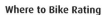

Prospect Park has extensive auto-free hours. See Traffic above.

About...

Since Prospect Park is the second large city park designed by the team of Olmstead and Vaux, there's a debate as to whether Prospect is an imitation of Central Park (it's smaller), or a perfection of the ideas that they tried with that other park in Manhattan (the landscaping is arguably more impressive). Both have a zoo, both have bodies of water, both have ampitheatres that have free concerts in the summer. Importantly for cyclists, both have interior roads that are great for cycling day or night year-round.

Riding in Prospect Park is so pleasant and so easy, it's easy to forget there's other riding in Brooklyn. If you want to ride alone, you can, if you want to link up with a group, you can. Fast; yes, slow; yes, day; yes, night; yes. There's even a mailing list for those who use Prospect Park as their main training ground.

Prospect Park isn't flat, but there's only one hill and it's fairly gentle both on the way up and the way down. What is nice is that the road is almost never straight. It's always turning a bit to the left or a bit to the right, with a few sweeping turns thrown in for good measure. You're always thinking a bit about the road, which keeps you alert and interested in the ride. As with other large city parks, this is an all-purpose playground, so you can go for a ride of any speed, then picnic, play Frisbee, listen to a concert, nap by the lake, wander through the forest, experience a playground or two, and more.

Speaking as a cyclist who spends more time in Central Park, Prospect feels a bit small for me. The 3.4 miles goes by too fast. That written, the bustle of Central Park, and the tourists, are largely absent and these absences can be a big relief. Smaller crowds mean you have less to fear from the clueless wandering across

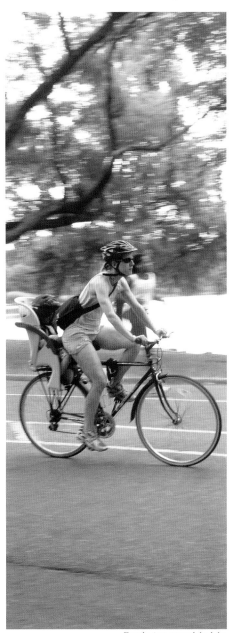

Family time around the lake.

the roadway. There's a more laid-back vibe in Prospect and it invites the cyclist to linger longer, whether riding or hanging out.

Ride Log

Perimeter Loop

0.0 Start at Grand Army Plaza. Bear right around the grassy island.

0.7 Check out the Prospect Park Bandshell on your right.

0.9 If you turn right at this grassy island, you'll ride out of the park to Bartel-Pritchard Circle.

1.7 Bear left to stay on park road. If you bear right, you'll go out to Ocean Parkway.

2.2 If you go right, you'll go out to Parkside Ave.

2.4 If you turn left into the parking lot, you'll find bathrooms in the locker room.

2.6 If you take this right, you'll find another bathroom

P1 Prospect Park Carousel
P2 Lefferts Homestead Historic House Museum
P3 Prospect Park Zoo
P4 Brooklyn Botanic Garden (including Japanese Hill and Pond Garden, Cherry Esplanade & Cranford Rose Garden)
P5 Nellie's Lawn
P6 Eastern Parkway-Brooklyn Museum
P7 Brooklyn Public Library
P8 Soldiers and Sailors Memorial Arch
P9 Grand Army Plaza
P10 Prospect Park Bandshell
P11 Pavilion Theater
P12 Park Circle
P13 Kate Wollman Prospect Park Rink
P14 The Nethermead

building on the left.

3.4 Finish at grassy island by Grand Army Plaza.

Southern Loop

0.0 Start at the intersection of 16th St and Prospect Park Southwest. Enter park. Turn right.

0.5 Bear left around grassy island.

1.5 Turn left off of perimeter road just as you're heading into the woods. This road is alternatively called Nethermead Arches or Central Dr. It isn't marked.

2.1 Coming to end of road. Turn left and immediately turn right.

2.1 End at 16th St and Prospect Park Southwest.

Northern Loop

0.0 Start at the end of East Lake Dr where it runs into Flatbush Ave next to the Prospect Park Zoo. Ride into the park.

0.2 Bear right onto the park Dr.

0.9 Park road goes left. Grand Army Plaza is on right.

2.1 Turn left. This is unmarked, though it's the only road on the left you'll come by. This is alternatively called Nethermead Arches or Central Dr.

2.7 Cross the park drive. If you turn left, you'll start another lap.

2.9 End at Flatbush Ave.

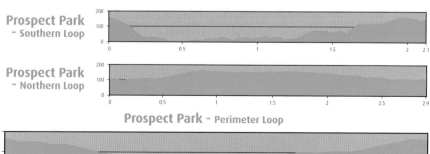

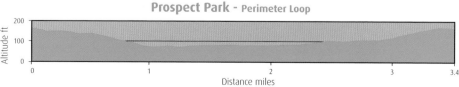

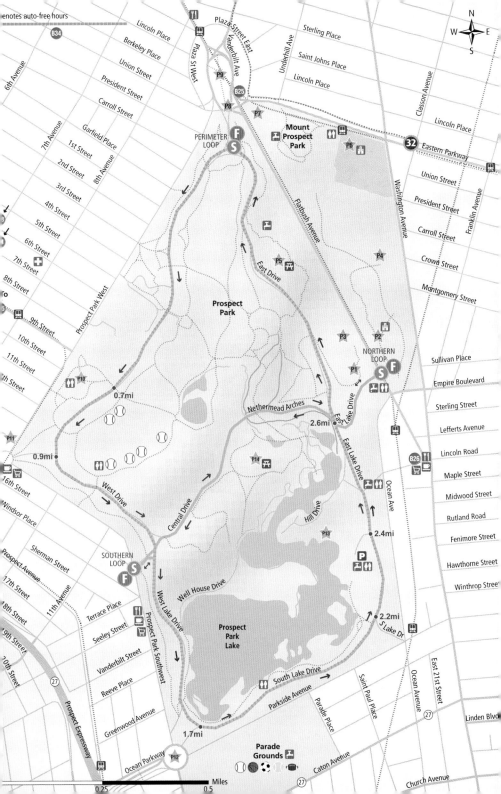

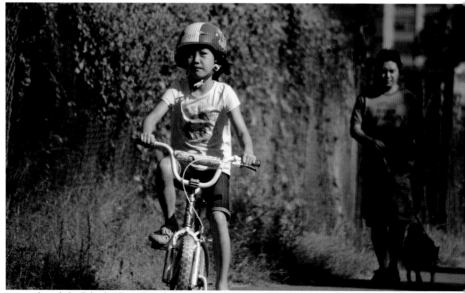

At ease through the Columbia Street Waterfront District.

Photo Matt Wittmer

At a Glance

Distance 8.6 miles   **Total Elevation** 255'

Terrain

Pretty flat. Start by descending, finish by climbing. In between, lots of flat followed by one gradual uphill and one fast descent.

Traffic

On bike paths much of the way. Most of the streets are fairly quiet.

How to Get There

The closest train station is the Brooklyn Bridge stop on the A and C lines, though several train lines converge on downtown Brooklyn, which is nearby.

Food and Drink

Traditional Brooklyn Pizza is Grimaldi's, which is either at the start or finish of the ride. It's fairly well-known, so the wait can be long.

Side Trip

The Waterfront Museum and Showboat Barge, in Red Hook, is a museum on a restored barge that tours New York Harbor. Simple, but fun, educational, and it's always great to be on the waters of New York Bay.

Links to ⑧

Where to Bike Rating

 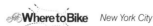

About...

Red Hook is an area that links New York to its industrial past. Mostly, it still survives because of neglect, as the Brooklyn Queens Expressway cuts it off from the rest of Brooklyn and no subway goes there. It's still a land of cobblestone streets, docks, and warehouses. Gentrification is slowly coming to the area, which is both good and bad. It is getting "cleaned up," acquiring hip eateries and a massive Ikea store, but also getting more crowded and losing some of its original flavor. Go now so you can tell people you knew it when.

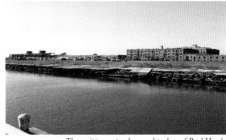

The gritty yesterday and today of Red Hook.

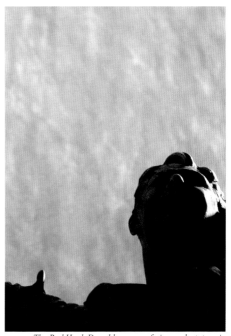

The Red Hook Doughboy, one of nine such statues in N.Y. parks. Photo Matt Wittmer

Starting on the edge of downtown Brooklyn, you immediately ride away from it all, zipping downhill to the Brooklyn waterfront. Long the home of shipyards, this ride takes you from the recently upgraded to the recently rediscovered, as you ride along improved waterfront parkland on the Brooklyn Bridge Greenway, then move onto industrial Red Hook.

Red Hook is a sight; warehouses, light industry, heavy industry, beat down buildings, quirky homes and storefronts, housing projects, and gentrifying forces all jumbled together. Just as it seems like you've gone back in time, you notice that the old warehouse you're passing is a fancy Fairway supermarket, and then two turns later you're confronted with the behemoth that is Ikea. Once past Ikea, you're back to industrial Red Hook, with the Gowanus Industrial Park on a pier alongside the Columbia Street Esplanade, where you'll find guys fishing and hanging out. Seen from above, this is the hook of Red Hook.

Once you turn around and start heading back, you'll pass the new and the old. First, the hip Red Hook Community Farms, an urban agrarian outpost bent on local agriculture. After that, you'll see the Red Hook Recreation Area, a depression-era Works Progress Adminis-

tration development with a massive public pool, one of 11 such pools in the city.

Once past the park and onto Clinton Street, you'll quickly pass under the highway and start climbing into tonier Brooklyn, riding into Carroll Gardens before making a left, riding downhill and returning to the waterfront.

Back along the water, you'll be riding north and will have views of downtown Manhattan and the Brooklyn Bridge before turning right, and climbing back up to the heights from which you started.

Brooklyn

Ride Log

0.0 Start on Cadman Plaza West across from subway entry.

0.1 Bear left onto Old Fulton St.

0.4 Enter Brooklyn Bridge Park at Furman St. Bear left to get on bike path.

0.9 Bear left to stay on path. Someday, you'll be able to go straight.

1.0 Turn right on Furman St bike path.

1.1 Turn right onto Joralemon St.

1.2 Bear left to get on bike path.

1.4 Bike path briefly ends at Atlantic Ave. Go straight.

1.5 Turn right onto Columbia St bike path.

1.9 Turn right to follow bike path onto Degraw St.

2.0 Bike path ends at Van Brunt St. Turn left.

2.3 Turn right onto Hamilton Ave to get to Imlay St. Turn left onto Imlay.

2.7 Imlay ends. Right on Pioneer St, then left onto Conover St.

3.1 Left onto Reed St.

3.2 Left onto Van Brunt St.

3.3 Right on Beard St.

3.4 Right onto bike path.

4.0 Cross Columbia St. Continue on bike path.

4.4 Columbia Street Esplanade ends. Make U-turn.

5.1 Turn right on Bay St.

5.5 Turn left on Clinton St.

5.8 Cross under Gowanus Expressway.

6.5 Turn left on Kane St.

6.8 Turn right onto Columbia St bike path. Now retracing ride back to start.

7.1 Left on Atlantic Ave.

7.2 Enter park. Stay on bike path.

 P1 Brooklyn Historical Society
P2 Brooklyn War Memorial
P3 Bargemusic
P4 Pier One
P5 Brooklyn Heights Promenade
P6 Brooklyn Bridge Park Pier 6
P7 Brooklyn Collective
P8 Bamboo Bike Studio

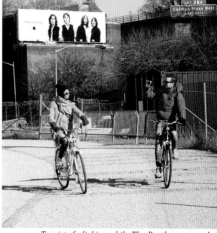

Tourists frolicking while The Beatles contemplate

7.4 Follow path onto Joralemon St.

7.5 Turn left onto Furman St bike path.

7.6 Turn left onto Montague St.

7.7 Turn right onto bike path.

8.2 Park ends. Ride straight onto Old Fulton St.

8.6 Bear right onto Cadman Plaza West.

8.6 End at Cadman Plaza West and Brooklyn Bridge subway station.

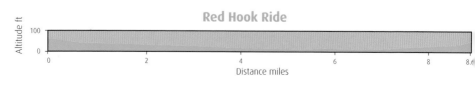

Red Hook Ride

Altitude ft

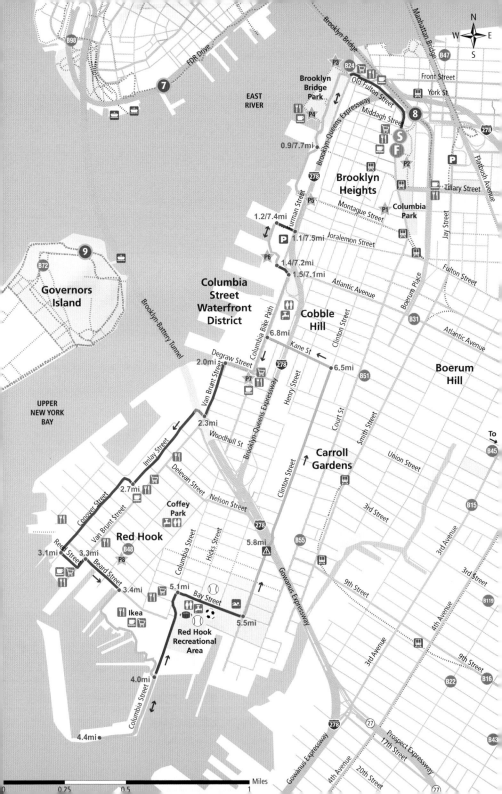

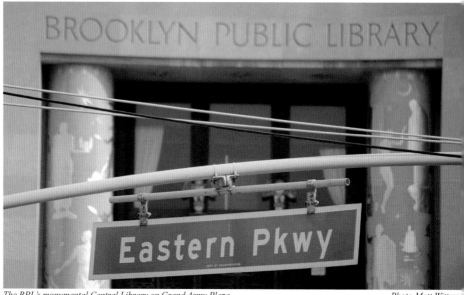

The BPL's monumental Central Library on Grand Army Plaza.   Photo Matt Wittmer

At a Glance

Distance 5.7 miles   **Elevation Gain** 188′

Terrain

Flat. Decent pavement most of the way.

Traffic

Just about the entire ride is either on a bike path or bicycle lanes. You'll encounter potentially heavy traffic on Eastern Parkway for a block or two, but otherwise, traffic should be light.

How to Get There

Take the 2, 3, 4, or 5 trains to the Crown Height-Utica Avenue station. You're on the route, a few blocks from the start. There's also a LIRR stop on Nostrand Avenue a few blocks north of the route.

Food and Drink

The short stint on Vanderbilt Avenue, right in the middle of Prospect Heights is where you'll find a rich selection of food choices, bars, cafés, restaurants, ice cream. American, ethnic, nouvelle. An impressive selection.

Side Trip

The Brooklyn Museum of Art. Big, lots of art, housed in a beautiful Beaux-Arts building; 560,000 square feet of space, and several large permanent collections.

Links to

Where to Bike Rating

About...

Eastern Parkway might read like something you've heard of before, and you're right, you have, but that's thanks to Eastern Parkway. Conceived in 1866, it is the world's first parkway. It was built for pleasure, for taking a scenic trip through Brooklyn either to or from Prospect Park. This was supposed to be the beginning of a system of parks and parkways. Now, it's a busy thoroughfare that just goes to Queens. But thanks to thoughtful design back then, there have always been paths for human-powered transit.

The Eastern Parkway is an impressive avenue. Wide, tree-lined, and zoned to keep commercial uses away from this thoroughfare. This ride takes in all but one block of the embodiment of Calvert and Vaux's vision of a parkway leading to a park.

You start at the eastern end of the parkway, by Lincoln Terrace Park, on the Brooklyn-Queens Greenway. You'll notice that you're on a hill that runs east-west. It's really a moraine, and it's the same geological feature that separates northern Long Island from southern. There is something easy-going about riding on Eastern, even if the traffic is pretty hectic alongside you. That there are few commercial concerns, and no shortage of interesting apartment architecture to enjoy might be part of the equation. That you're protected by not only curbs, but trees helps with this. For cyclists, this represents a dilemma; it would be nice to have more protected, tree-lined roads for riding, but it would be bad to have more roads like the parkway for driving.

Once at Grand Army Plaza, you skirt the traffic circle by taking a bike path around to Vanderbilt Avenue, the commercial center of Prospect Heights. The only difficulty of this street is finding a single place to eat.

Turning right onto Dean Street you get a long,

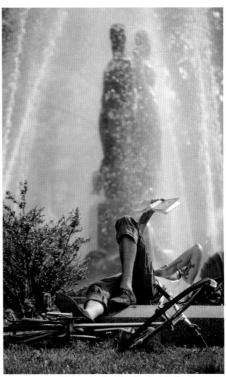

Kicking back with a book at Bailey Fountain.
Photo Matt Wittmer

Brooklyn

straight road lined with brownstones and a bicycle lane. The hope seems to be that this will become a major bicycle transit route in the future, as Bergen Street, paralleling Dean to the south, also has a bike lane that runs the length of the street.

Dean takes you a quiet way through Crown Heights (Eastern Parkway is the busy way), a neighborhood with a strong Caribbean flavor, a fact reflected not only in the restaurants, but also the offerings found in the delis. The road is straight and wide and not popular with drivers, making it great for riding.

In terms of feeling a neighborhood, you're much more in the place when riding Dean than you are on Eastern. It's easier to get a feel for the style and rhythm of life. Unfortunately, just as it's all flowing well, you're at the end of Dean, and it's a right, left, and right, and you're shooting downhill back to the park where you started.

Ride Log

0.0 Start at the edge of Lincoln Terrace Park by the intersection of Eastern Parkway and Buffalo Ave. Bike path is on south side of parkway.

1.9 Path ends at Classon Ave. Cross street and turn left to continue on Eastern Parkway.

2.4 Turn right on Plaza St East.

2.6 Turn right on Vanderbilt Ave.

2.9 Turn right on Dean St.

5.1 Dean ends. Turn right on Rochester Ave.

5.2 Turn left on St. Marks Ave.

5.3 Turn right onto Buffalo Ave.

5.7 Finish at Buffalo and Eastern Parkway.

P1 Eastern Parkway-Brooklyn Museum
P2 Brooklyn Public Library
P3 Brooklyn Botanic Garden (including Japanese Hill and Pond Garden, Cherry Esplanade & Cranford Rose Garden)
P4 Prospect Park Zoo
P5 Soldiers and Sailors Memorial Arch
P6 Grand Army Plaza
P7 KAI Studio
P8 Grant Square
P9 Brooklyn Children's Museum
P10 Weeksville Heritage Center

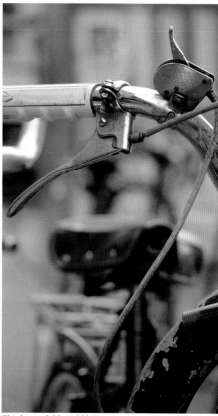

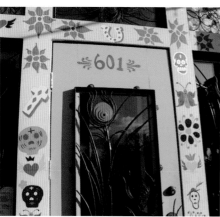

One of the many colorful eateries along Vanderbilt.

This borough likes old bikes.   *Photo Matt Wittmer*

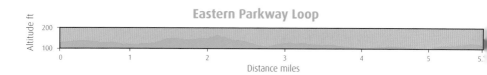

Eastern Parkway Loop

Altitude ft

Distance miles

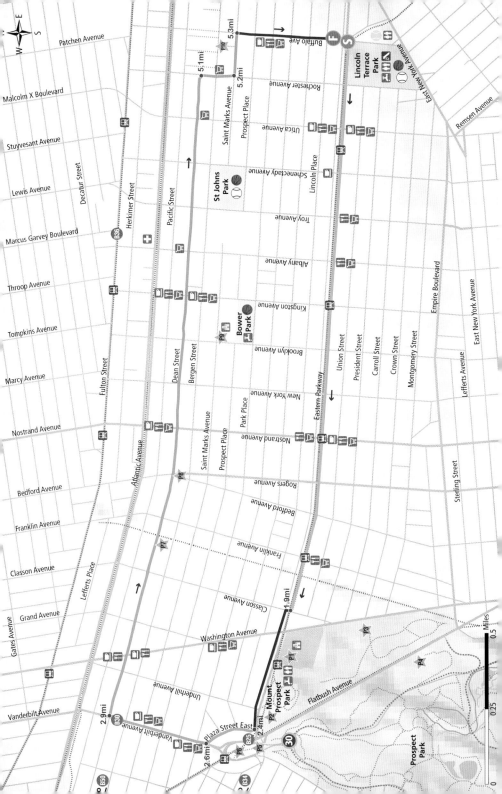

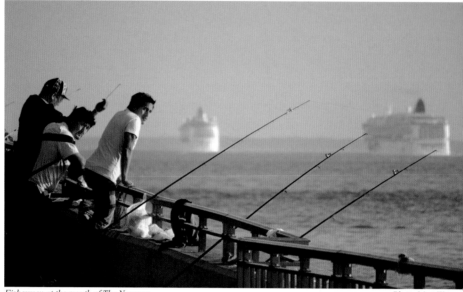

Fishermen at the mouth of The Narrows.

Photo Matt Wittmer

At a Glance

Distance 8.2 miles   **Elevation Gain** 350′

Terrain

Mostly flat. The route descends from the ridge to the water and climbs back up.

Traffic

Light. Much of the ride is on bike paths. For the rest of the ride, the streets are mostly quiet.

How to Get There

Take the R Train to the Bay Ridge Avenue stop.

Food and Drink

Both Fourth Avenue, where the ride begins and ends, and Third Avenue, where the ride passes, are crowded with choices. The eateries at Third Avenue are more diverse, more interesting, and have a more casual atmosphere, all good for taking the time to enjoy your food.

Side Trip

Hanging out on the pier and fishing is a fine pastime But checking out the Harbor Defense Museum in For Hamilton is a great way to educate yourself about the important task of defending waterways. The museum itself is located in a former defense bastion and is stocked with artifacts from World War II, when the Germans periodically tried invading, all the way back to the Revolutionary War (during which New York was an important battleground).

www.harbordefensemuseum.com

Where to Bike Rating

About...

While New York City is generally known as a home for immigrants and transients, a place for people on the move looking to move, Bay Ridge is known for having families that stay through multiple generations. This might contribute to the comfort level that you can feel in the air. Comfort or not, the riding is good. Simple, straightforward, pretty surroundings, and great views.

I thought of Bay Ridge as "gritty" for years. That was before I took this ride. The route starts out on the edge of a busy commercial strip, but by taking a side street, you quickly leave that world behind. In a few blocks, you're on a bike path and that you climbed out of a subway station minutes earlier is largely forgotten. Pass Owl's Head Park on your right, make the left on Shore Road, and you have stately houses on your left and New York Bay on your right. The view over the water, taking in the Verrazano Narrows and the bridge of that name, with Staten Island in the background is impressive enough that it's easy to not notice the Belt Parkway buzzing below.

At the end of Shore, you turn right onto a sidewalk to ride over the highway and drop down to Shore Road Park. You're effectively riding back from where you came, with the water now on your left, and straight ahead is New Jersey and Upper New York Bay. Once at the northern end of the path, turn left to enjoy Pier 69.

Turn around and head out. Once you climb out of the park, turn right and you're on Shore road again. Take it to 83rd Street, where you'll turn left, venture into the neighborhood. Once you get to Narrows, the first intersection, stop and turn left and check out the home

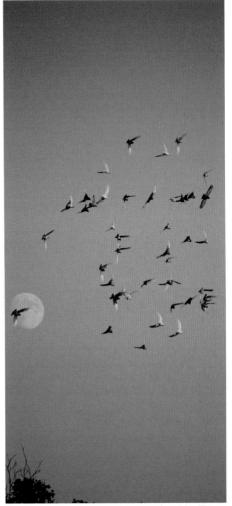

City birds circling at sundown.   *Photo Matt Wittmer*

known as The Gingerbread House. It's worth a look.

Back on 83rd. Pop out on Third Avenue. Third Avenue is a good place for a break. Several cozy cafés and eateries line the block between 83rd and 84th where you'll turn right again and make it to Ridge Boulevard.

Ridge is yet another quiet street and will take you back north through the neighborhood. Near the end, you'll turn right on Senator, make your way back to Fourth Avenue, and the ride is already done.

Ride Log

0.0 Start at the corner of 68th St and Fourth Ave. Head northwest.

0.1 Jog a little to the right to stay on 68th.

0.7 Turn left on Shore Rd.

2.9 Turn right onto Fourth Ave. Get onto overpass sidewalk to go over Belt Parkway.

3.0 Start heading north alongside water.

5.1 Turn left to ride onto pier.

5.2 End of pier. Make U-turn.

5.3 Go under highway and then exit park. Turn right onto Shore Rd.

6.2 Turn left on 83rd St.

6.7 Turn right on Third Ave.

6.8 Turn right on 84th St.

6.9 Turn right on Ridge Blvd.

7.8 Turn right on Senator St.

8.1 Turn right on Fourth Ave.

8.2 End at Fourth Ave and Bay Ridge Ave.

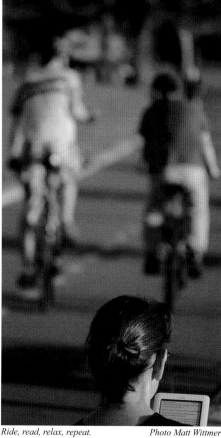

Ride, read, relax, repeat.   *Photo Matt Wittmer*

 P1 Narrows Botanical Garden
P2 Monastery Square
P3 69th Street Pier
P4 Gingerbread House

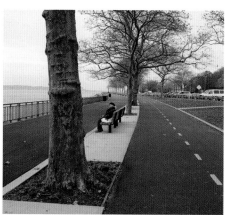

A quiet morning by the Verrazano Narrows.

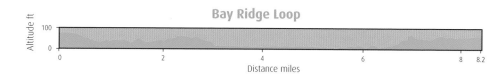

Bay Ridge Loop

Altitude ft

Distance miles

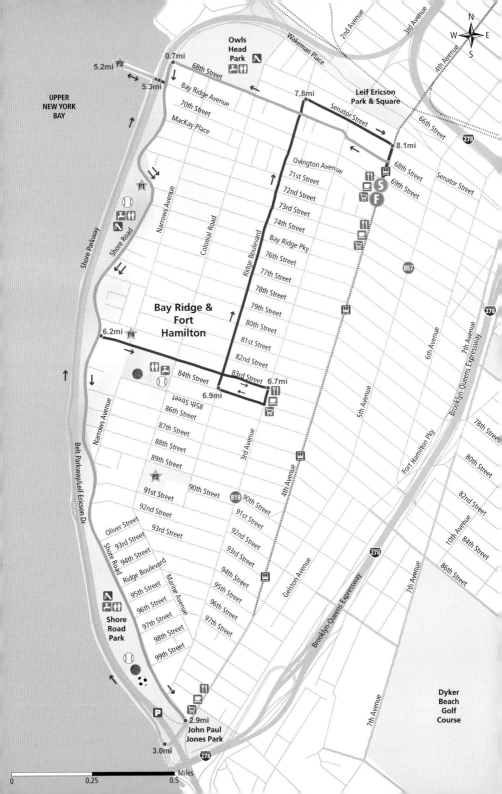

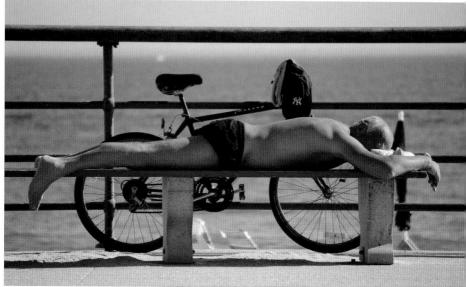

It doesn't get much better than this.

Photo Matt Wittmer

At a Glance

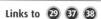

Distance 18.1 miles   **Elevation Gain** 426′

Terrain

Flat; the only rises are bridges. But just because it's flat, doesn't make it easy. The winds around Jamaica Bay can be strong. Expect the ride to be breezy.

Traffic

Light. Mostly on bike paths and protected bike lanes.

How to Get There

The easiest way to get there is to take the L Train to the end of the line, the Canarsie-Rockaway Parkway Terminal. Ride down Rockaway Parkway to the Canarsie Pier. Otherwise, you can take the A Train to Howard Beach, Broad Channel, or Beach 90th.

Food and Drink

Canarsie Pier has food trucks in the summer. There are also restaurants along Broad Channel.

Side Trip

Jamaica Bay Wildlife Refuge visitors center in Broad Channel is a great stop if you want to not only see the bay up close, but also get advice on what to look for and where.

Links to 29 37 38

Where to Bike Rating

About...

Jamaica Bay Wildlife Refuge, which this ride circles, is part of the Gateway National Recreation Area and a bird sanctuary, one of the largest in the Northeast, because of its position on the Atlantic Flyway, a prime migratory route. With its diverse habitats, over 300 different species have been observed stopping by for a break en route to points north and south.

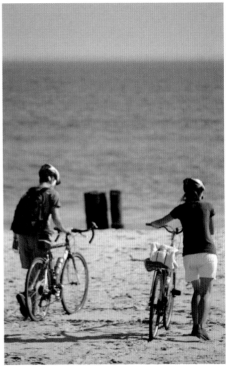

Another nice idea.   *Photo Matt Wittmer*

At many a concert on Central Park's Great Lawn, the city parks commissioner has spoken about the danger of releasing helium balloons (traditionally used as picnic site markers at park events) into the air. Balloons have been known to float over to Jamaica Bay, where they present a dietary temptation as well as a major health hazard to shore birds. It's only a mildly effective scare tactic, but it aroused this author's curiosity about the place.

First, it's a huge body of water to have inside a city; 18 miles around. I don't know how they know that prevailing winds would take balloons there, but there is lots of open space and few places for people.

This ride starts and finishes at Canarsie Pier, which is convenient for those who want to drive, as it has a huge parking lot, with benches and picnic tables scattered around. You head out of the parking lot and immediately turn right. The route is pretty simple: all you're doing is skirting the bay.

The opening and closing sections are along the Belt Parkway, a busy highway. Look right and you'll see three former landfills looking more and more like parks. The second, Fountain Avenue, has a notorious history as a dumping ground for organized crime.

Once past the new parks, you'll turn right off the

Belt and do a brief tour of Howard Beach, Queens. At the end, you'll turn onto Cross Bay Boulevard, which is just that—it takes you across the bay. After the first bridge, you'll be able to get off the road and ride on a bike path through much of Broad Channel. The path is a straight line paralleling the road with the Gateway grounds on both sides. Once you get to the end of the park, it's a short tour of Broad Channel, a seafaring community, and then over the bridge to the Rockaways.

The Rockaway portion is probably where the wind will be at its most fierce and, unfortunately, you're on the road for much of it. A bike path is planned for here and it will be a relief when it comes.

The last portion is over the Gil Hodges/Marine Parkway Bridge and takes you back to federal land, which you'll be on past Floyd Bennett Field and back to Canarsie, where you will have earned whatever treat you decide to pick up.

Ride Log

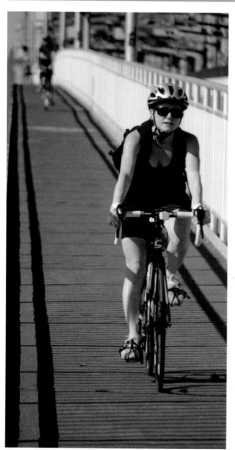

Descending the Marine Parkway-Gil Hodges Memorial Bridge over Rockaway Inlet.
Photo Matt Wittmer

0.0 Start at the Canarsie Pier. Head northeast on the bike path.

3.0 Turn right on 84th St.

3.1 Turn left on 157th Ave.

3.5 Turn right on 91st St.

4.4 Turn left on 165th Ave.

4.5 Turn right on Cross Bay Blvd.

8.2 Turn left at 21st Rd. Look for bridge bike path that goes along the eastern side of the Cross Bay Bridge.

9.0 Turn left at Beach 92nd St and then left again to get on bike path.

9.3 Bike path ends. Turn right to continue going southwest on Beach Channel Dr.

12.7 Go under Gil Hodges Bridge to get to path on western side of span.

13.0 On Gil Hodges Bridge.

14.0 At Aviation Rd, an entry to Floyd Bennett Field, cross Flatbush Ave to follow bike path on other side of road.

15.2 Bike path bears right to follow Belt Parkway.

18.1 Finish at Canarsie Pier.

P
P1 Canarsie Pier
P2 Fountain Avenue
P3 Jamaica Bay Visitors Center
P4 September 11th Memorial Park
P5 Rockaway Artists Alliance Studios 6 & 7

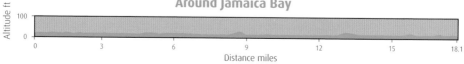

Altitude ft

Around Jamaica Bay

100

0

0   3   6   9   12   15   18.1

Distance miles

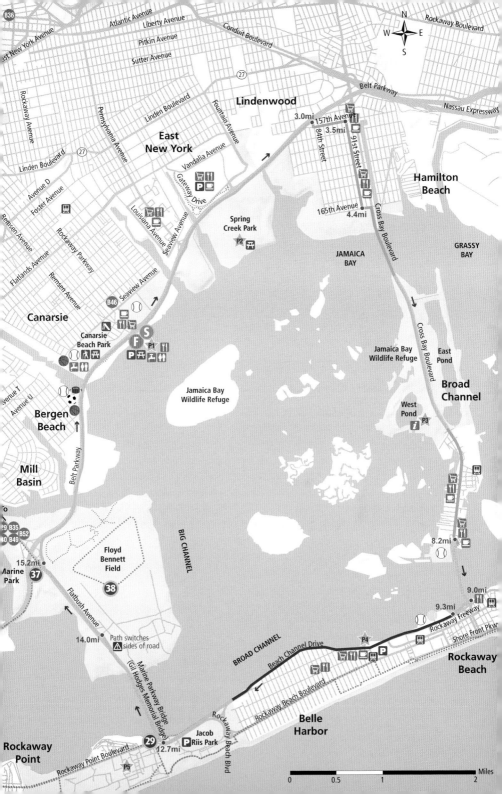

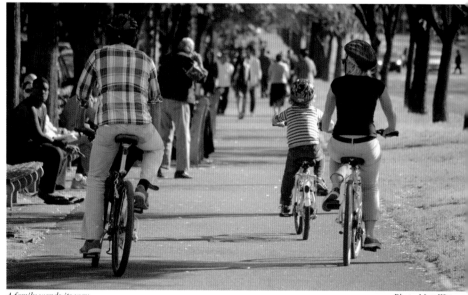

A family wends its way.   Photo Matt Wittmer

At a Glance

Distance 7.7 miles   **Elevation Gain** 105′

Terrain

Flat. Half the route is on a bike path.

Traffic

Light. Pedestrians will be your only worry on the bike path.

How to Get There

You can ride south on the Ocean Parkway bike path from Prospect Park to get to the ride. You can also take the B or Q trains to the ride start on Avenue H. Or get pretty close by taking the F Train to 18th Avenue or the 2 or 5 trains to Brooklyn College.

Food and Drink

Check out Salud at 1308 Avenue H. It's close to the start, or finish. Organic Mexican with a New Agey vibe. The Mexican hot chocolate is excellent.

Side Trip

The Brooklyn Center for the Performing Arts. Brooklyn has its own cultural and literary traditions that, in many ways, can be argued eclipses Manhattan's. And this center makes a point of celebrating its home borough. It used to be a home of Yiddish theatre, now it's focusing more on Brooklyn-based writers.

Where to Bike Rating

About...

Ocean Parkway has a place in bike history. It is the first bike path in the United States; so designated in 1894. Ocean, like Eastern Parkway before it, is the brainchild of park architects Olmstead and Vaux. And in this way, looks similar, broad central roadway flanked by greenspaces on both sides and smaller roads and then buildings. The road runs from the southern tip of Prospect Park to Brighton Beach, almost five miles in total.

There's the grand vision of city planners and then there's the reality. Ocean Parkway is the fully-executed vision of a parkway joining Prospect Park to another great open space, Brighton Beach. The Brooklyn that the parkway was built in was largely rural in 1880. Now, it is both urban and suburban in many flavors. Could the planners envision today's Brooklyn? Knowing then what we know now, would they have designed differently?

The ride starts in a suburban stretch of Avenue H. Roll east to Brooklyn College and the ride starts to feel more urban. Roll down the Bedford Avenue bike lane and the neighborhoods change. It's two-and-a-half miles, straight and flat, along Bedford, but with all there is to see along the road, this stretch of Bedford feels much longer.

Avenue Y's name gives you the feeling that you're coming to the end, and indeed, you're just about at Brighton Beach. But it's only a small stretch of avenue and then you get to step back in history to enjoy the Ocean Parkway bike path.

First the bicycle and then the car were game-changers. There were horse races and chariot races on the parkway, and there were bridle paths along the park-

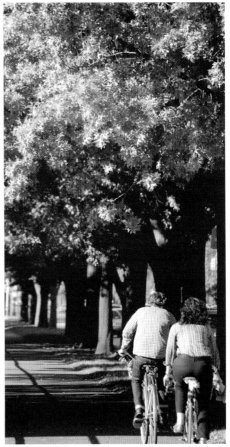

Smooth sailing.   *Photo Matt Wittmer*

way until the 1970s. If you experience the parkway in a car today, hard to say if you'll appreciate the beauty, as you'll probably be paying too much attention to traffic.

The contrast with riding a bike is dramatic. You get to experience the vision of the plan, have an easy-going ride in a pleasant open space, and observe how various housing booms built up the area.

The only problem is that too soon it's over. In another two-and-a-half miles Avenue J comes up fast. Too fast. Our preference would be to go over to the eastern edge of Ocean Parkway and ride back to do it again, but bike riding is only permitted on the western side. Taking H and restarting to down Bedford is a possibility.

Brooklyn

Ride Log

0.0 Start at Ave H and E 15th St.

0.2 Turn right on Ocean Ave.

0.4 Turn left on Ave I.

0.7 Turn right on Bedford Ave.

3.3 Turn right on Ave Y.

4.4 Turn right on Ocean Parkway bike path.

6.9 Turn right on Ave J. Cross Ocean Parkway. Turn left onto Ocean Parkway side road.

7.2 Turn right on Ave H.

7.7 Finish at start: Ave H and E 15th St.

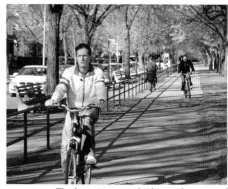

The design is supposed to keep pedestrians and cyclists separate ...

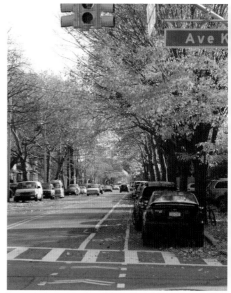

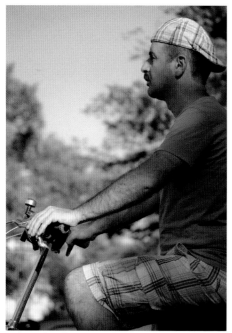

Stylin' and profilin' on a foldy.   *Photo Matt Wittmer*

... And when you're off the path, you have your own lane through suburbia.

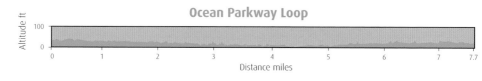

Ocean Parkway Loop

Altitude ft

Distance miles

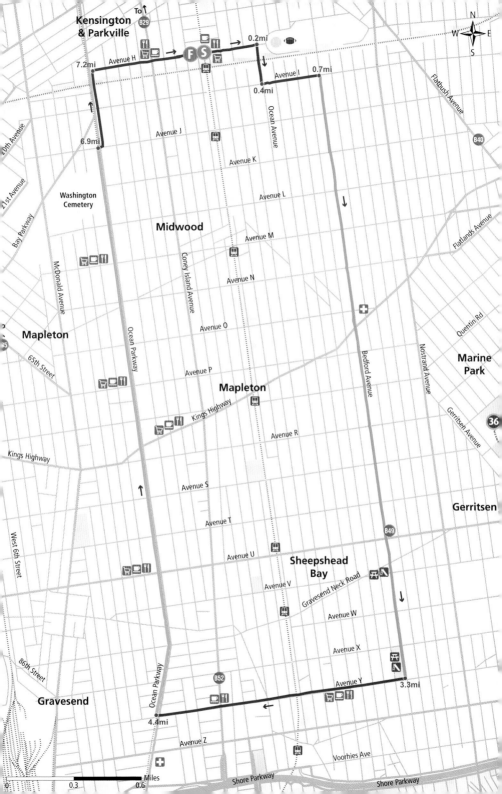

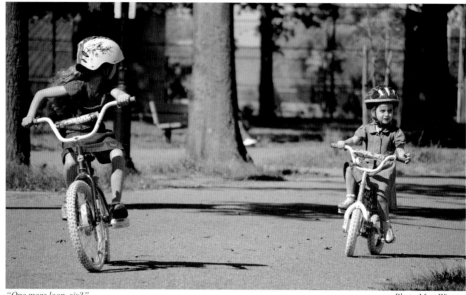

"One more loop, sis?"

Photo Matt Wittmer

At a Glance

Distance 0.9 mile　　**Elevation Gain** 4′

Terrain
Flat oval track with good asphalt.

Traffic
None. Bike path the entire way.

How to Get There
Take the B or Q train to Avenue U and ride along U until you get to the park.

Food and Drink
Go a few blocks east of the park on Avenue S and you'll find both food and coffee. Pizza Emporium gives you the time and atmosphere to savor the day and some slices.

Side Trip
Check out the Carmine Carro Community Center at the top of the park, which should be open by the time this book is published. The building is the first "green" Parks Department building, with solar panels on the roof for electricity, planted greenery on the roof for insulation and rainwater absorption, and geothermal wells for heating and cooling.

Links to

Where to Bike Rating

About...

Marine Park is Brooklyn's largest city park. The oval rides around a tiny portion of it. While this little section seems like a peaceful suburban idyll, a green space similar to countless others in countless other places in the country, this one was part of a bulwark against creeping industrialization. There had been talk about turning nearby Jamaica Bay into a deep water port and that would have meant dredging the adjacent Rockaway Channel, but this plan was nixed and locals donated land to the city with the stipulation that it be turned into public parkland.

The Marine Park Oval is one of the quickest rides in this book and the shortest in Brooklyn. Like most of the other time-friendly rides, this one is entirely on parkland. Of the brief rides, this is probably the best of all for new cyclists and children. It's flat, compact; there's no chance of crossing car traffic, and somewhat protected from the wind. The other traffic you'll encounter here will not be driving, riding, or running fast. At this distance, someone learning to ride a bike can pretty much get off whenever, wherever and can easily walk back to where they came. And there is little fear of cars, buses, even speeding cyclists coming too close.

Another nice feature of riding in a wide-open oval are the good sight lines. You can leave a kid, or parent, on a bench or playing somewhere and see them while still feeling entirely independent. With all the space, someone can be playing baseball, Frisbee, soccer, you name it, and still keep an eye out for the cyclist, or vice versa.

And there are lots of places to stop. Benches all the way around. And if you want to have the ride as part of an afternoon-athon, you can play cricket, baseball, softball, basketball, tennis, bocce here, as well as taking the measure of the playground in the northwest

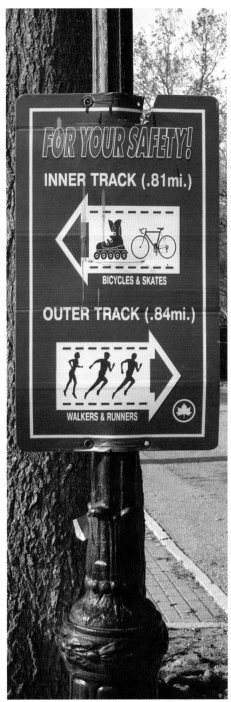

The Parks Department tries to keep order.

Brooklyn

Ride Log

0.0 Start at parking lot by E 32nd St and Ave S. Turn left to get on path.

0.9 Finish lap at parking lot.

 P1 Lott House
P2 Salt Marsh Nature Center
P3 Carmine Carro Community Center

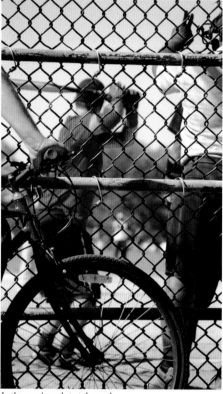

In the ump's pocket at the oval.
Photo Matt Wittmer

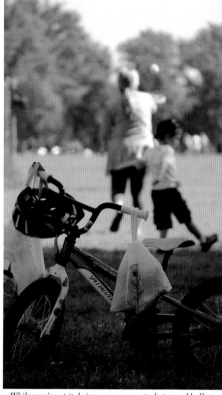

While you're at it, bring your racquets, bats, and balls too.
Photo Matt Wittmer

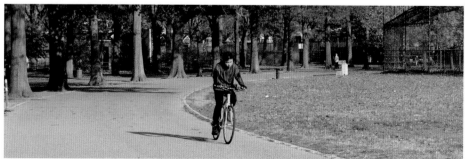

This rider looks like he's been putting in the laps!

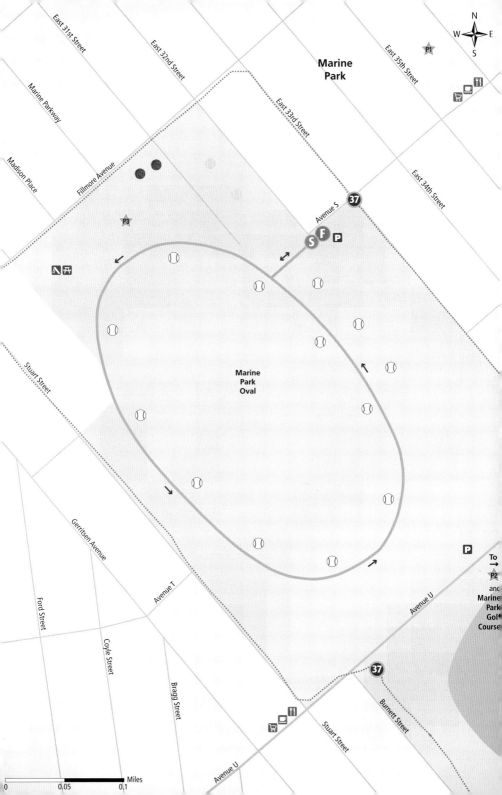

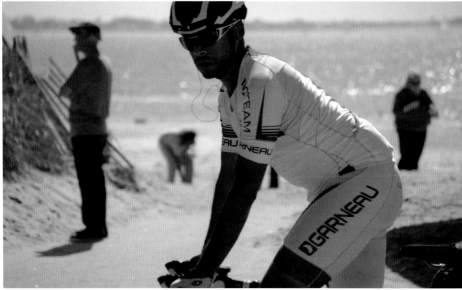

Ready when you are.   Photo Matt Wittmer

At a Glance

Distance 6.6 miles   **Elevation Gain** 121′

Terrain

Flat, with two rises. The bike path on Flatbush is made of cement blocks, so it might feel a bit rough. Otherwise, the roads are in good condition.

Traffic

Mostly light. More than half the ride is on bike paths, but you'll have to contend with a few highway interchanges.

How to Get There

Take the B or Q train to Avenue U and ride along U until you get to the park.

Food and Drink

Go a few blocks east of the park on Avenue S and you'll find both food and coffee. Pizza Emporium gives you the time and atmosphere to savor the day and some slices.

Side Trip

Visit the Salt Marsh Nature Center just south of Avenue U. It is not only a home to bird watchers, but also a center for environmental education.

Links to 34 36 39

Where to Bike Rating 🚲🚲

About...

Gerritsen Inlet, an inlet to Jamaica Bay, is home to saltwater marshes and one of the areas designated "forever wild" by the Parks Department. It is fed by Gerritsen Creek, which you can't see anymore, as it is now an underground storm drain. It still empties into the inlet, feeding the habitat and helping host a diverse ecosystem. The inlet, and the value of protecting it was the reason for the creation of Marine Park.

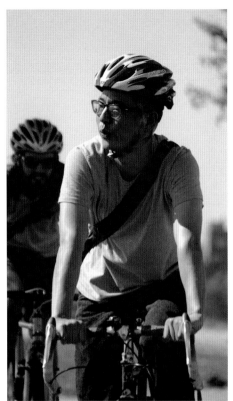

Approaching Plumb Beach.   *Photo Matt Wittmer*

This ride goes around the two biggest parks in Brooklyn, the federal government's Gateway National Recreation Area and the city's Marine Park. Both are efforts to preserve natural habitats, particularly fragile wetlands in a sprawling metropolis. Both are succeeding.

You start at the northern end of Marine Park, right next to the Marine Park Oval described in the previous ride. From here, you're basically going to circumnavigate Marine Park. The far end includes riding along Gateway grounds.

The Gerritsen Inlet is straight ahead. You ride down 33rd and when you get to Avenue U, it's across the street and beyond the grass. So you weave left, then right, then left, then right onto Flatbush Avenue. Flatbush, the outgrowth of a footpath hundreds of years old almost feels like a highway here, so make sure you turn onto the bike path. At the moment, it looks like a sidewalk and you can barely see the painted lines for bikes on it, but that's where it is.

Ride over the Belt Parkway overpass, and turn right. You're still in Marine Park, but Gateway's Floyd Bennett Field, also a site of a ride, is across the street.

You'll be riding next to the Belt Parkway for a spell. The cars are boring, but once you get to the in-

let bridge, you'll start to get great views of the water and the Rockaways. Plumb Beach, which is on your left, is part of Gateway. Not a huge beach, but looking out over the water while relaxing on sand is always peaceful.

When you get to Sheepshead Bay, it's time to turn right and start heading back to the northern end of Marine Park. Knapp Street can feel a bit crowded for the first few blocks, but it settles down. Before you know it, you'll be at Allen Avenue. Turn right and traffic will just about disappear. When you get to Gerritsen, you're in the midst of sleepy suburbia, a world away from the bustle of the Belt Parkway. You'll have a bike lane on a pretty quiet street that runs back to the water. You can then do a 180 and ride back to where you made the detour, and then follow the edge of Marine Park back to the oval, around the oval and to your starting point.

Brooklyn

Ride Log

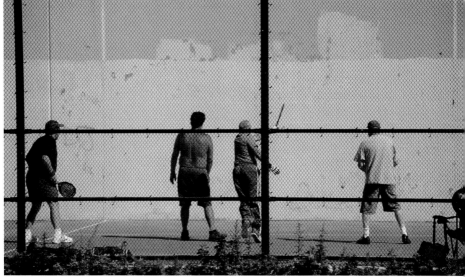

Paddleball match at Marine Park. Photo Matt Wittmer

0.0 Start at the corner of Ave S and E 33rd St. Head southeast along park edge.

0.3 Turn left on Ave U.

0.6 Turn right on Ryder St.

0.8 Turn left on Ave V.

0.9 Turn right on Hendrickson St.

1.0 Turn right on Flatbush Ave. Bike path is sidewalk here.

1.8 Go straight over Belt Parkway overpass.

2.2 Turn right onto Belt Parkway bike path.

4.1 Turn right on Knapp St. Knapp will start going right then turn left.

4.9 Turn right on Allen Ave.

 P1 Lott House
P2 Salt Marsh Nature Center
P3 Carmine Carro Community Center
P4 Plumb Beach
P5 Amity Little League Stadium

5.1 Turn right on Gerritsen Ave followed by immediate left onto Ave X.

5.2 Road turns left and becomes Burnett St.

5.7 Turn left on Ave U and then right onto Stuart St.

6.2 Turn right on Fillmore Ave.

6.5 Turn right on E 33rd St.

6.6 Finish at start, Ave S and E 33rd St.

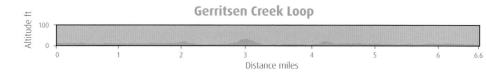

Gerritsen Creek Loop

Altitude ft

Distance miles

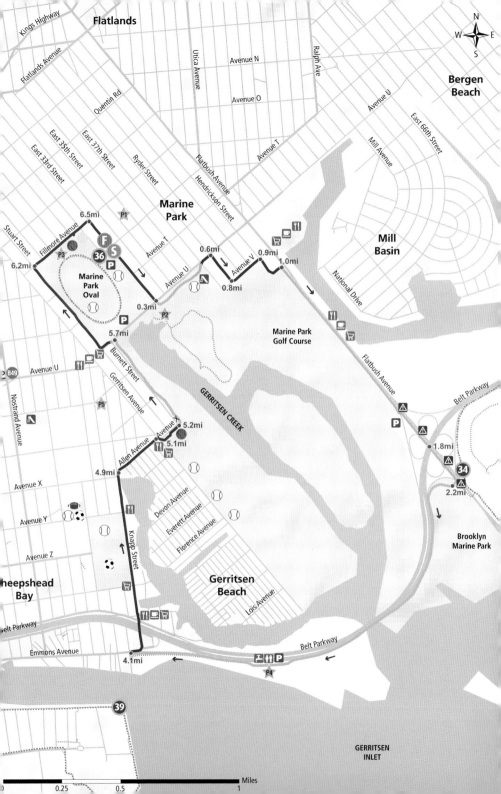

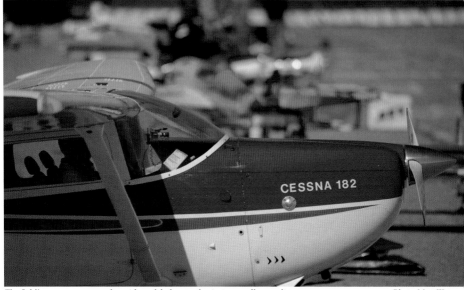

The field's runways are popular with model plane enthusiasts as well as cyclists.

Photo Matt Wittmer

At a Glance

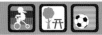

Distance 2.3 miles   **Elevation Gain** 9.3′

Terrain

Flat. The runways seem to have their original pavement, which seem to be cement and chip blocks. This surface is consistently on the rough side of things and the seams come at constant intervals.

Traffic

None.

How to Get There

Take the 2 or 5 train to the Flatbush Avenue-Brooklyn College Terminal, then ride southeast on Flatbush Avenue to FBF. Flatbush is pretty busy when you first get on the street, but the traffic thins out fairly quickly.

Food and Drink

There are often food trucks by the Aviator Sports Com-

plex. Otherwise, you have to either ride northwest along Flatbush a ways or ride to The Rockaways.

Side Trip

FBF is in the midst of a re-imagining to bring in more visitors. Hangar B, which houses historic aircraft is worth a visit and the Ryan visitor center is in the midst of being transformed to its former glory, when it was an integral part of the active airfield.

Links to 34

Where to Bike Rating

About...

Floyd Bennett Field was New York City's first municipal airport. From 1930-39, it was the center of aviation in N.Y.C. and site of many record-setting flights. In 1939, La Guardia Airport opened and FBF became a Naval Air Station, which it remained until being decommissioned in 1971. Since then, it has become part of the Gateway National Recreation Area, along with Jamaica Bay, The Rockaways, and Sandy Hook, N.J. It's now a home to sports facilities, hiking trails, a model airplane field, campsites, a NYPD helicopter unit, and a Marine Corps Reserves site.

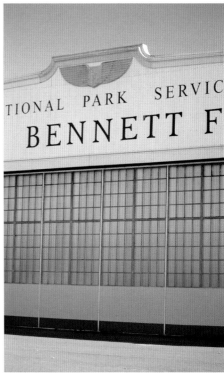

The façade of historic Hangar 8.   *Photo Matt Wittmer*

There is something otherworldly about riding in FBF. While there are roads on the edges of the park, most people ride the runways. References to the movie Mad Max crop up. After being in a city with lots of buildings and trees, in a region with lots of hills and few straight roads, the incredibly wide runways of the place and little vegetation taller than humans is a striking anomaly. If you go to Floyd by bike, whether it's taking Flatbush from downtown Brooklyn, or riding the bike paths from Canarsie, riding the narrow paths of the adjacent greenways, the change in scenery is jaw-dropping.

Until you go, it's hard to appreciate how dramatic the change is. When was the last time you rode your bike on an abandoned, dead-flat, absolutely straight 12-lane highway that has nothing but fields on either side? And it's just about always windy—it's an airfield.

FBF is a great place to ride if you want room, if you want to be alone, if you want quiet. You'll get lots of it all. The narrowest runway is three or four car-widths wide, and it's fairly short. Then they get wider and wider. It's so wide, you might even have trouble holding a straight line.

All of this might seem like criticism of FBF. It isn't. Floyd is so different from everywhere else it needs to

be explained. There's a stark beauty to it. Fondness grows on return trips.

Our first experience at Floyd was bike racing. Many people believe racing on pancake flat roads is necessarily easy. Races here can be amongst the hardest in the region. We appreciated the difficulty but had some trouble getting used to the location. As we went back, we found ourselves liking the place more and more.

There are Tuesday and Thursday night races in the spring and summer. There are also occasional weekend races starting in March and running into October.

But racing only takes up an hour or two occasionally. The runways are available pretty much all the time. A hard rain might briefly flood them, but the water recedes quickly. Snows even disappear fast, and they don't plow. It's just about always clear and usually empty. Bring your friends, your family, there's room for everyone to ride.

Ride Log

0.0 Start at southern corner of airfields. Head northwest on wider runway.

0.5 Turn right onto widest runway.

1.3 Turn right onto narrow runway.

1.8 Turn right onto wide runway.

2.3 Finish at start, the southern corner of the airfield.

P1 Community Garden
P2 Hangar Row
P3 Ryan Visitor Center
P4 Aviator Sports and Recreation Complex
P5 Hangar B
P6 Raptor Point
P7 Model Airplane Field

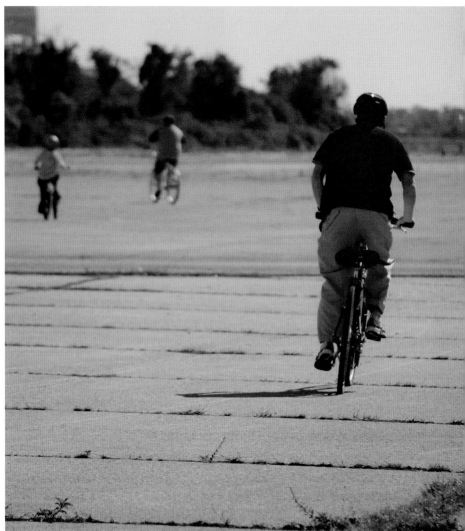

Room to roam.   *Photo Matt Wittmer*

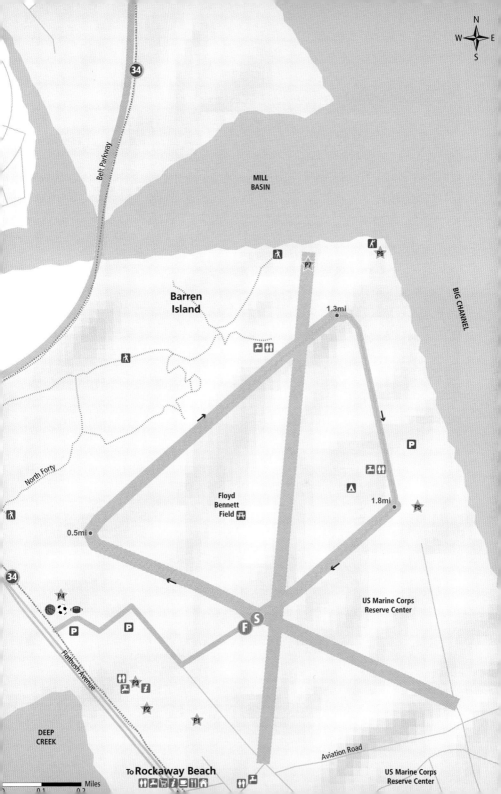

N
W · E
S

34

Belt Parkway

MILL
BASIN

P7

P6

BIG CHANNEL

Barren
Island

1.3mi

North Forty

Floyd
Bennett
Field

1.8mi

P5

0.5mi

34

P4

P

P

F S

US Marine Corps
Reserve Center

Flatbush Avenue

P3

i

P2

P1

DEEP
CREEK

Aviation Road

To Rockaway Beach

US Marine Corps
Reserve Center

Miles

0.1

0.2

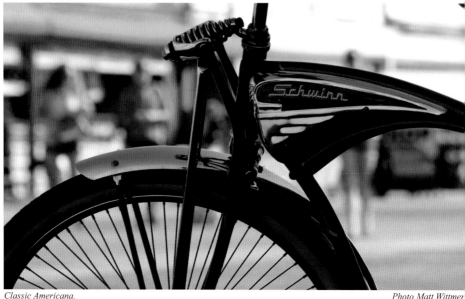

Classic Americana.

Photo Matt Wittmer

At a Glance

Distance 9.6 miles **Elevation Gain** 98′

Terrain

Flat, with a rise or two to get onto a bridge and the boardwalk. The roads are a mix, while the boardwalk is in excellent condition.

Traffic

From multi-use paths to city streets, you get the busy, the light, and in between. The boardwalk, while a multi-use path, qualifies as all three. Technically, cycling is only permitted on the boardwalk from 5am to 10am. But take that as a guideline for summer weekends. During the week and the winter, foot traffic will be light.

How to Get There

The D, F, N, and Q trains all stop at Coney Island-Stillwell Avenue, which is where the ride begins.

Food and Drink

Lots of food, from typical city fare of pizza, Chinese, Russian and the humble sandwich, to the usual beach fare of hot dogs, sausages, and sweets; Coney Island is diverse. Still, you owe it to yourself to stop by the very first Nathan's Famous at the corner of Surf and Stillwell, catty-corner from the start and finish of the ride.

Side Trip

In the summer, catch a game at MCU Park, home of the Brooklyn Cyclones. Minor league baseball has a rough-hewn charm that the majors can't offer.

Links to 37

Where to Bike Rating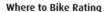

 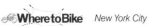

About...

While the name originates from Dutch, meaning Rabbit Island, the place is known for the beach and amusement parks. The wide beach is impressive. Unbelievably, the amusement parks were almost always hated by "respectable people." Said people's efforts have finally, after more than 130 years, paid off. During the late nineteenth and first half of the twentieth centuries, Coney Island was the largest "amusement area" in the United States. There were three separate amusement parks. Now, there is only one, Luna Park, a recent amalgam of survivors, and it's tiny. So, too is the commercial area of the boardwalk.

There is so much going on in New York, so many things to do and see and consider, that sometimes you can't see the big things. The Coney Island Loop seems to highlight this aspect of the city for us.

We'll start by paraphrasing an old Yogi Berra line; the beach is so crowded hardly anyone goes there. The beach is pretty big, like 100 yards deep and running the length of the (former) island. Thousands of people can go to the beach and there's still room for thousands more. And the amusement parks were so big that they scared city officials with all that vulgar entertainment for the masses.

But lost in the mix is the train station where the ride starts. It's the largest elevated subway station in North America, and it was rebuilt several years ago.

But the ride. You start by heading east on Neptune, which was probably the northern edge of the island before city officials decided to fill in part of the gap between this island and the rest of Brooklyn. Not the most scenic; it winds around several large housing complexes. But once the houses have gotten smaller, you're at the start of Sheepshead Bay and the riding is about to get much quieter.

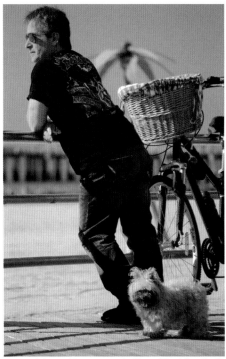

A dog and its owner on the Coney Island Boardwalk.
Photo Matt Wittmer

Quieter, yes, but maybe not easier. The closer you get to the water, the windier it gets, and you'll be hugging the coast in three directions. You loop around Manhattan Beach, then take a dip into Brighton Beach, before hitting the beach itself.

Once on the boardwalk, you're taking it to the end. It will usher you past Russian restaurants, the New York Aquarium, Luna Park, empty lots where amusements once stood, the disappearing commercial boardwalk strip, and MCU Park before turning left and riding to the end of Steeplechase Pier. If you're short on time, just turn around and ride out to Surf Avenue, you're just a few blocks away from where you started.

But the western segment of beach is less crowded, so check it out. At the end, you'll be at Sea Gate, one of the few gated communities in the city. Skirt it and start coming north on Neptune, back to the start.

Once back in the heart of Coney, celebrate with a few dogs.

Brooklyn

Ride Log

P1 Nathan's Famous Frankfurters
P2 Manhattan Beach Park
P3 Seaside Park
P4 New York Aquarium
P5 The Cyclone Roller Coaster
P6 Luna Park
P7 Deno's Wonder Wheel Amusement
P8 MCU Park: Home of the Brooklyn Cyclones
P9 The Parachute Jump
P10 The Steeplechase Pier
P11 Leon S Kaiser Playground

0.0 Start at the corner of Stillwell Ave and Surf Ave. Head north.

0.2 Turn right on Neptune Ave.

2.0 Turn right. Ride on bridge over inlet to Sheepshead Bay.

2.1 Turn left on Shore Blvd.

3.0 Turn right on Seawall Ave.

3.3 Turn right. Follow Seawall.

3.7 Turn right on Perry Ave.

3.8 Turn left on Oriental Blvd.

4.7 Turn right at Gerald H. Chambers Square, then the first left on Brighton Beach Ave.

4.8 Turn left on Brighton 14th St.

5.0 Turn right on boardwalk.

6.5 Turn left on pier.

6.7 U-turn at end of pier.

7.0 Turn left on boardwalk.

7.9 Boardwalk ends. Turn right on West 37th St.

8.2 Turn right on Neptune Ave.

9.4 Turn right on Stillwell Ave.

9.6 Finish at start, the corner of Stillwell and Surf.

Vintage experience. *Photo Matt Wittmer*

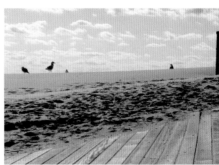

The year-round beach residents enjoying their sun and sand

Coney Island Loop

Altitude ft

Distance miles

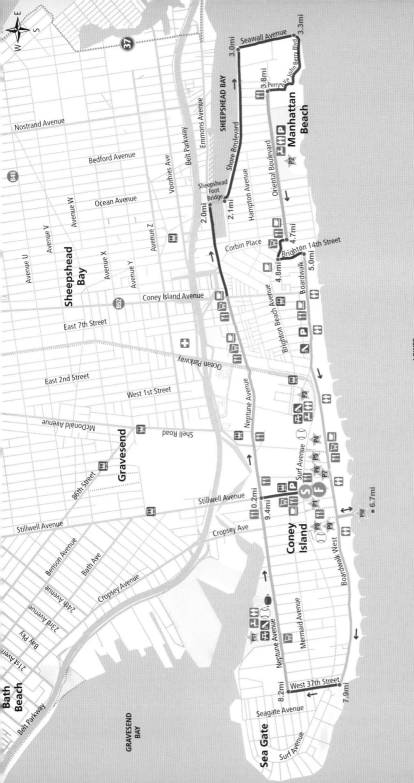

Staten Island

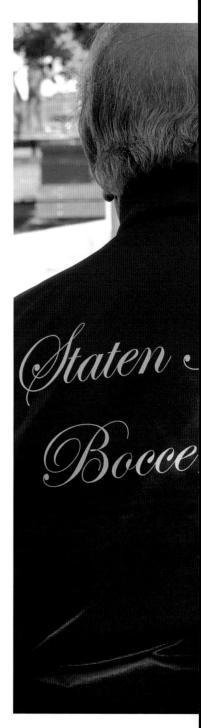

The saddest thing about preparing to master the roads and routes of Staten Island was how dedicated cyclists who lived in the borough told me the riding wasn't good. I appreciated the honesty, noted the blasé humor as an affect of weary cyclists, but was worried about the riding prospects. From afar it struck me as strange: this is the most thoroughly suburban county in the city, and that would, at least in my mind, promise good roads that are quiet most of the time. Not that my own experience prior to this book showed that to be the case.

After riding the length of the island several times, seeing the northern and southern edges, riding the perimeter, climbing the tallest hill, making my way past industrial zones and landfill, I can see where there's quite a bit of good riding. But at the same time, I see the limitations that someone who lives and breathes cycling must feel. It's hard to fit in a long ride on the island without experiencing the frustrations of riding on overburdened roads. Too many cars traveling too fast on narrow roads between too many lights.

The good thing is that for cyclists gaining their footing, the riding detailed here keeps you away from car traffic and offers up simple, short routes that anyone should be able to accomplish. And, as most of the rides are close to one another, when you get more fit and ambitious, you can link the rides together into more interesting and more challenging efforts.

Another plus is that riding in Staten Island makes you a pioneer. The more you're out there, the more you convince your family and friends and co-workers to ride, the more cyclists will get space for riding and the easier it is for the city to create and retain bike routes around the place. I can only imagine it's going to get better on Staten Island in the future. Not only with more places to ride, but more places to connect to, as the Bayonne Bridge is an easy escape to New Jersey and several greenway routes are planned alongside the waterways leading north from Bayonne.

The picaresque figure in me sees ways to combine various routes through all five boroughs and New Jersey for epic odysseys, starting or finishing at Conference House Park, the southernmost tip of both the city and state.

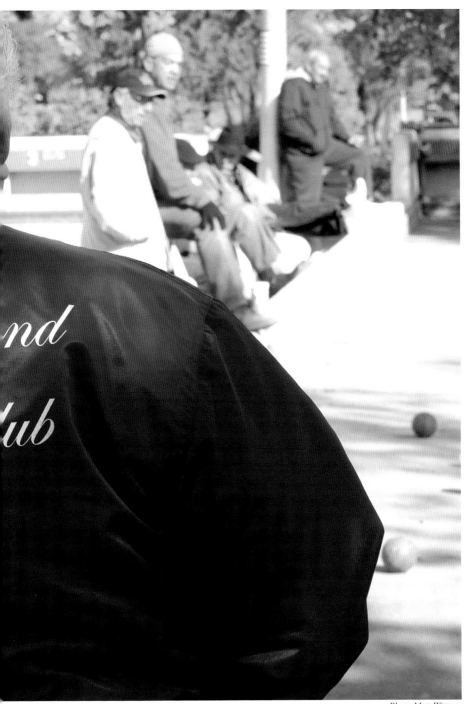

Photo Matt Wittmer

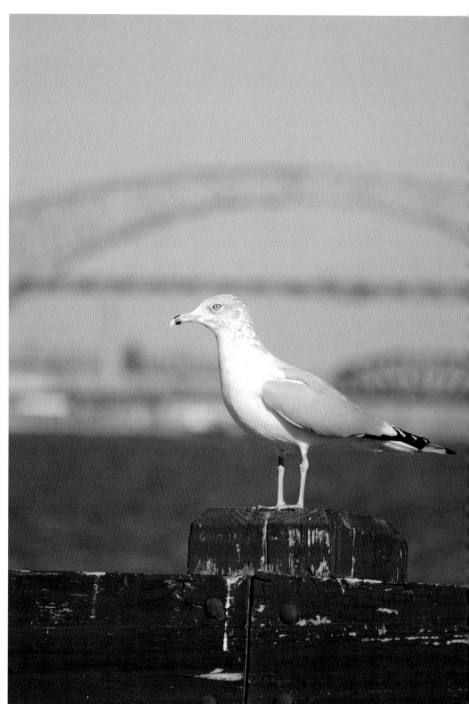

Photo Matt Wittmer

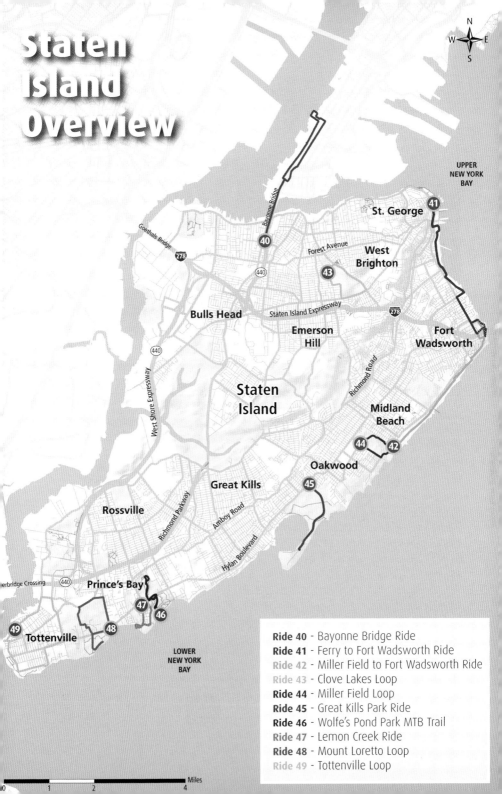

Staten Island Overview

N
W   E
S

UPPER NEW YORK BAY

St. George   ④①

West Brighton

Forest Avenue

④⓪

④③

440

Goethals Bridge

278

Bayonne Bridge

Bulls Head

Staten Island Expressway

278

Emerson Hill

Fort Wadsworth

440

West Shore Expressway

Staten Island

Richmond Road

Midland Beach

④④ ④②

Oakwood

④⑤

Great Kills

Rossville

Richmond Parkway

Amboy Road

Hylan Boulevard

erbridge Crossing   440

Prince's Bay

④⑦ ④⑥

④⑨ ④⑧

Tottenville

LOWER NEW YORK BAY

Ride 40 - Bayonne Bridge Ride
Ride 41 - Ferry to Fort Wadsworth Ride
Ride 42 - Miller Field to Fort Wadsworth Ride
Ride 43 - Clove Lakes Loop
Ride 44 - Miller Field Loop
Ride 45 - Great Kills Park Ride
Ride 46 - Wolfe's Pond Park MTB Trail
Ride 47 - Lemon Creek Ride
Ride 48 - Mount Loretto Loop
Ride 49 - Tottenville Loop

Miles
0   1   2   4

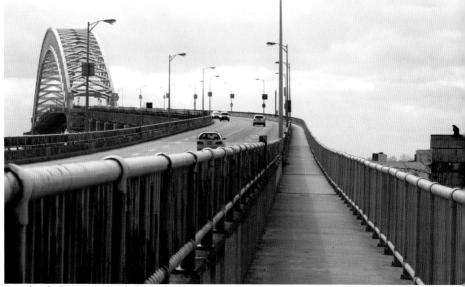

Ascending the Bayonne Bridge, the hill on the ride.

At a Glance

Distance 6.7 miles   **Elevation Gain** 201′

Terrain

One big hill climbed both ways, with a few rises in Bayonne. Good road surfaces.

Traffic

Almost three miles of the ride are on the bridge, where you'll only encounter the occasional cyclist. At the start of the Bayonne side, it could be a little busy, but then it will remain sleepy the rest of the way.

How to Get There

If you're riding from the Staten Island Ferry, you take Richmond Road around the northern edge of the island and make a left once you pass under the bridge.

Food and Drink

There are some places to stop by the start/finish in Staten Island, but Kennedy Boulevard in Bayonne is where you've got more choices.

Side Trip

Both City and Mayor Dennis P. Collins parks offer great spots for relaxing and views of the water.

Where to Bike Rating

About...

The Bayonne Bridge, though not one you hear about often, is actually the fourth longest through-arch bridge in the world, at 5,778 feet. The Sydney Bridge in Australia is a better-known, if shorter, version. Rather than the deck suspended from cables attached to cables, aka suspension bridges, the deck is suspended from cables hanging off a steel arch.

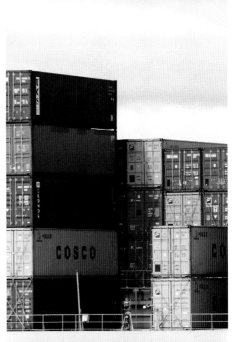

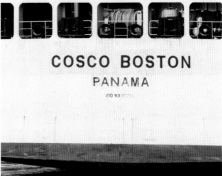

COSCO BOSTON
PANAMA

A cargo ship breaches The Narrows.   *Photo Matt Wittmer*

The Bayonne Bridge is one of three bridges linking Staten Island to the mainland United States, and is the only one you can legally ride over. On the other side of the island is the Verrazano Narrows Bridge, and that span is only rideable one day a year, when the Five Boro Bike Tour rides from Brooklyn to Staten Island. So this is the only chance to enjoy the peace and beauty of bridge riding in this borough.

And, at 1.4 miles each way, it is also among the longest, uninterrupted car-free stretches in Staten. Yes, it's a hill to climb both ways, but there is a descent both ways, too, and the views are excellent.

Once in Bayonne, you're taking largely sleepy streets through the port town that has the distinction of being both on Newark and Upper New York bays. Your destination is Veterans Park, a lap of the big field, and a view of Newark Bay.

After the park lap, it's back to quiet city streets for your return. There's a suburban vibe even though the streets display an urban population density.

Bayonne is very much a place in transition. There's the Hudson Bergen Light Rail Terminus on Eighth Street, which is bringing people closer to both Jersey and New York cities. It's also a way to get to the ride. And if you're looking for more riding, there's an effort underway to link the bike path that starts on the Hud-son River by Hoboken through Jersey City all the way south to Bayonne. It's years away, but it will be great when it finally comes to fruition.

Before you know it, it's time to walk the stairs to the start of the Bayonne Bridge again. It's a remarkable, if subtle, structure.

Staten Island

Ride Log

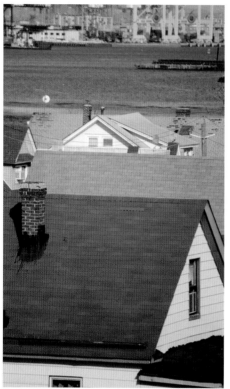

Rooftop view off the Bayonne Bridge.   *Photo Matt Wittmer*

0.0 Start at the intersection of Morningstar Rd and Hooker Pl. The start to the Bayonne Bridge bike path is on the northeast corner. Ride onto the bridge.

1.4 Stop bike. Dismount. Descend stairs. Turn right onto W Fourth St.

1.5 Turn left onto John F. Kennedy Blvd.

1.7 Kennedy Blvd becomes Cr-501/Kennedy Blvd.

3.0 Turn left onto W 26th St.

3.2 W 26th jogs left then right.

3.3 Enter Veterans Park. Turn right to take Park Rd around the park.

3.7 Park Rd becomes West 25th St.

3.8 Turn right on Ave A.

5.2 Turn left on W Fourth St.

5.3 Turn right onto the Bayonne Bridge. Stop. Dismount. Climb stairs.

6.7 Finish at the start, Morningstar Rd and Hooker Pl.

P1 Faber Pool and Park
P2 Bergen Point
P3 Below the Bridge Indoor Skate Park
P4 Bayonne Museum
P5 City Park

Bayonne Bridge Ride

Altitude ft

0 1 2 3 4 5 6 6.7
Distance miles

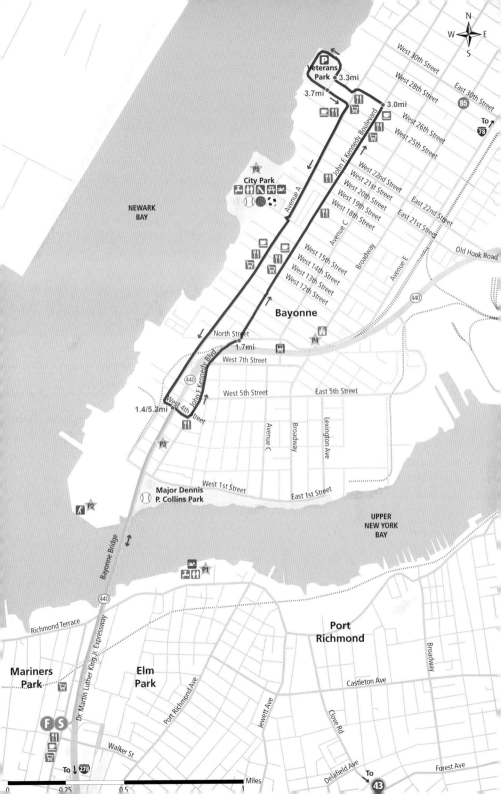

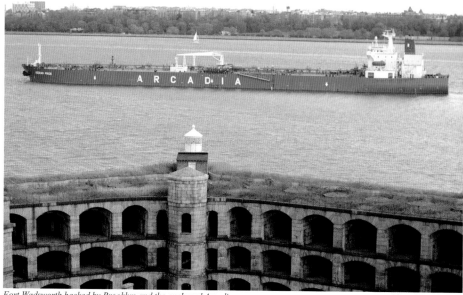

Fort Wadsworth backed by Brooklyn and the anchored Arcadia.

Photo Matt Wittmer

At a Glance

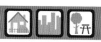

Distance 7.5 miles   **Elevation Gain** 410′

Terrain

Hilly. You first descend quickly to the water, but then climb away from the water to the fort, descend to the water on the turnaround, and reverse the action on the way home.

Traffic

Mostly light. The start and finish will present the busiest streets, but most of the riding is on quiet side streets.

How to Get There

The Staten Island Ferry takes you right to the start. You just need to ride uphill to get out. This could change as more bike paths are created.

Food and Drink

You've got plenty of cafés and restaurants by the ride start in St. George. They're sleepy most of the time, as they depend on the commuter traffic coming and going from the ferry. You'll also pass through a downtown-y area once you turn back on Bay Street by the fort.

Side Trip

Alice Austen House. It's a landmark structure, built in 1690 and restored to how it looked in the early 20th century. Austen, who spent most of her life in the house, known as Clear Comfort, was a photographer who documented life in the late 19th and early 20th centuries. The house also houses a collection of her photographs.

Links to

Where to Bike Rating

About...

This loop, while an out-and-back, should serve as a gateway to most of the rides on Staten Island. It runs along the shore, and, so long as you keep the water on your left, you can start here and ride all the way to Tottenville, and take in Staten Island rides 42, 44, 45, 46, 47, 48, and 49. This route starts as one of the most urban and industrial of the rides laid out in Staten Island, but the payoff, Fort Wadsworth, is bucolic.

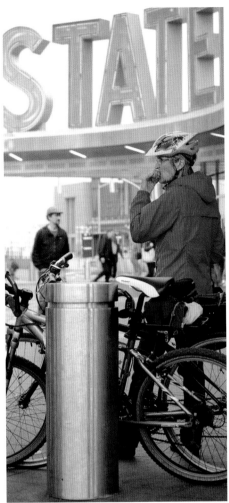

Lower Manhattan's Whitehall Ferry Terminal.
Photo Matt Wittmer

We start with riding from the ferry itself as many people reading this book will be coming from other parts of the city. The problem with starting at the ferry is that it's a major transit point for locals. That means there can be quite a bit of car traffic when you're leaving the ferry terminal if you happen to go at the wrong time.

That's why this course quickly skirts the busy thoroughfare of Bay Street and takes you down to the water. Quiet industrial roads like Front Street show a working city, and give a brief glimpse into the island's seafaring past. But once you feel like you've got the rhythm down, you turn and are suddenly thrust into a suburban downtown that almost as quickly gives way to Fort Wadsworth.

Wadsworth is part of Gateway National Recreation Area, much like Floyd Bennett Field, is a decommissioned military installation. Gateway, which is part of the National Park Service, has their area headquarters in Wadsworth. All the same, it still houses military personnel, so some of the grounds are off limits to the public.

At the far end of the ride, you loop under the Verrazano Narrows Bridge and ride past the lower fort,

Battery Weed. Weed, originally Fort Richmond, was built in the mid 19th century to protect New York City from naval attack.

Once past it, you climb up to get onto Mont Sec Avenue, an officers' row, before turning back to retrace your route back to the ferry.

After riding on quiet and largely abandoned streets most of the way, the turn onto Bay Street is a bit disconcerting, but it means you're only a few blocks from finishing the ride.

Staten Island

Ride Log

 P1 Staten Island Museum
P2 Borough Hall
P3 National Lighthouse Museum
P4 Cromwell Recreation Center
P5 Garibaldi Meucci Museum
P6 Alice Austen House Museum
P7 Fort Wadsworth
P8 Battery Duane
P9 Battery Weed

0.0 Start at the entrance to the Staten Island Ferry. It's the intersection of Lighthouse Plaza, Staten Island Ferry Viaduct, Nick Laporte Pl, Richmond Terrace, and Bay St. Head southwest on Bay.

0.5 Turn left on Hannah St.

0.6 Hannah bears right onto Murray Hurlbert Ave/Front St.

1.8 Front turns right. Then immediately turn left onto Edgewater St.

2.3 Turn right onto Hylan Blvd.

2.5 Turn left onto Bay St. (yes, the same Bay St.)

3.1 Enter Fort Wadsworth. Bay becomes New York Ave.

3.4 Turn left onto Tompkins St.

3.6 Turn right onto Hudson Rd.

3.8 Make 160-degree turn onto S. Weed Rd.

4.0 S. Weed becomes N. Weed.

4.2 Left onto Mont Sec Ave.

4.4 Turn right onto Bay St.

5.0 Turn right onto Hylan Blvd.

5.2 Turn left onto Edgewater St.

5.9 Turn right onto Front and then Front immediately turns left.

7.0 Turn left onto Hannah St.

7.1 Turn right onto Bay St.

7.5 Finish at the start, at the ramp to the Staten Island Ferry.

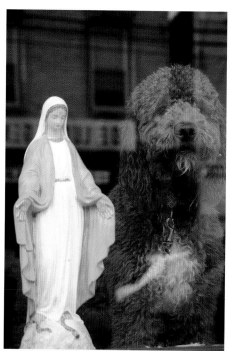

Storefront scene in Shore Acres.   *Photo Matt Wittmer*

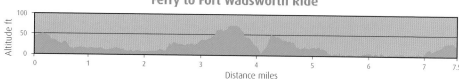

Ferry to Fort Wadsworth Ride

Altitude ft

Distance miles

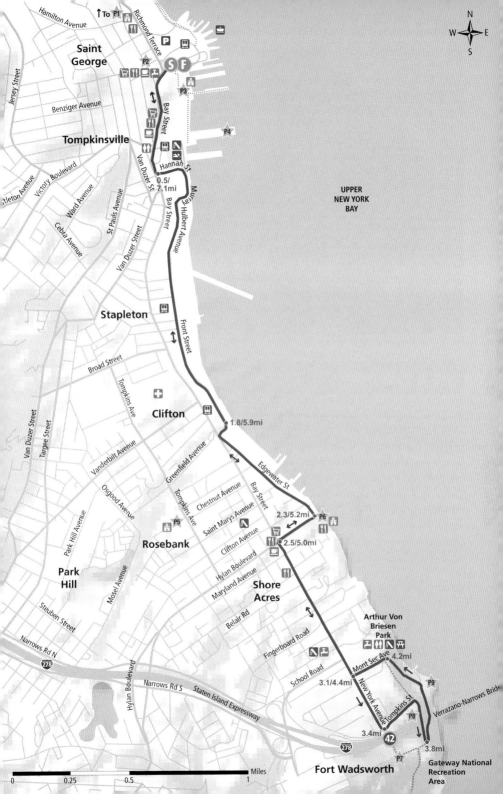

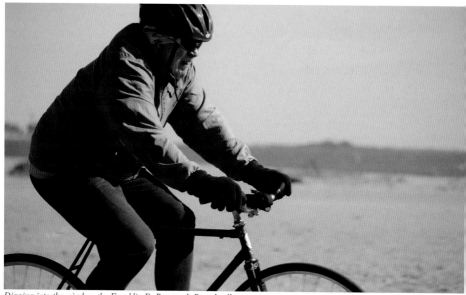

Digging into the wind on the Franklin D. Roosevelt Boardwalk.

Photo Matt Wittmer

At a Glance

Distance 7.5 miles **Elevation Gain** 305′

Terrain

Largely flat, with one ascent to the halfway point and one descent back to the water.

Traffic

Almost non-existent. Most of the way is on a bike path or in Fort Wadsworth. You'll have to watch for pedestrians along the path and cars at one or two places.

How to Get There

You can always take Ride 41 to Fort Wadsworth and do this ride or you can get to Miller Field by Hylan Avenue, which is one of the most-traveled thoroughfares in Staten Island.

Food and Drink

From Miller Field, you can easily ride to the Hylan Commons mall on Hylan Avenue and New Dorp Lane. There are also delis along New Dorp facing Miller. If

you do the ride, there are places to stop along Father Capodano Boulevard, which runs parallel to the ride, in Midland Beach and across from FDR Boardwalk and beach.

Side Trip

Fort Wadsworth. While the fortifications were long-ago retired, they are still impressive structures. The one along the water is Battery Weed, and the one above is Battery Duane. And if the weather's nice, take a break and relax on the beach or ride to the end of the pier attached to the FDR Boardwalk.

Links to

Where to Bike Rating

About...

This ride links two sectors of the Gateway National Recreation area, which means both were once defense installations. Miller Field was an Air Force base, both with runways for planes with wheels, and ramps for planes with pontoons. The runway remains because unlike Floyd Bennett Field, the strip was grass, not pavement.

Miller Field is an immense patch of grass, and circumnavigating it is its own ride. I'd hate to mow it! But it's also a good starting point for a ride as it takes the beach bike path all the way up to Fort Wadsworth, linking the ride from the ferry, creating a nice 15-mile loop from the ferry, a nice day's outing.

Since this ride spends most of its distance right next to a beach, expect that the ride can feel pretty windy. It's not a bad thing; if you get a tailwind, you'll get a nice easy ride, and if you get a headwind, you'll have to either ride slower or work a bit harder. The good thing about riding along the beach is little traffic. At the height of summer heat, expect the path to get crowded, otherwise you'll have much of the ride to yourself. At a certain point on your ride north, the boardwalk begins and it should mean a nice separation between pedestrians and cyclists, but you lose a view of the water for a while.

With so little to worry about in terms of safety, the ride goes by very quickly. Even when the bike path ends and you enter the forts' grounds, there are very few cars to worry about. The forts appear just after riding under the massive Verrazano Narrows span, a contrast of modern and early American history.

The forts really are something to behold. Not only were they an essential part of protecting New York Harbor from invasion starting in the 17th century, but

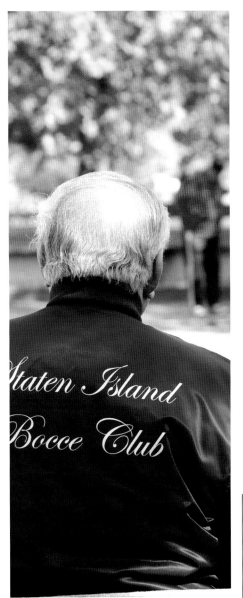

An island tradition.   *Photo Matt Wittmer*

the structure was built for another era, so there are tunnels that go through the place in all sorts of directions.

While we prefer stopping by Battery Weed for the views, there are plenty of picnic areas, playgrounds, and miles of sand to relax on.

Staten Island

Ride Log

0.0 Begin at the start of the bike path at the eastern edge of Miller Field. It's right by a parking lot and the start of Friar Capodanno Blvd. Head northeast with the water on your right.

2.1 Passing The Vanderbilt. Briefly on a parking lot road.

2.7 Bike path ends. Turn right on USS North Carolina Rd.

3.2 Turn left on Hudson Rd.

3.3 Turn right on New York Ave.

3.4 Turn right on Tompkins St.

3.6 Turn left on Hudson Rd.

3.8 Turn right on N Weed Rd.

4.2 Go straight onto Hudson Rd.

4.3 Turn left on USS North Carolina Rd.

4.8 Turn left onto bike path.

5.3 Passing The Vanderbilt. Briefly on a parking lot road.

7.5 Finish at the start, the end of the bike path at Miller Field.

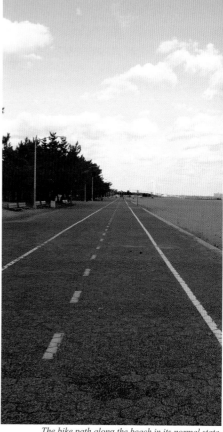

The bike path along the beach in its normal state.

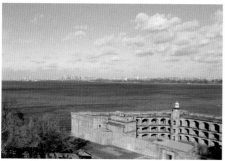

Battery Weed with Bay Ridge, Manhattan and Jersey City in the distance.

P1 Fort Wadsworth
P2 Battery Weed
P3 Battery Duane

Miller Field to Fort Wadsworth Ride

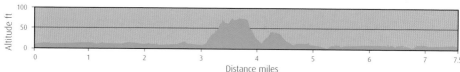

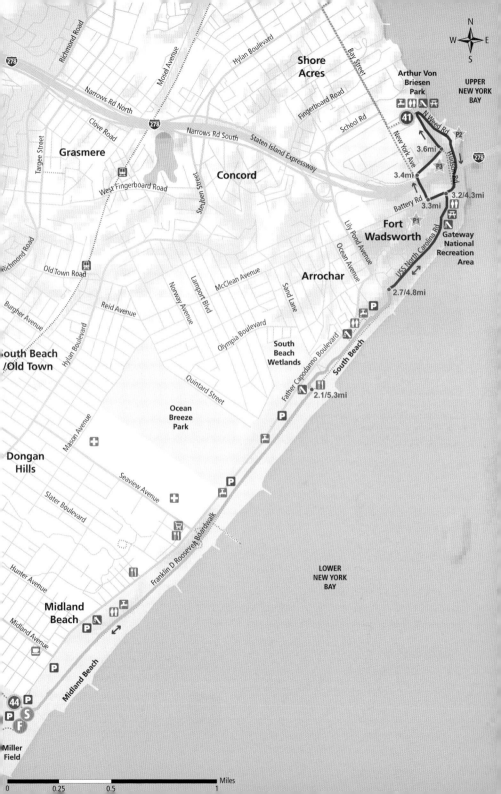

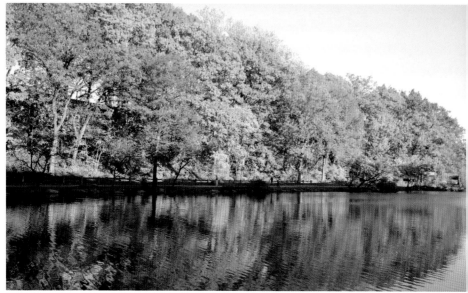

Fall color at Clove Lake.

Photo Matt Wittmer

At a Glance

Distance 2.5 miles   **Elevation Gain** 259′

Terrain

Hilly, with decent roads.

Traffic

Mixed. It has the potential to be both devoid of cars and busy with traffic.

How to Get There

The easiest way to get here from the ferry is Victory Boulevard the whole way, though it's a busy road. A less direct, but more pleasant route is to take Richmond Terrace to Broadway which will take you there.

Food and Drink

You can find several choices at the intersection of Clove Road and Victory Boulevard. Still, the standout of the pack is the Indian Clove restaurant on the east corner.

Side Trip

Clove Lakes Park is a city facility with many attractions; lakes, ice rink, hiking trails, playgrounds, and more. Not the least of which are the freshwater wetlands designated "Forever Wild" by the Parks Department. The park is also a common resting place for the peripatetic monarch butterfly, which usually makes an appearance in June.

Where to Bike Rating

About...

The lakes of Clove Lakes Park are, like much of the city, constructed nature. There was a Clove Brook that ran down to Kill Van Kull through the valley that cleft between Emerson and Grymes hills, but it was dammed starting in 1683. There were several dams built here, most of them to create enough water pressure to mill both grain and wood. The Clove Lake was created in 1825 to supply water pressure to a grist mill.

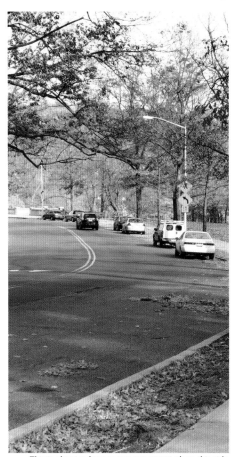

This is about as busy as you can expect along this ride.

Challenging is in the eye of the beholder. This fairly simple route is one of the more strenuous rides we've mapped in Staten Island. Not that you can't find hillier; you can always ride over Todt Hill, directly south of this ride, if you're looking for long ascent. The top of Todt, at 410 feet above sea level is the highest point in the city and the highest point on the Atlantic Coastal Plain.

Still, while the rises might be challenging, the length of this ride makes it doable for just about everyone. The nice thing is that it gives up a challenge in small doses. This loop not only curves, but dips and rises over the distance. Because the elevation changes are on the straights, it's hard not to be hyper-aware of the changes, possibly thinking they are greater than they appear.

To us, the surprises of the ride have more to do with the change that occurs shortly after the start of the ride. Clove Lakes Park, at the starting point, seems like many a small urban park, with a nice little patch of forest, and pretty ponds. But turning onto Clove Road, that sense of the park shifts. You realize how big the park really is. Clove runs along the longest edge of the park and Victory Boulevard the second-longest, and it can feel like the park goes on forever. But just as it is starting to feel infinite, you turn off of Victory and onto a quiet side street, which returns you pretty much to what you started with, and hugging the perimeter on lightly-traveled roads is what you've got in front of you.

While we don't want to push the idea of "training" on to everyone, this is a good ride for just that. With very few turns, and almost no intersecting roads, this is a ride you can do over and over and over again. And because of the few places you might need to stop, it's great for timing your efforts and seeing how your fitness measures up between when you first rode it and your next attempt..

Staten Island

Ride Log

0.0 Start at the corner of Slosson and Martling avenues. Head east on Martling.

P1 New York Army National Guard
P2 War Memorial Ice Skating Rink
P3 Barrett Park & Staten Island Zoo

0.2 Turn right on Clove Rd.

1.2 Turn right on Victory Blvd.

1.8 Turn right on Royal Oak Rd. Turn left on Rice Ave.

2.2 Turn right on Slosson Ave.

2.5 Finish where you started, the corner of Slosson and Martling.

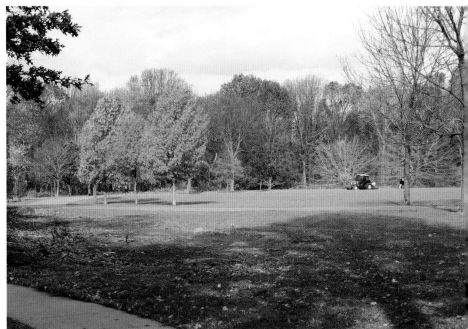

Plenty of paths for walking when you're done riding.

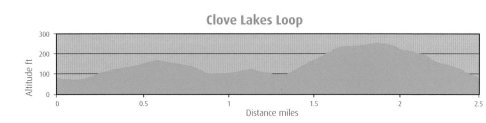

Clove Lakes Loop

Altitude ft / Distance miles

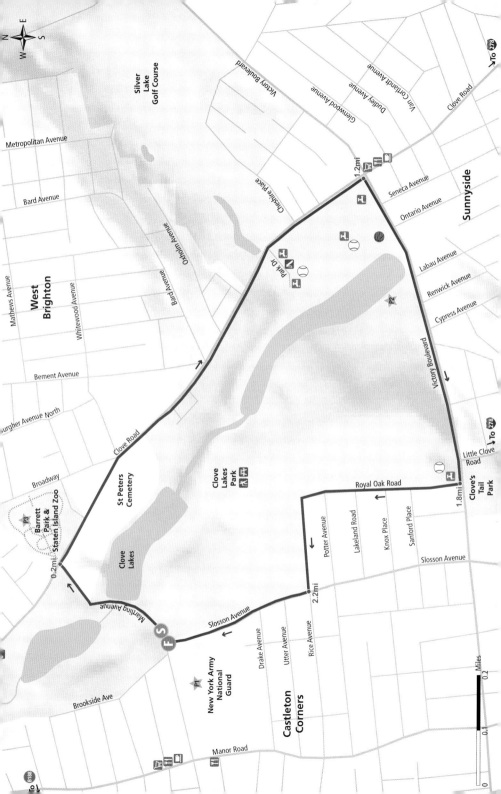

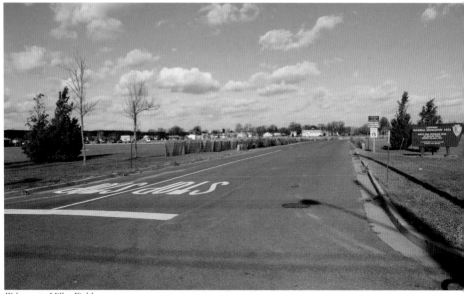

Welcome to Miller Field.

At a Glance

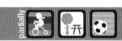

Distance 1.8 miles   **Elevation Gain** 15′

Terrain

Flat. About half the pavement is in good condition, about half is a bit rough.

Traffic

Light. Two-thirds of the ride is in a park, the other third is a lightly-traveled street.

How to Get There

It's easy to follow the ride from the ferry to the fort, and then the fort to here. Or, you can take the Staten Island Railroad to the New Dorp stop and ride New Dorp Lane to the field.

Food and Drink

There are some delis on the ride, but there are plenty of food choices along Hylan Boulevard.

Side Trip

The movies. Hylan Plaza has the UA Hylan Plaza Five, five screens for your viewing enjoyment. There is always a great feeling associated with watching movies at a theatre in daylight; it feels even more like hookey than bike riding.

Links to 42

Where to Bike Rating

About...

Miller Field, yet another reminder of New York's military past, is moving into the past as it moves into the future. It's currently a huge grassy expanse, over 187 acres; somewhat between its military use as an airstrip and its previous life as a farm. The farm, built by the Vanderbilts, was a freshwater wetland before it was a farm. You can still see remainders of the wetland in the northwest corner today. The Swamp White Oak Forest, its soil formed from glacial outwash, spends part of the year flooded.

This is an easy family ride. One of the easiest on this island. You don't need directions, you don't need a map: you just ride around the field. It's short, so if you're learning how to ride, teaching someone to ride, or just starting out using cycling as part of your fitness routine, this ride asks very little of you and allows you to stop pretty much whenever you want. Perfect for beginners; the only problem is you have to go around the field counter-clockwise rather than clockwise because the north end has one-way traffic, a directive we cyclists must follow.

There is some car traffic, but it's mostly people coming and going from their parking spot. They're going slow and will have their heads up. And on nice days, the field itself will have a decent level of activity, but as it is a fairly vast field, even when it's crowded, it isn't crowded.

If you want to take a break before riding more, there are benches. If you want to go to the beach, it's at the end of New Dorp Lane or just before you turn past the entry to the Franklin D. Roosevelt Boardwalk. You can drop people off to play on the field (baseball, football, Frisbee, soccer, etc) and get a good ride in all by yourself. If you're bringing kids, there's a playground on

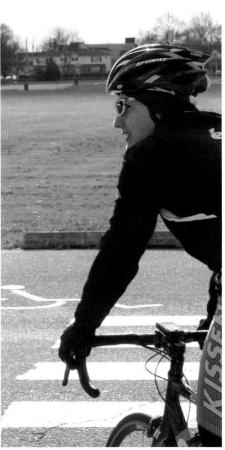

Rolling out for an easy spin around the park.

site. Considering the shopping nearby, the ride can be integrated into your errands.

If you're feeling like making this part of a larger ride, you can link up with most of the rides we have outlined in Staten Island.

The ride is simple. It gives you a chance to use your creativity to build whatever you want around it.

Staten Island

Ride Log

0.0 Start at the intersection of Mill Rd and New Dorp Ln. Take New Dorp toward the water. The park is on your left.

0.6 Turn left on Cedar Grove Ave.

0.9 Turn left as Cedar Grove turns left.

1.2 Turn right to get on bike lane around parking area

1.4 Bike path merges on to park road.

1.5 Park road turns left. Follow road.

1.8 Finish at the start. Mill Rd and New Dorp Ln.

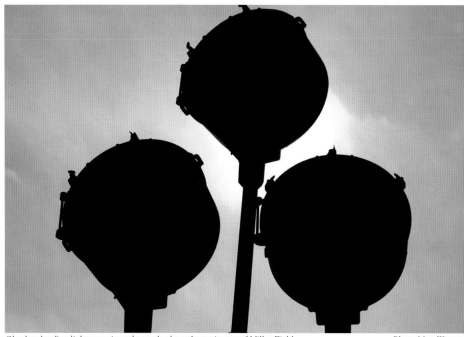

Obsolete landing lights remain at the ready along the perimeter of Miller Field.　　　*Photo Matt Wittmer*

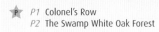

P1　Colonel's Row
P2　The Swamp White Oak Forest

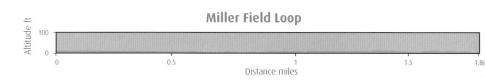

Miller Field Loop

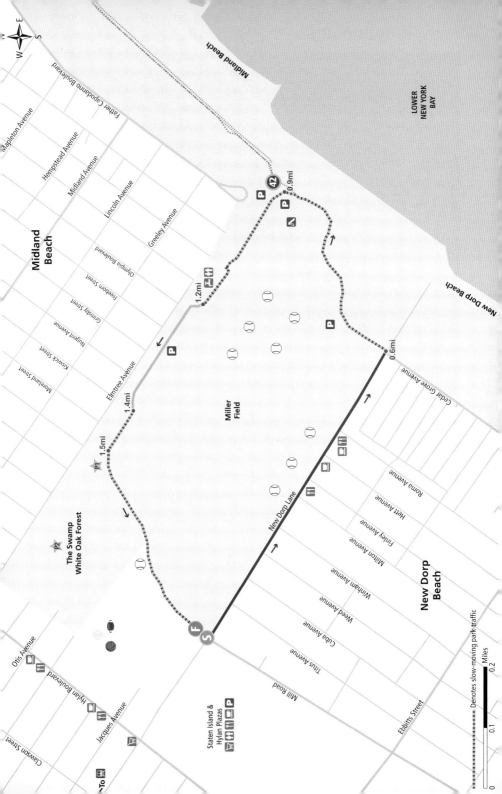

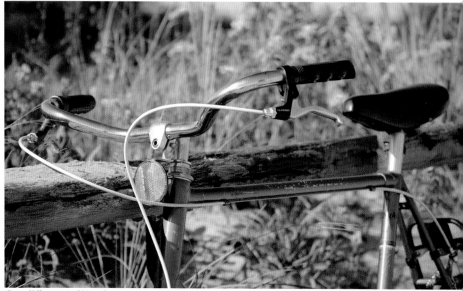

Great Kills is one of 11 parks comprising Gateway National Recreation Area.

Photo Matt Wittmer

At a Glance

Distance 3.4 miles   **Elevation Gain** 45′

Terrain

Flat. Road and paths are in generally good condition.

Traffic

Light. The park road is a dead-end street, so there's no through traffic. And the second half of the ride is on a multi-use path.

How to Get There

This park is less than three miles down Hylan Boulevard from Miller Field, so if you can get there, you can get here. You can also take the Staten Island Railroad to the Bay Terrace stop, and ride less than a mile to the park. You can take your boat to Nicholas Marina and rent a slip for the day.

Food and Drink

There's a seasonal snack bar on the beach, but for more vittles, you'll need to ride further down Hylan to the Bay Terrace neighborhood.

Side Trip

The Jacques Marchais Museum of Tibetan Art is by the lighthouse on the ridge to the west of the park. It's designed to feel like a Tibetan monastery, complete with fieldstone buildings evoking Tibetan architecture, a pond, and meditation areas.

Where to Bike Rating

 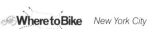

About...

Great Kills Park, the southernmost section of Gateway National Recreation Area within New York City, is, like much of the city; constructed nature. There was an island, Crooke's Island, and then the northern section of the channel, between Crooke's and Staten islands was filled in creating a peninsula and the Great Kills Harbor, which has marinas on both sides of it, and plenty of room for protected sailing.

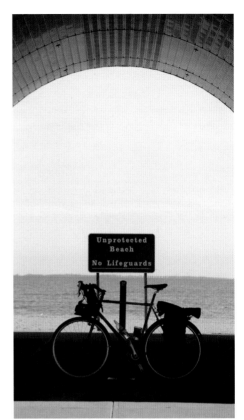

Here off-season? The beach might be yours alone.
Photo Matt Wittmer

If you're wondering about the name, it's derived from old Dutch, as are many place names in Staten Island; it basically means "many streams" or "channels" and the area indeed has a bunch.

Having ridden around Staten Island, there's a great feeling you get when turning off Hylan Boulevard, a fairly busy street by Great Kills, and getting on to Buffalo. It's like turning into a private driveway. And as much of this island feels quite crowded, it is a welcome respite.

Great Kills Park is the fifth ride along Staten Island's Atlantic coast. Like the others, it has a big virtue in that car access is extremely limited. While you're riding on an access road for the first half, the road dead ends shortly after the turnaround.

But you'll be on a bike path back to the start for the rest of the way. And if riding near car traffic makes you uncomfortable, you can ride the bike path both ways.

If the distance of the ride isn't quite enough for your fitness level or time, do a second lap, and when you get to the turnaround, keep on going. First to the parking lot at the end of Buffalo Street, then do a U-turn, ride back to the first turnaround, and then go left. That will also take you to another parking lot. Two laps of the loop plus these detours boosts your mileage up to about eight miles.

This ride can also be a part of a larger route, one that starts at Miller Field, Fort Wadsworth, or even the ferry itself. Conversely, you can start at Tottenville and head north along Hylan here. You can always reverse course to get back or take the train. It's free to ride once you're away from the ferry terminal and the Tompkinsville stops.

Ride to the southernmost point of the island and you come across the osprey platform at the southern tip of the peninsula. If you think riding a bike takes time, get a gander of these birds. They winter in the Caribbean or South America and visit Great Kills in April and May en route to points north. In summertime, some of the birds hang out at Great Kills because the fishing is good and the climate agreeable. You can see them sitting in tree branches eating their catch.

Staten Island

Ride Log

0.0 Start at the parking lot on Buffalo St just inside the park entrance on Hylan Ave. Ride southeast.

1.7 Turn left into parking lot. Bike path starts between the parked cars and the dune. Get on bike path.

3.4 Finish at the start. The parking lot on Buffalo just inside the park entrance.

 P1 Nichols Great Kills Marina
P2 Crooke's Point
P3 Great Kills Beach
P4 Seaside Wildlife Nature Park

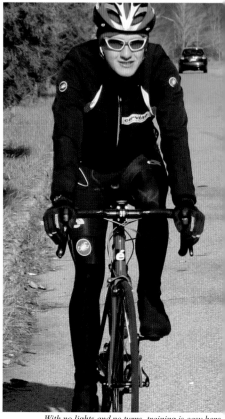

With no lights and no turns, training is easy here.

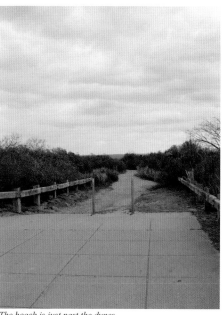

The beach is just past the dunes.

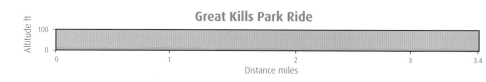

Great Kills Park Ride

Altitude ft

Distance miles

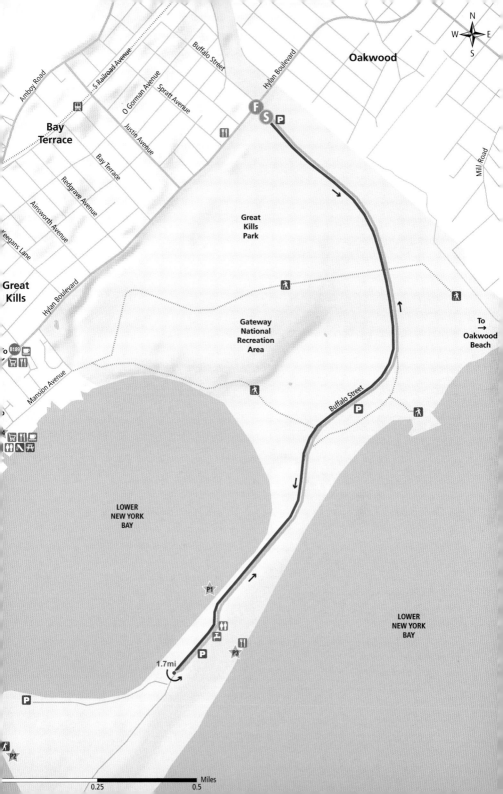

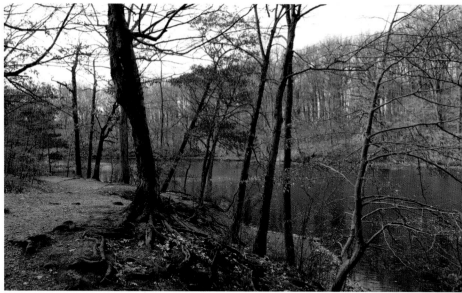

Wolfe's Pond is peaceful and quiet.

At a Glance

Distance 2.8 miles   **Elevation Gain** 182'

Terrain

Flat. There are a few short hills, but the rest of the terrain changes are small dips. Most of the ride is on trails, which are a little rocky and rooty, but should be fine for novice mountain bikers.

Traffic

There's a short stretch on Hylan Boulevard, which is a road, but the rest is on trails, and these will probably be lightly traveled by cyclists and walkers.

How to Get There

If you want to ride, all you need to do is get to Hylan Boulevard and it will take you. If you're taking the Staten Island Railroad, get off at the Huguenot station. If you're driving, there is plenty of parking.

Food and Drink

There's nothing at the park. The new nearest outposts for eats are by the Huguenot and Prince's Bay train stations. Prince's Bay has more choices.

Side Trip

While we detailed a simple route that beginner mountain bikers should be able to ride, we suggest trying all the trails before going home. And if it's a nice day, bring some charcoal and meat and grill up some flesh, then walk down to the beach and enjoy the pastime of sitting still with a vast expanse in front of you.

Links to 47

Where to Bike Rating

About...

This park, at 302 acres one of the city's largest on Staten Island, has enough stuff for more than a day's worth of activities for the entire family. Besides the mountain bike trails, there are walking trails, a beach, a playground, a war monument, a roller hockey rink, basketball courts, tennis courts, grills for barbecuing, picnic tables, a beach on the Atlantic, a forest, and freshwater ponds.

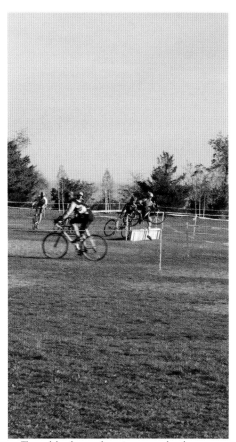

The park has become home to an annual cyclocross race.

This is one of three officially-sanctioned MTB trails in N.Y.C. We cover all three in this book. Of the three, this seems the least used. While the trails on the ocean side of Hylan Boulevard are well-tended and seem to have signs of regular use, at least by pedestrians, the trails in the North Forest, on the bay side of Hylan, rarely encounter a knobby tire. There are four miles of trails in all; most are considered "beginner", some are "intermediate", and one is "expert". That written, a mountain bike without suspension should be able to handle everything these trails have to offer.

The intermediate trails seem a bit narrower and have steeper pitches both up and down, but these pitches are short, so even if you have to get off your bike, it will only be for a short time, and nothing is long enough that you'll really pick up speed. To us, these trails are excellent for skills-building, and as just about everyone can improve their riding skills, we say take the time to learn how to ride everything.

Riding around the trails on the south side of Hylan is fairly easy and straightforward, though you do have to encounter typical MTB obstacles like roots, rocks, steep drops, and fallen trees. The trickiest obstacle seems to be of the moving kind. People walking on the same trails you're riding. We're all for sharing trails, we don't see it as a problem, just wanted to alert you.

As we mention earlier, this is a place where you can stay all day. The city gets a rap as not having much "nature" within its borders. Hopefully, you know by now this is false. There is an amazing diversity of natural habitats and wild creatures. This park is one of the many you should be checking out for its nature. The pond of the title is a freshwater pond that is mere feet from the Atlantic. Across Hylan, you will find Acme Pond, not a possession of Wile E. Coyote, home to diverse wildlife, including toads, painted turtles, snapping turtles, and red backed salamanders. The flora around the pond is similarly diverse, with white oaks, pin oaks, hickory trees, sour and sweet gum trees, red maples, and more, and the fauna living in it includes downy woodpeckers, green herons, and flickers.

Staten Island

Ride Log

 P1 Prince's Bay Beach
P2 Seguine Mansion

0.0 Start by the bathroom at the end of the parking lot in the park. There is a trailhead just north of the building. Ride into the woods.

0.3 Trail ends at Hylan Blvd. Cross street and make left turn.

0.5 Turn right into woods at trailhead. Continue on trail. You're now starting to head back to where you entered this section of park.

1.7 Trail ends at Hylan Blvd. Cross street. Enter park at trailhead on other side. Follow trail to the left. Turn right onto trail you first headed out on.

2.2 Trail splits. Take the right turn. You'll now have Wolfe's Pond on your right.

2.5 Trail turns left, away from pond.

2.8 Finish at the start.

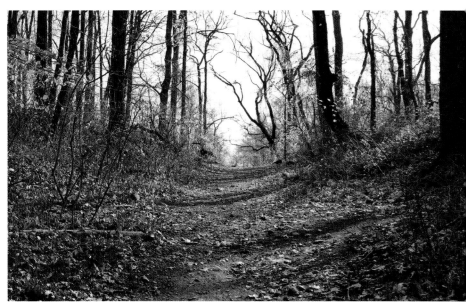

There are a few short hills, but as they're pretty smooth, they shouldn't require a dismount.

Wolfe's Pond Park MTB Trails

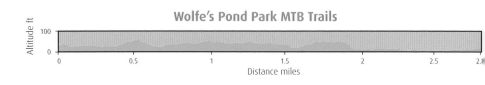

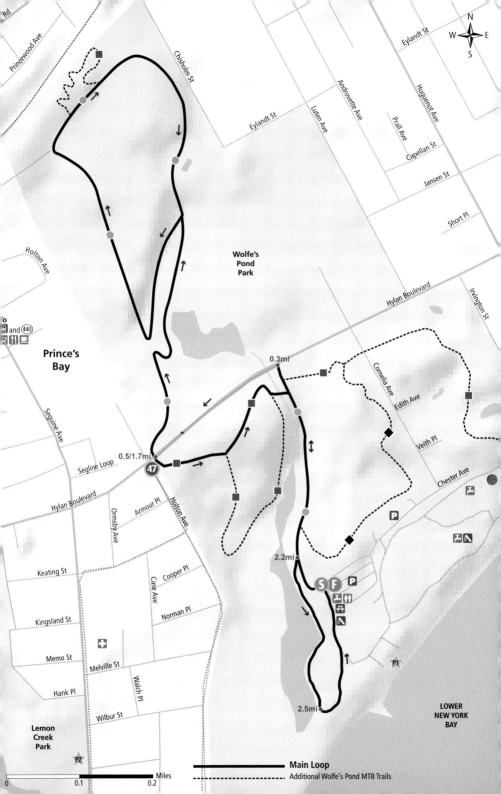

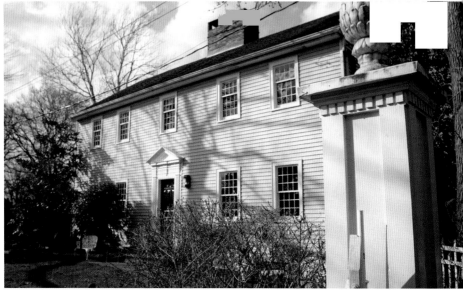

A historic home on the Seguine Mansion grounds.

At a Glance

Distance 1.8 miles   **Elevation Gain** 64'

Terrain

Flat. The wind will provide the resistance, not the terrain. Mostly paved roads in good condition, with some riding on fine gravel.

Traffic

Light. This ride takes place entirely on residential roads and parkland. You'll see few cars and no one should be speeding.

How to Get There

This is yet another ride off of Hylan Boulevard, so any ride you do that bracket this main thoroughfare will get you to Lemon Creek. You can also take the Staten Island Railroad to Prince's Bay and ride toward the Atlantic on Seguine Avenue to get to the start.

Food and Drink

This is a ride through a residential neighborhood, so your best bet is to find repast at the two shopping centers just past the Prince's Bay SIR stop.

Side Trip

Schedule a horseback ride at the Seguine Equestrian Center. There's quite a bit of terrain to choose from.

Links to 46

Where to Bike Rating

About...

This is a neighborhood ride. The neighborhood is Prince's Bay, sometimes Princess Bay. In the late 19th century, this was a fishing village and the oysters pulled out by local oystermen, "Prince's Bay Oysters" had international renown. As all of the ride is south of Hylan, and bounded on one side by Wolfe's Pond Park and on the other by Lemon Creek, there is very little car traffic, and no through traffic.

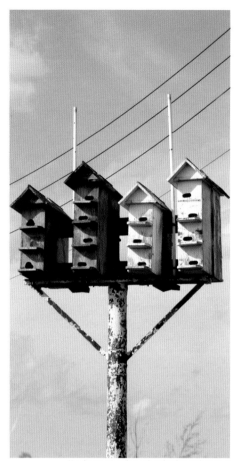

You know it's urban when birds get their own high-rise condos.

As neighborhood rides go, this is a very easy one. It's the ideal ride for anyone who wants to get a feel for riding on open streets in a low-pressure environment thanks to the minimal traffic. Good for kids, too.

Starting out, you have Wolfe's Pond and the park which shares the name on your left. If you took the mountain bike ride, you would be on the other side. For some reason, it seems more believable that the pond is freshwater when viewed from this side.

At the end of Holten, you have the southern section of Lemon Creek Park in front of you. We guide you onto a path that runs parallel to Purdy Place, but we expect that in time you'll be able to ride into the park and along the water around to Prince's Bay. Keep your eye out as this detour could be pretty excellent.

Either way, the ride takes you out to the edge of the peninsula and the mouth of the bay. If you stop for a moment and scan the distant shore, you should see the John Cardinal O'Connor Lighthouse. Formerly the Prince's Bay lighthouse, the beacon looks out over the bay.

At this point, you're more than halfway done. Before saddling up, look north. You'll see the Princess Bay Boatmen's Association and the Lemon Creek

Boatmen's Association marinas. They line Lemon Creek, and they wind around saltwater marshes, which provide an unmatched filtration system as well as protection from erosion. They were under threat at one time, but people came to their senses and let them be. To give you a sense of how far in they go, the marshes reach the SIR tracks.

There are now basically two more roads on the ride. Easy breezy, fairly straight lines with little traffic. Our preference would be to first, go for another loop, then roll through the rest of the streets, as there aren't many, and maybe moving on to another ride before calling it a day.

Staten Island

Ride Log

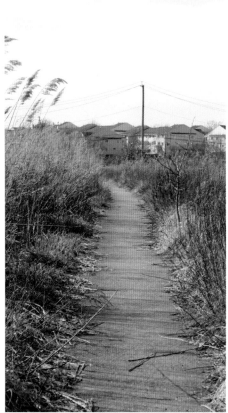

Riding through reeds reminds that the city isn't all that urban.

0.0 Start at the corner of Hylan Blvd and Holten Ave. Have the park on your left as you head toward the water.

0.5 Turn right onto Purdy Pl and then make an immediate left onto a bike path.

0.7 Bike path ends. Turn left onto Seguine Ave.

0.8 Enter Lemon Creek Park by Johnston Terrace. Turn right then left to get onto path. Follow path in a clockwise direction.

1.2 Path ends. Leave park and turn left on Seguine Ave.

1.5 Turn right on Keating St.

1.7 Turn left on Holten Ave.

1.8 Finish at start, the intersection of Hylan and Holten.

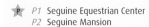

P1 Seguine Equestrian Center
P2 Seguine Mansion

Lemon Creek Ride

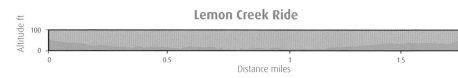

Altitude ft

100

0

0   0.5   1   1.5   1.8

Distance miles

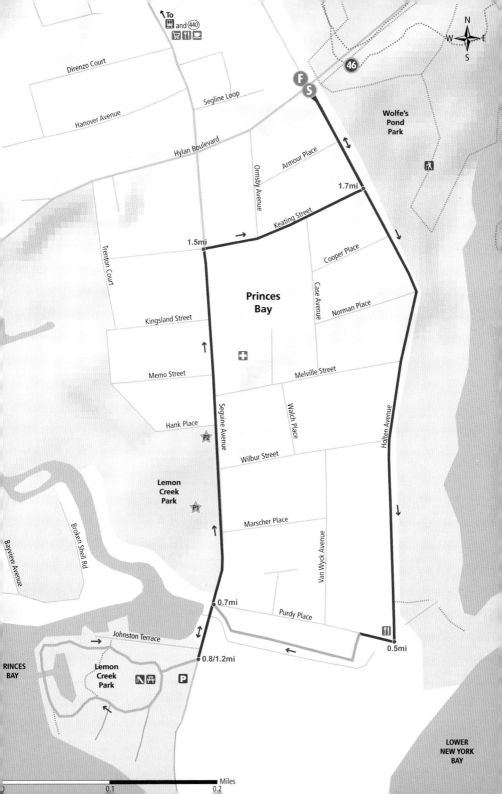

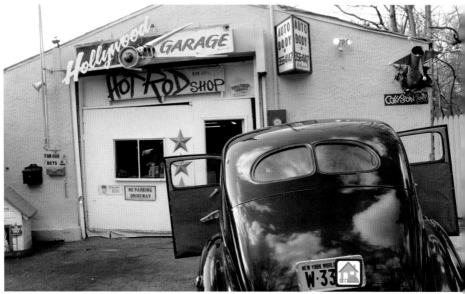

Vintage cars can be observed behind the forest.

At a Glance

Distance 3.8 miles   **Elevation Gain** 196'

Terrain

Flattish. One hill up to the lighthouse on the bluffs, otherwise, you have some rises during the ride.

Traffic

Light. Over half the ride is on parkland and dedicated bike lanes. The Mount Loretto Unique Area is often closed to car traffic, as is Kenny Road. Amboy Road is narrow and can be busy at times.

How to Get There

The ride uses Hylan Avenue, but thankfully, Hylan is pretty empty by the time it gets out here. You can also take the Staten Island Railway (SIR) to the Pleasant Plains station and ride pretty quickly to the start.

Food and Drink

Not much to find, though what's available is just beyond the northern edge of the ride, mostly situated around the train station.

Side Trip

Mount Loretto Unique Area. Check out the area south of Hylan. There are a number of footpaths as well as three roads. Of note are the bluffs above the Raritan Bay, the only red clay bluffs in the city.

Where to Bike Rating

Parts of Mount Loretto have auto-free hours. See Traffic above.

About...

Mount Loretto Unique Area, as it is officially known, is a New York State Park. But it's a new one, having been purchased from the mission of the Immaculate Virgin in 1999. The Mission ran the largest orphanage in New York State, serving both boys and girls, and was a working farm as well as a school. Times have changed and the state purchased the land to keep it out of the hands of developers.

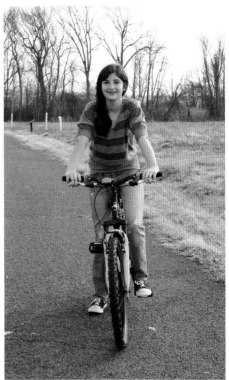

Kayla out for an afternoon spin.

While there is a working farm in Queens, it's surrounded by highways and busy roads. This loop gives you a sense of what a more agrarian Staten Island might have looked like, from an era before the bridges attached this little island to the New York archipelago and Jersey.

Mount Loretto takes you on a tour of the Pleasant Plains section of Staten Island, an area once dominated by the orphanage for which this ride is named. The land both north and south of Hylan between Sharrot and Cunningham was once orphanage property. The kids living on the grounds allegedly grew their own food, milked their own cattle, collected their own eggs, and even made their own clothes. Whether or not this was a good thing, we'll let others decide, but when the grounds, some 400 acres in total, were bought in 1871, kids as young as six years old were living on the streets of New York City. The mission owned a ten-story building in Greenwich Village before they bought and built up this space.

Now that the grounds are in state hands, the area can possibly return to what it looked like before it was farmed. The 194-acre tract south of Hylan is a combination of grasslands, wetlands (both freshwater and tidal), and coastal shoreline. All are popular with animals, and both birdwatchers and butterfly fans that

spend time in Mount Loretto will find plenty to tell their friends about. It could be a quirk of geography, but the shoreline, which is a mile long, is supposedly the last undeveloped shoreline in the state.

When riding around the area, you'll find that the Unique Area seems to be a transplant from a much more rural community. Flanders came to mind for us, thanks to the church building that stands on the grounds north of Hylan.

But even with the large public park, the reality of suburbia intrudes, but only after taking in the Unique Area and turning onto Amboy Road. Even though Amboy feels narrow and crowded, there are few houses and almost no cross streets until you make the turn off it and start heading back to the start. In all, there is very little of this ride where public parkland isn't on one or both sides of the road you're pedaling down. And that makes the riding good.

Staten Island

Ride Log

0.0 Start at the circle inside the parking lot by the intersection of Sharott Ave and Hylan Blvd. Head out to Hylan and turn left.

0.5 Turn left on Kenny Rd. This brings you inside the park.

0.8 Turn left on Monsignor Rd. Make U-turn.

1.4 Turn right on Kenny.

1.7 Cross Hylan.

1.9 Turn left. Almost immediately, you'll be at a T-intersection. Turn right.

 P1 Mount Loretto Unique Area
P2 John Cardinal O'Connor Lighthouse

2.0 Turn left at T-intersection.

2.1 Turn right at T-intersection.

2.5 End of park. Turn right on Amboy Rd.

3.0 Bear right on Bedell St.

3.1 Turn right on Sharrott Ave.

3.8 Cross Hyland Blvd and finish at the start.

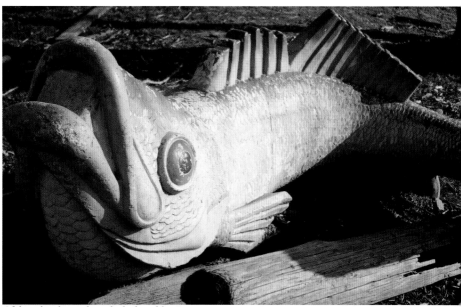

A fish ready to be caught marks the foot of the pier.

Mount Loretto Loop

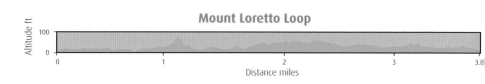

Altitude ft

Distance miles

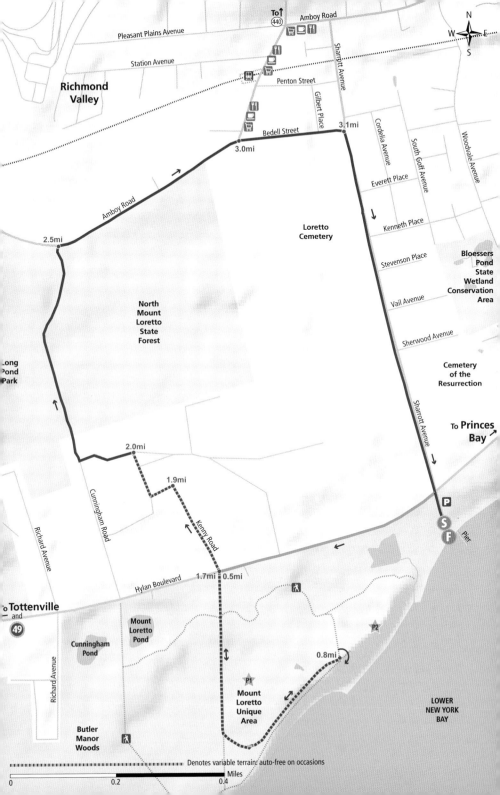

Tottenville Loop

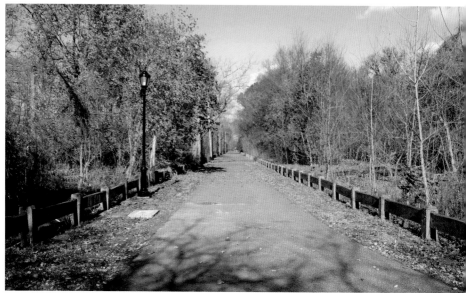

Conference House Park offers quiet paths for walking and riding.

At a Glance

Distance 5.0 miles   **Elevation Gain** 269′

Terrain

Flat. With mostly good, if narrow, roads.

Traffic

Light. This is the southern tip of Staten Island and not many people live here and no one is passing through. There's a short park section toward the end, but the open roads are usually pretty quiet.

How to Get There

Just keep going south. You can follow the Atlantic side on Hylan Boulevard or Arthur Kill Road or take the Staten Island Railroad to the Tottenville Terminal.

Food and Drink

Town Deli and Pizza is a comfortable stop shortly after the start, or you can choose from any number of food options by the Page Avenue and Amboy Road intersection.

Side Trip

Conference House is an overlooked bit of Revolutionary War History. It was the site of the Staten Island Peace Conference, which took place here in 1776. The house is the only pre-Revolutionary manor house surviving in the city.

Where to Bike Rating

About...

Tottenville, once known as Bentley Manor, is the southernmost community in New York State and Conference House, the southernmost point. There's even a South Pole. If you roam around the streets, you'll find a number of Victorian homes, reflective of the fact that this area was settled far earlier than the rest of southern Staten Island.

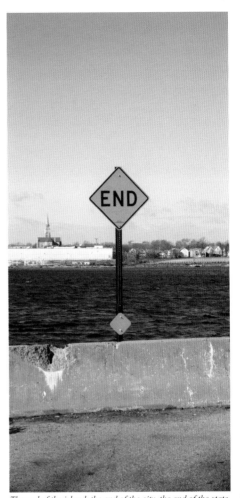

The end of the island, the end of the city, the end of the state, with the Arthur Kill and New Jersey beyond.

Because it's the far end of a small island, Tottenville is almost by definition sleepy. While the Outerbridge Crossing is only a little north of the northern edge of the ride, most of that traffic is heading north and east, not south. And this makes it one of the best places to ride on the island. Between the quiet streets and home density, there's a sense that just about every day is a holiday weekend, as if much of the population is sleeping in, on vacation, or watching television.

We assumed when we first got out of the train terminal that this feeling would quickly go away. It didn't. The western shore of Tottenville used to be fairly industrial, heavy with shipbuilding. Those days seem long gone, and marinas have taken up the space. Industry is across the Arthur Kill in New Jersey and this portion of the eastern edge of the Garden State is littered with refineries.

Meanwhile, Arthur Kill Road, the street you head out on seems to get a tiny bit busier on the way to Richmond Valley Road. But then traffic drops off, briefly picks up on Page Avenue, Amboy Road seems to also have a little more car density, then drops off again. Leaving the road to us pretty much for the rest of the loop.

The best part of the ride was the section through Conference House Park. There's a bridge over a small creek. Stopping there for a few minutes, sitting silently, nobody else in sight, and without the hum of a busy nearby street, nature seemed to come alive, with ducks paddling through and plenty of calls in the air.

Conference House Park is a fine place to stop. Not only is the titular house there, but there are two 19th century homes as well. When investigating old digs gets tired, you can stop and admire the Arthur Kill, the Raritan Bay, and New Jersey Coast by sitting in the Russell Pavilion, located right on the beach at the very end of Hylan Boulevard.

Staten Island

Ride Log

0.0 Start at the Tottenville SIR terminal at the end of Bentley St. Head away from the water. Take the first left on Arthur Kill Rd.

0.2 Turn right onto Main St, then immediately turn left to get back on Arthur Kill.

0.8 It might look like a fork in the road. Bear left to stay straight on Arthur Kill. Turn right on Richmond Valley Rd. Turn right on Page Ave.

2.3 Turn right on Hylan Blvd.

2.8 Turn left on Sprague Ave.

3.1 Turn right on Surf Ave.

3.2 Turn right on Loretto St, then immediate left on Billop Ave.

3.6 Entering Conference House Park.

3.8 Turn right on Surf Ave.

4.0 Bear left on Satterlee St.

4.2 Exit park at Hylan.

4.6 Turn left on Amboy Rd followed by an immediate right on Hopping Ave.

4.9 Turn left on Bentley.

5.0 Finish at the start, the Tottenville SIR terminal.

 P1 Conference House
P2 Russell Pavilion
P3 Ward House
P4 Rutan-Beckett House
P5 Biddle House

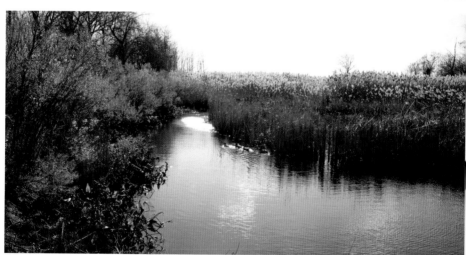

Salt water marshes help make the city a place rich in biodiversity.

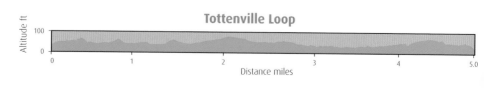

Tottenville Loop

Altitude ft

Distance miles

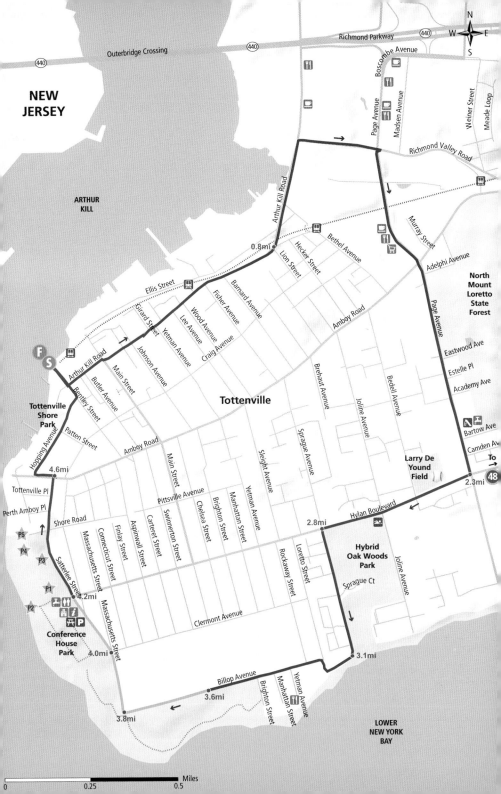

Northern New Jersey

New Jersey comes in for lots of derision from New Yorkers. For city cyclists, it's the sixth borough, thanks to much more hospitable riding environments than those in southern Westchester. Ambitious riders see the George Washington Bridge as the gateway for all things north, as the road riding can be most excellent, with empty roads and plenty of hills.

One of the reasons I like riding in Jersey is that it's easy to add a little to a ride to make it a little longer if I'm feeling good or have more time. Likewise, it's easy to subtract a little if I'm running late. Another is that it's easy to put together flat rides if I'm feeling tired or hilly rides if I'm feeling good. The valleys generally seem to run parallel to the Hudson River, in a nearly north-south axis, while the hills often come when you're riding east-west.

The holy grail for developing fitness cyclists is to pedal-through Bergen County to Nyack, N.Y., grab sustenance at a café, and ride home. We've detailed that ride, though it's on a route that is much more than the out-and-back 9W plan most cyclists imbibe. An intermediate step to Nyack is riding River Road, at the southern tip of the Palisades Interstate Park System, it is hilly and virtually car-free, so you've got a great escape just across the bridge. Northern New Jersey is rather hilly, lots of short, steep rises, and plenty of hills that take five minutes to climb. well.

If you're averse to hills, or long distances, or are looking for easy, scenic places to ride that aren't in the five boroughs, we've got that, too, running along the west bank of the Hudson from Jersey City north to almost the George Washington Bridge.

Greenways aren't just popular in New York City; Jersey is getting in on the act as well. There are plans for multi-use paths to start in Bayonne, just across the bridge from Staten Island and run up both the west side of the city along the Newark Bay to the Hackensack River and on the south side along Kill Van Kull to join up with Liberty State Park. There will also eventually be a bike path from the George Washington Bridge south to Weehawken, further expanding car-free road cycling options.

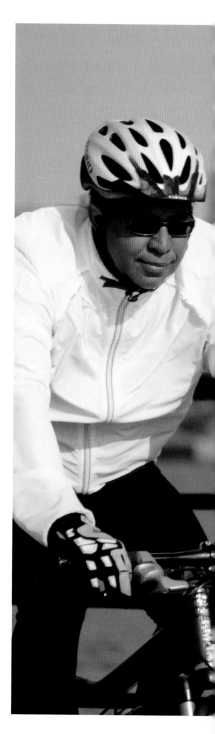

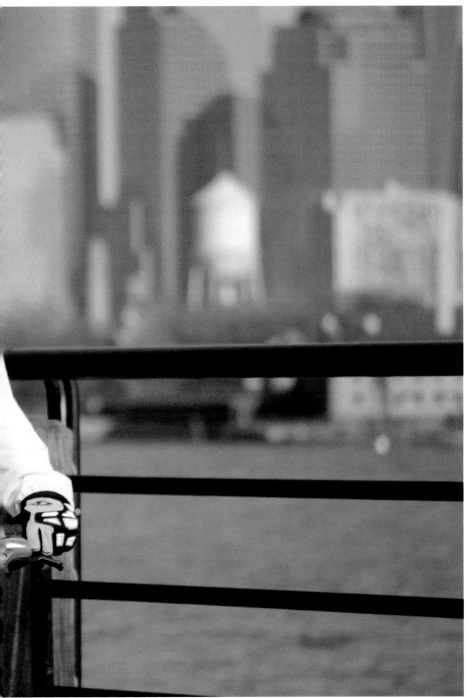

Photo Matt Wittmer

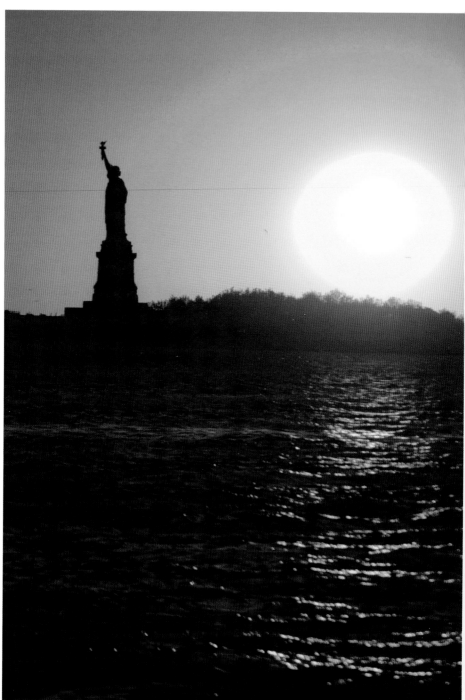

Photo Matt Wittmer

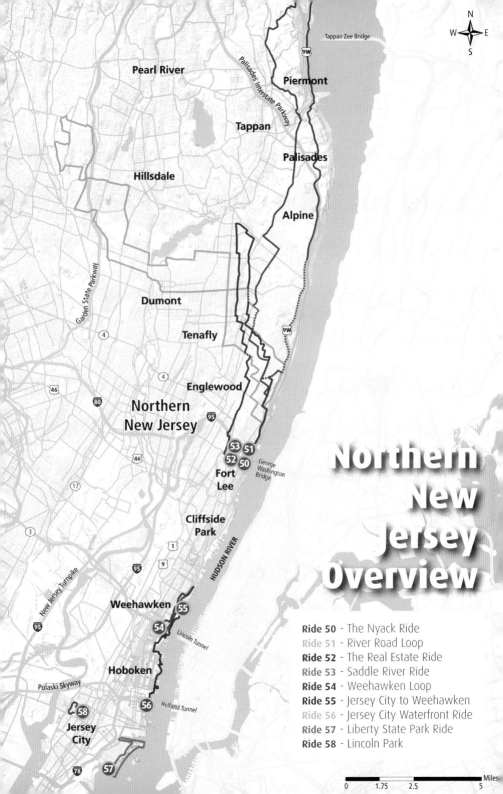

N
W   E
S

Tappan Zee Bridge

Pearl River

Piermont

Palisades Interstate Parkway

Tappan

Palisades

Hillsdale

Alpine

9W

Garden State Parkway

Dumont

Tenafly

9W

4

Englewood

Northern
New Jersey

80

95

53 51

52 50

46

Fort
Lee

George
Washington
Bridge

17

Cliffside
Park

1

9

3

HUDSON RIVER

95

Northern New Jersey Overview

New Jersey Turnpike

Weehawken

55

54

Lincoln Tunnel

95

Hoboken

Pulaski Skyway

56

Holland Tunnel

58

Jersey
City

57

78

Miles
0   1.75   2.5   5

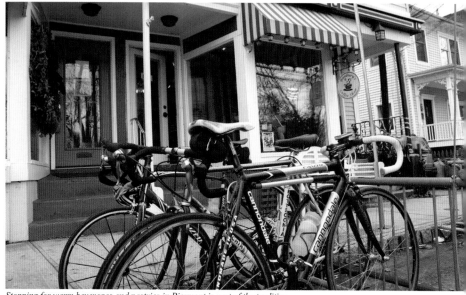

Stopping for warm beverages and pastries in Piermont is part of the tradition.

At a Glance

Distance 42.6 miles   **Elevation Gain** 2248′

Terrain

Very hilly with a variety of road surfaces. As with any ride in N.J., expect the road surfaces to range from pristine to in need of replacement. Most are decent, with some cracks and patches..

Traffic

Moderate to light.

How to Get There

The ride starts and finishes at the Jersey side terminus of the George Washington Bridge Bike Path. The path starts just west of the intersection of Haven Avenue and West 178th Street in Manhattan. Most take 177th and then make a right onto Haven to get there. The 1 and A trains stop right by the bridge. You can also easily take the West Side Greenway Bicycle Path to either 158th or 181st streets and then ride to the bridge from there.

Food and Drink

At the northern end of the ride, you pass through Nyack and Piermont. Popular attractions for cyclists are the Runcible Spoon Bakery in Nyack and the Piermont Community Market and Bunbury's Coffee Shop in Piermont. All three have bike racks on the street directly out the front.

Side Trip

Forty-three miles and great coffee shops and you need a side trip? If visual art is your thing, stop by the Hopper House in Nyack: **www.hopperhouse.org**. You can also get an unbelievable view of the Hudson River if you ride to the end of the pier in Piermont.

Links to

Where to Bike Rating

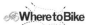

About...

For many New Yorkers, the journey to becoming a cyclist is complete when they ride to Nyack, stop for a snack, and ride home. At 43 miles plus whatever it takes to get to the George Washington Bridge, the ride is not insignificant, and you get a bit of everything, fast descents, stiff climbs, super vistas, and a sense of going somewhere. Much of the ride is on State Bike Route 9, which, while it doesn't afford a special bike lane, does give you decent signage.

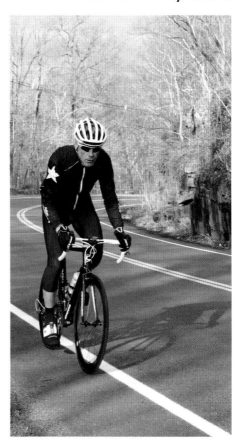

Climbing stateline hill on 9W can present a challenge.

There's something special about riding to and from Nyack. Maybe it's that for most New Yorkers it means you've ridden at least half a century, 50 miles, and that feels significant. Maybe it's that Nyack is a quaint town with a shabby-chic vibe popular throughout the Hudson Valley. Maybe it's that the to and from of the ride does a great job of removing you from the city as the housing gets less and less dense, feeling like you're far, far removed from everything and then you go over a hill and you're dropped into Nyack. On the way back, you ride through another sleepy town and then have 10 miles of nothing but woods on both sides of the road before you pop out of the country into Tenafly.

Another good thing about the ride is that on both the out and the back, you spend many miles riding with very few intersections and not many traffic lights; the uninterrupted quality makes the riding feel easier.

There's also the preparation factor. While this ride is a goal in and of itself, and the point of riding can be just to ride more, there are plenty of people who are training for events, be they bike trips or races. This route offers them training for those things.

Finally, there's the ride back over the George Washington Bridge. On a clear day, with most of Manhat-tan Island spectacularly laid out to your right, it's hard not to feel triumphant; that you rode, you conquered, and now you're heading for a victory lap and a well-deserved meal.

Notes about the ride: this route is set up to have distinct out and back sections, though many just ride north on 9W, hit Nyack or Piermont, then ride home on 9W. The initial drop from Englewood Cliffs to Tenafly takes you through quiet suburban neighborhoods where you'll see few cars. It's a bit tricky the first time you do it, but it's easy to remember. On the way back, you are taken off 9W near the end of the road because that's where the traffic is most concentrated. The back roads of Tenafly and Englewood Cliffs only take a few extra minutes to navigate, but are much more peaceful.

Northern New Jersey

Ride Log

0.0 Start out at Jersey end of GW Bridge Bike Path. Turn right onto Hudson Terrace.

2.2 Turn left onto East Palisade Ave. Go through light.

2.3 Turn right onto Floyd St.

2.7 Turn left onto Chestnut St.

2.8 Turn right onto Summit St.

3.0 Turn left onto Lyncrest Rd.

3.4 Turn right onto Woodland St.

4.2 Turn left onto Churchill Rd.

4.9 Turn right onto Leroy St. Then immediately turn left onto Woodland Park Dr.

5.4 Turn right onto Engle St.

6.5 Turn left onto Hudson St.

6.7 Turn right onto County Rd (CR-501).

9.0 Bear left to stay on CR-501.

9.8 Bear right to stay on CR-501. It is now Piermont Rd.

13.4 Cross into New York State. Piermont Rd is now Route 340.

14.3 The route bears left onto Valentine Ave.

14.5 End of Valentine. Turn left onto Orangeburg Rd (Route 340).

14.7 Turn right onto Hickey. Take immediate left onto Kings Hwy.

16.3 Turn right onto Route 303.

16.5 First right. Mountainview Ave. Turn right. Road immediately turns left and becomes Greenbush Rd.

17.9 Greenbush runs into Route 303. You'll be on 303 for 97 feet, then you bear right onto Greenbush.

18.4 Turn right onto Bradley Parkway.

19.1 Bear right to stay on Bradley Hill Rd.

19.5 Bear left to stay on Bradley Hill.

19.7 Turn left onto South Highland.

19.9 Turn left to stay on South Highland.

20.2 Cross the light and ride onto 9W North.

20.2 Turn right onto High Ave.

20.6 Turn left onto South Midland Ave.

21.7 Stay straight at fork in road.

22.2 Turn right at end of Midland onto Larchdale Ave.

22.5 Turn right onto North Broadway.

24.3 Nyack Bicycle Outfitters is on right.

24.31 Runcible Spoon Bakery is on left.

24.4 Turn left onto Main St.

24.5 Turn right onto Piermont Ave.

25.6 Cross under Tappan Zee Bridge.

28.0 Entering downtown Piermont. Piermont Bicycle Connection is off to your left. Ahead are eateries on both your right and left including Piermont Community Market.

28.1 Bunbury's Coffee Shop is on right.

28.1 Piermont Ave becomes Ferdon Ave.

28.5 Turn left onto Rockland Rd.

29.1 Turn left onto Route 9W South.

30.0 Palisades Market is on your left.

30.4 Start climbing up to the state line.

31.1 State line. Cross back into New Jersey.

31.4 Start climbing again.

34.5 On left is entrance to the Palisades Park; you're joining up with the River Rd Loop also detailed here.

38.7 Turn right onto Sage Rd.

38.9 Turn left onto Johnson Ave.

39.2 Turn left onto Van Wagoner Dr.

39.3 Turn right onto Floyd St.

40.3 Turn left onto East Palisade Ave.

40.6 Turn right onto Hudson Terrace.

42.6 Finish at George Washington Bridge bike path.

The Nyack Ride

Please note: the profile for Ride 50 is depicted in 200ft vertical increments due to unusually high elevation.

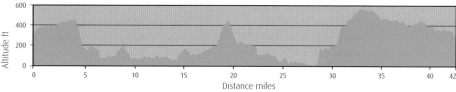

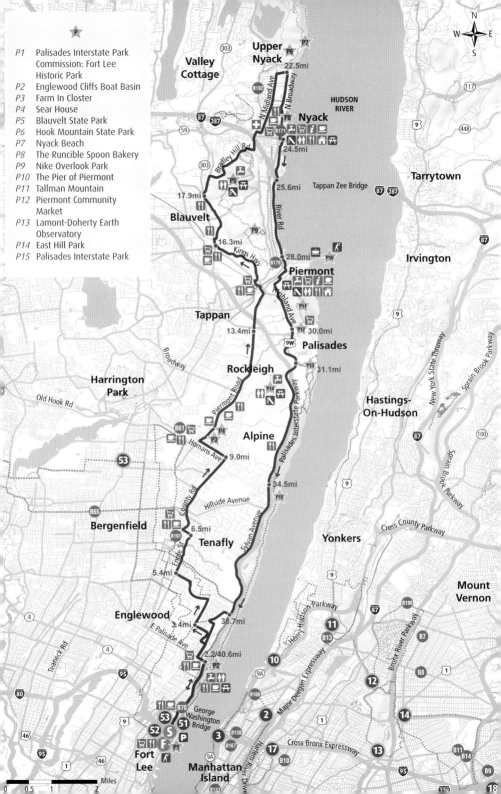

P1   Palisades Interstate Park
     Commission: Fort Lee
     Historic Park
P2   Englewood Cliffs Boat Basin
P3   Farm In Closter
P4   Sear House
P5   Blauvelt State Park
P6   Hook Mountain State Park
P7   Nyack Beach
P8   The Runcible Spoon Bakery
P9   Nike Overlook Park
P10 The Pier of Piermont
P11 Tallman Mountain
P12 Piermont Community
     Market
P13 Lamont-Doherty Earth
     Observatory
P14 East Hill Park
P15 Palisades Interstate Park

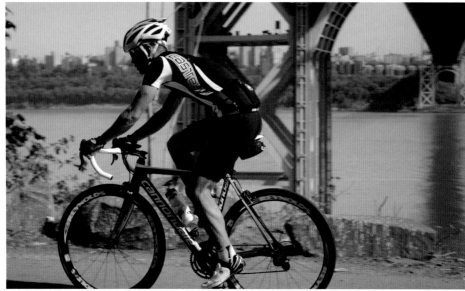

Henry Hudson Drive dives downhill beneath the George Washington Bridge.

Photo Matt Wittmer

At a Glance

Distance 16.6 miles   **Elevation Gain** 1325'

Terrain

Very hilly with a variety of road surfaces. River Road can have boulders and branches and lots of divots.

Traffic

Light to none for most of the first half of the ride. Light to moderate, with about a mile somewhat busy on the way back.

How to Get There

The ride starts and finishes at the Jersey side terminus of the George Washington Bridge Bike Path. The path starts just west of the intersection of Haven Avenue and West 178th Street in Manhattan. The 1 and A trains stop right by the bridge.

Food and Drink

This ride almost entirely bypasses commercial establishments. There are vending machines by the bath-rooms in Palisades Park. There's a café that's open in the spring and summer at the Englewood boat basin. And the Strictly Bicycles shop on the route in Fort Lee has the standard cyclist fare as well as a coffee bar.

Side Trip

The Kearney House, located at the far end of the Alpine Boat Basin, is a home from the 18th century, and a pleasant little diversion from riding as well as an excellent regional history lesson. Open May through October on weekend afternoons.

Links to

Where to Bike Rating

Henry Hudson Drive has extensive auto-free hours.

About...

When city cyclists go "over the bridge," Henry Hudson Drive (aka River Road) is probably the first place they ride. They go for good reason. The road is 8.4 miles long and chances are you'll see more bicycles than cars, and even then, you'll see only a few cyclists. Fitness types love the mile-long hill at the northern end of the drive. And 9W, the road you'll be riding on most of the way back has a huge, decently-paved shoulder.

While this ride is definitely not flat, River Road is such a pleasant place to ride that most people we know will go out here even when they're feeling beat. The views are awesome, whether it's seeing the bridge shooting out of the ground and overhead; looking across at the settlements known as Upper Manhattan, The Bronx, and Yonkers across the majestic Hudson River; checking out the waterfalls en route; or watching hawks cruise above.

One cool, scary feature of riding along River Road is the park you're riding in. You're pretty much riding with a steep rock wall to one side and a steep drop-off to the river on the other. This terrain seems to have prevented commercial development, but that's not the whole story. Once privately held, the land was residential—divided into little villages—and was used for quarrying and logging. This history, combined with the area's geology, might have made it more prone to the occasional landslide.Not frequent enough that you should be worried about getting caught in one, but enough that they do lead to occasional road closures. Personally, I like that nature overwhelms a place so close to New York City, where man has totally dominated for years.

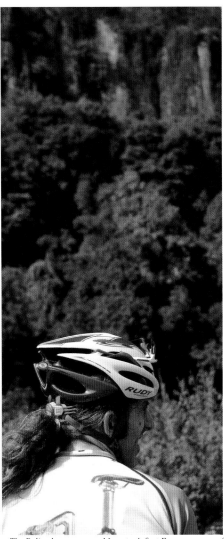

The Palisades appear on Mercator's first European map of the New World. Photo Matt Wittmer

9W, the road you'll be taking back, is the closest thing to a country bicycle highway in the area. With generous shoulders and few intersections, it's very easy to ride here with minimal concern of or interference from car traffic. Come out to 9W on a summer weekend morning and you could see hundreds of cyclists pass. Many are headed to Nyack or Piermont (we have a ride that goes to both places).

Northern New Jersey

Ride 51 - River Road Loop

Ride Log

0.0 The New Jersey entrance to the George Washington Bridge Bike Path. Turn left onto the sidewalk. It's actually less. You'll ride through an intersection and a bike path will appear. Ride onto the path.

0.5 Bike path ends. Make left onto Henry Hudson Drive into Palisades Interstate Park. Gate will be closed in the winter. You can lift your bike over the gate and continue riding.

1.4 Go around circle. If you take the road on the right, you'll drop down to the Ross Dock picnic area.

2.9 Go around circle and start heading uphill. On your right is the Snack Shack, open Tuesday through Sunday in the summer. If you go straight, you'll be at the Englewood Boat Dock picnic area.

3.2 Go straight down the hill. The gate is sometimes closed in the winter. While the road to your left looks inviting, it is off-limits to cyclists.

7.7 Go around the circle and start heading uphill. To the right is the Alpine Boat Basin, home of Kearney House. The climb is about a mile long and takes you up the Palisades.

8.8 Henry Hudson Dr T's into Route 9W. Turn right, and you get on Bike Route 9, which will eventually take you to Montreal. Turn left, and you stay on this loop and start to head back to the bridge.

14.5 Make a left at the light off of 9W onto East Palisades Ave. On your left is the Royal Cliffs Diner.

14.5 Right onto Hudson Terrace. If you go straight, you'll encounter that beautiful road verboten to cyclists.

16.6 Back at the entrance to the George Washington Bridge bike path.

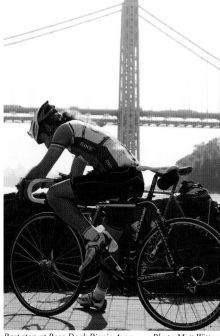

Rest stop at Ross Dock Picnic Area.   *Photo Matt Wittmer*

P1 Palisades Interstate Park Commission: Fort Lee Historic Park
P2 Ross Dock Picnic Area
P3 Englewood Cliffs Boat Basin
P4 Grassy Hangout on water's edge
P5 Alpine Boat Basin
P6 Kearney House
P7 Palisades Interstate Park
P8 Flatrock Nature Center

River Road Loop

Please note: the profile for Ride 51 is depicted in 200ft vertical increments due to unusually high elevation.

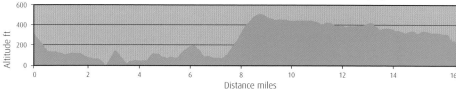

Altitude ft

Distance miles

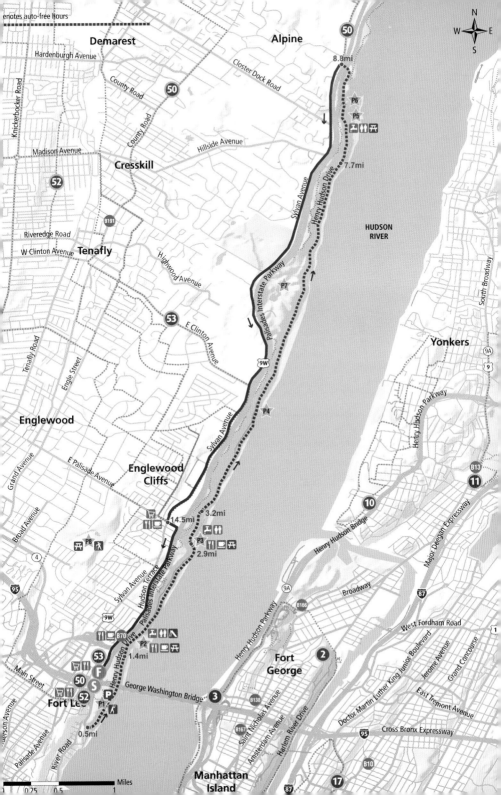

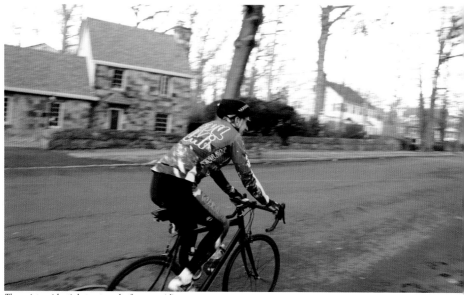

The quiet residential streets make for easy riding.

At a Glance

Distance 20.9 miles   **Elevation Gain** 1134′

Terrain

Hilly with a variety of road surfaces.

Traffic

Very light to moderate.

How to Get There

The ride starts and finishes at the Jersey side terminus of the George Washington Bridge Bike Path. The path starts just west of the intersection of Haven Avenue and West 178th Street in Manhattan. The 1 and A trains stop right by the bridge.

Food and Drink

Café Lamaison, 140 Main Street, Fort Lee, is a stop among cyclists, though on this route it's more at the start than at the finish. Café Angelique, 1 Piermont Road, Tenafly is much closer to the end of the ride. Both have ample outdoor seating.

Side Trip

Historic Fort Lee is just south of the George Washington Bridge. Turn left at the first light you encounter after turning left onto Hudson Terrace. See the view that soldiers had of the river and the easy lines to cannonball passing ships.

Links to

Where to Bike Rating

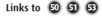
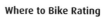

About...

The main difficulty of this ride is staying on course. There are lots of turns, but the reason for all the turning is to link together as many quiet suburban residential streets as possible. While there is significant climbing, just about all of it comes at the end, and most of the climbing is on quiet streets, so you can paperboy it if you need to and nobody will notice or care.

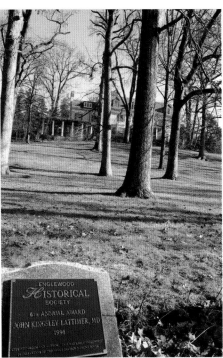

There are houses and there are houses.

Years ago, a friend and I, when we were interested in going extra slow, used to take on what he termed "real estate rides". Essentially, we'd ride around fancy suburban neighborhoods, trying to find the quietest, leafiest streets with the biggest houses. We found that high median home value areas generally had curvy streets that didn't go anywhere. There was no reason for people to drive through the neighborhoods as people who weren't either going home or leaving home would not be able to go through quickly on said roads.

This ride wends and winds through several towns looking for similar roads. Many of these streets do go somewhere, but they aren't the kind of going somewhere streets that people wanting to drive fast from Point A to Point B are going to want to traverse.

I think you'll find that the highest home prices on this route are in Englewood, Englewood Cliffs, and Tenafly, not that the other neighborhoods are any less charming.

Near the end, when you start climbing up from Tenafly, the first road, East Clinton Avenue, is the hardest and one of the busier streets of this ride. Once you make a right and quick left onto Stonehurst, the streets will be nearly abandoned for the rest of your climbing.

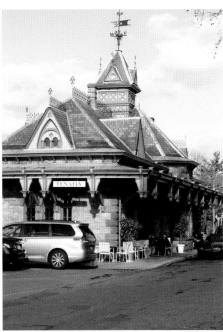

Tenafly's restored train station has a café inside.

Ride 52 - The Real Estate Ride

Ride Log

0.0 Start at the George Washington Bridge bike path. Make a left onto Hudson Terrace.

0.1 Not even. Turn right onto Bruce Reynolds Bvld.

0.1 Turn left onto Central Rd.

0.3 Turn right onto Main St. Go through downtown Fort Lee. Turn right onto Jones Rd.

1.7 Tricky downhill left hand turn.

1.8 Turn right onto Ridgeland Terrace.

2.0 Turn right onto Jones Rd.

4.0 Cross Palisades Ave. Jones turns to Brayton St.

4.1 Turn left onto Chestnut St.

4.3 Turn right onto Lydecker St.

4.6 Bear left onto Davison Pl.

4.8 Bear right onto Whitewood Rd.

5.3 Turn right onto Engle St.

5.6 Turn left onto Elm St.

5.8 Turn right onto Dean Dr.

6.1 Turn left onto Westervelt Ave.

6.3 Turn right onto George St.

6.5 Turn left onto West Clinton Ave.

6.7 Turn right onto Foster Rd.

6.9 Roosevelt Commons is in front of you. Bathrooms. Turn left onto Tenafly Ave.

7.0 Turn right onto Jefferson Ave.

8.4 Cross Grant Ave. Jefferson turns into Merrifield Way.

8.6 Turn left onto Brookside Ave.

9.1 Brookside T's onto Hardenburgh Ave. Turn left.

9.1 Turn right onto Palisade Blvd.

9.3 Turn left onto Madison Ave.

9.4 Turn right onto Columbus Rd.

10.4 Turn right onto High St.

10.9 Turn right onto Durie Ave.

11.0 Turn left onto Demarest Ave.

11.3 Turn right onto County Rd.

12.0 Merge onto Piermont Rd.

12.7 Bear right to remain on Piermont Rd.

14.5 Turn left onto Central Ave.

14.6 Turn right onto County Rd.

15.0 Turn left onto Clinton Ave. Climb hill to light.

15.3 Turn right onto Engle St.

15.3 Turn left onto Stonehurst Dr. You're going to star some stair-step climbing through Tenafly up to Engle-wood Cliffs.

15.9 Turn left onto Leroy St.

16.2 Turn right onto Devon Rd.

16.4 Turn left onto York Pl.

16.7 Turn right onto Oxford Dr.

16.9 Turn left onto Buckingham Rd.

17.1 Turn right onto Woodland St. The climbing is done.

17.9 Turn left onto Johnson Ave.

18.2 Turn right onto Van Wagoner Dr.

18.4 Turn right onto Floyd St.

19.4 Turn left onto East Palisades Ave.

19.5 Pass Royal Cliffs Diner.

19.7 Turn right onto Hudson Terrace.

20.2 Strictly Bicycles shop on right.

20.9 End of ride.

The Real Estate Ride

Please note: the profile for Ride 52 is depicted in 200ft vertical increments due to unusually high elevation.

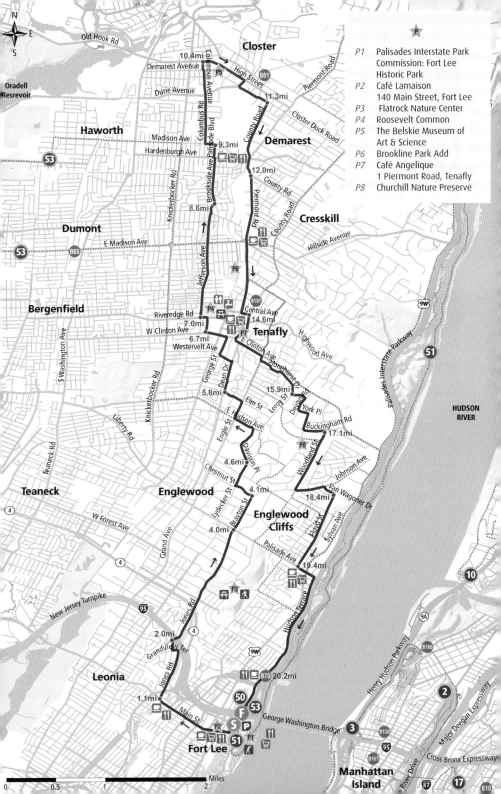

Closter

Demarest

Cresskill

Tenafly

Haworth

Dumont

Bergenfield

Teaneck

Englewood

Englewood Cliffs

Leonia

Fort Lee

Oradell Resrevoir

HUDSON RIVER

Manhattan Island

Old Hook Rd

High Street

Demarest Avenue
10.4mi

Durie Avenue

Columbus Rd

Madison Ave
9.3mi
Hardenburgh Ave

11.3mi

Piermont Road

Closter Dock Road

County Road

Palisade Ave

Brookside Ave

12.0mi
County Rd

Hillside Avenue

E Madison Ave

8.6mi

Jefferson Ave

Piermont Rd

County Road

Central Ave
14.6mi

Knickerbocker Rd

P6

P4

Riveredge Rd

W Clinton Ave
7.0mi
6.7mi
Westervelt Ave

P7

E Clinton Ave

Highwood Ave

Stonehurst Dr

S Washington Ave

George St

Dean Dr

15.9mi
Leroy St

York Pl

Devon St

Buckingham Rd
17.1mi

Elm St

5.8mi

E Hudson Ave

Davison Pl

P8

Woodland St

Johnson Ave
18.4mi

Van Wagoner Dr

Engle St

Chestnut St
4.6mi

Liberty Rd

4.1mi

Lydecker St

Braxton St

Englewood Cliffs

Floyd St

Sylvan Ave

Knickerbocker Rd

W Forest Ave

4.0mi

Grand Ave

Palisade Ave

19.4mi

P3

Jones Rd

New Jersey Turnpike

Palisades Interstate Parkway

2.0mi
Grandview Ter

9W

Hudson Terrace

Jones Rd

Main St

1.1mi

20.2mi

P2

George Washington Bridge

P1

Henry Hudson Parkway

River Drive

Major Deegan Expressway

Cross Bronx Expressway

Miles
0   0.5   1   2

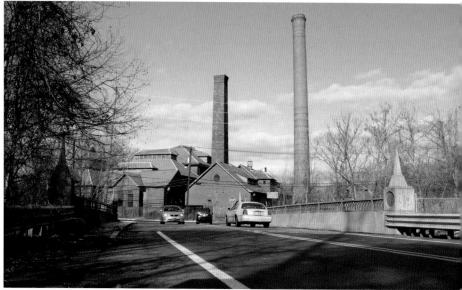

The past can loom over the present even in up to date suburban New Jersey.

At a Glance

Distance 42.7 miles   **Elevation Gain** 2999′

Terrain

Very hilly. The roads are mostly narrow and road conditions vary widely. There always seems to be some new pavement and some roads in need of patching or resurfacing.

Traffic

Moderate to light.

How to Get There

The ride starts and finishes at the Jersey side terminus of the George Washington Bridge Bike Path. The path starts just west of the intersection of Haven Avenue and West 178th Street in Manhattan. The 1 and A trains stop right by the bridge.

Food and Drink

This ride passes through several towns, and there are nice little cafés just off route in Englewood, Tenafly,

Hohokus, Westwood, Cresskill, and Dumont, but the easiest thing to do is finish the ride and head over to Main Street in Fort Lee or pick up a hot beverage at Strictly Bicycles.

Side Trip

This is the kind of ride where we wouldn't stop, but if you're looking for a break, the Arts Center of Northern New Jersey is between both the out and back segments in New Milford. Very much a people's art space, with events and a gallery space largely highlighting local work.

Links to

Where to Bike Rating

About...

When this area was carved up aeons ago, glaciers headed south, scraping out the Hudson River and creating lots of little river valleys that run roughly parallel to the Hudson. As a result, most of the flat roads around this area of northern N.J. run roughly north-south and the ridges are encountered when you go east-west. This ride goes northwest, tacking from north to west in short segments. When it comes back, it goes southeast, tacking back and forth as well.

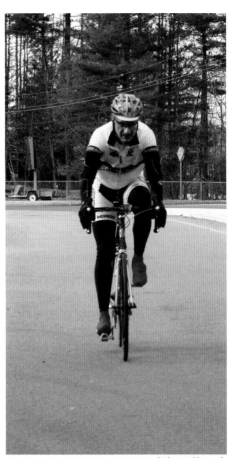

Riding to Haworth.

This is, in our opinion, the hardest ride in the book. Not only is it strenuous at over 2800 feet of climbing, but it can be confusing, with lots of turns. We think it's worth the effort to stay on the route and hump all the hills.

The 9W corridor is overused by area cyclists. It's easy, straightforward, has a reward of nice cafés in both Piermont and Nyack, and you can hit longer hills if you roam around Clausland mountain. But it gets boring and the longer hills favor one kind of riding.

We think the twists and turns, the passing through of small towns and over train tracks to have their own rewards. It shows that you're riding through places and not just taking a wooded corridor. Yes it means lights and some stops, but get on a good rhythm and a decent day and you'll make the lights.

The big benefit is the hills. There are countless short, leg-breaking rises. Several of them have grades topping around 14 percent. New Jersey can be pretty hilly and if you want to build strength or just get better at going uphill, giving yourself a steady diet can be a great way to improve.

The funny thing about the hills here is that most of the challenges are going up. There aren't many decents where you'll pick up considerable speed. The one long, fast descent is the drop on Clinton Avenue off of 9W at the start. If you're the daredevil type, sprint over the top and you'll pick up speed fast. Everyone else should move out in the road once their speed picks up to 30mph.

A secret of this ride is you can cut out several of the hills or even cut the ride short very easily. If you take a close look, you'll see the route loops back on itself several times and the return part of the trip is very close to the out part. Even with the final segment through Englewood, you're routed up the same ridge on three occasions and then take on a fourth. If you're tired, just choose one and soft-pedal the rest of the way back to the GWB.

Northern New Jersey

Ride 53 - Saddle River Ride

Ride Log

0.0 Start out at Jersey end of GW Bridge Bike Path. Turn right onto Hudson Terrace.

2.2 Turn left onto East Palisade Ave. Go through the light.

2.3 Turn right onto Sylvan Ave.

4.1 Left into E. Clinton Ave.

5.4 Turn right onto Engle St.

6.5 Turn left onto Hudson St.

7.3 Turn left onto Madison Ave.

10.8 Turn left onto New Milford Ave.

11.1 Turn right onto Kinderkamack Rd.

11.4 Turn left onto Ridgewood Ave.

12.8 Turn right onto Pascack Rd.

14.9 Turn left onto E. Glen Ave.

15.7 Turn right onto Van Emburgh Ave.

16.9 Turn left on Wearimus Rd.

17.2 Turn right on Wearimus Rd.

17.6 Turn left on Mill Rd.

18.3 Turn left on Jacquelin Ave.

18.6 Turn right on E. Saddle River Rd.

19.6 Turn right on Old Woods Rd.

20.2 Turn left on Chestnut Ridge Rd.

20.6 Turn left on Oak Rd.

21.4 Turn right on E. Allendale Rd.

21.6 Turn right on Woodcliff Lake Rd.

22.7 Turn right onto Overlook Dr.

24.6 Turn left onto Washington Ave.

26.3 Turn right onto Lafayette Ave.

P1 Palisades Interstate Park Commission: Fort Lee Historic Park
P2 Camp Merritt Memorial Monument
P3 Little Firehouse Theatre
P4 Demarest Farms
P5 Oradell Reservoir
P6 Art Center Of Northern New Jersey
P7 Flatrock Nature Center

28.4 Turn right onto Soldier Hill Rd.

29.4 Turn right onto Kinderkermack Rd.

29.8 Turn left onto Oradell Ave.

30.5 Turn left onto Grant Ave.

31.7 Turn left onto Haworth Dr.

32.0 Turn right onto Haworth Ave.

33.3 Turn right onto Knickerbocker Ave.

36.7 Turn left onto Ivy Ln.

37.9 Turn right onto Elkwood Terrace.

38.0 Turn left onto Lydecker St.

38.2 Turn left onto Speer Ave.

38.5 Turn right onto Highview Rd.

38.8 Bear left onto Thornton Rd.

38.9 Turn left onto Booth Ave.

39.3 Turn right onto N. Woodland St.

39.9 Turn left onto W. Palisades Ave.

40.2 Turn right onto Summit St.

40.5 Turn left onto Charlotte Pl.

41.3 Turn right onto Hudson Terrace.

42.7 Arrive at GWB bike path.

Saddle River Ride

Please note: the profile for Ride 53 is depicted in 200ft vertical increments due to unusually high elevation.

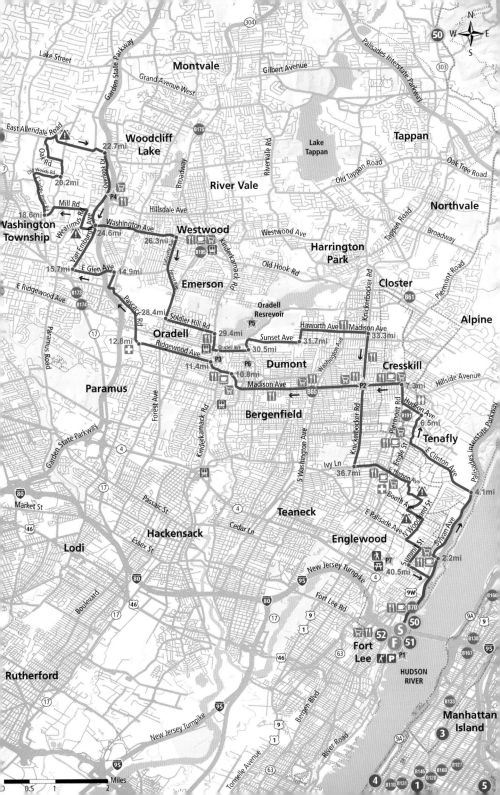

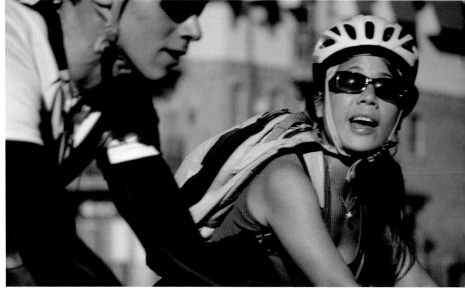

Cruising at a conversational clip.   Photo Matt Wittmer

At a Glance

Distance 4.9 miles   **Elevation Gain** 340′

Terrain

Flat roads with one good-sized hill to climb.

Traffic

From light to busy and everything in between.

How to Get There

The ride starts and finishes in front of the Port Imperial dock of the New York Waterway ferry service. You can take the ferry from Hoboken, Jersey City, or New York City. You can also take N.J. Transit or a PATH train to Hoboken and ride from there. And the Hudson Bergen Light Rail line has its northern terminus at Port Imperial as well.

Food and Drink

The easiest place to pick up sustenance is at the apartment complex just north of the ferry terminal.

Side Trip

The Hudson Riverfront Performing Arts Center (HR-PAC) is an active promoter of free outdoor concerts on the water. Generally, they're on summer evenings at 7pm at Lincoln Harbor Park.

Links to 55

Where to Bike Rating

About...

Weehawken is the site of a duel that changed the course of American history. In 1804, sitting Vice President Aaron Burr dueled former Secretary of the Treasury Alexander Hamilton. Hamilton was fatally wounded; a political grudge match like few others in America. The location of the site is not certain and probably has been both paved over and run through with train tracks. They didn't do history then like they do now.

The area beneath the Palisades is both the opening part of the ride and the most likely locale for the duel. The name Weehawken itself seems to be an Algonquin term that refers to the Palisades. The ride heads south along the Palisades, with the start of the light rail line on your right and parks and the Hudson on your left before an opening at what is just about the southern end of the stone cliffs, allows you to turn right and start climbing up to get to the top of the ridge.

As you begin the climb, you'll be riding alongside the entry to the Lincoln Tunnel. You won't have lots of cars to deal with as you're headed away from the tunnel on a road that is hard to access for tunnel traffic. But you will see the massive cliff above the tunnel entry and get a sense of how deep the tunnels burrow into the bedrock before starting under the Hudson River en route to Manhattan.

The transition from feeling like you're riding on a highway access road to suburbia is quick, you start moving away from the highway at the first light you see and once you're past the gas station, you're in a much quieter place.

Around two curves, you're at the top of the hill and riding north along the Palisades. The views across the water and up along the Hudson are excellent and you can see why the homes facing the water are coveted. It's also a good thing that there are parks along the cliffs; the rest of us can take in the views standing still, too.

My temptation is to slow down along this section. No need to ride fast when there's such a vista. The park benches and tables, statuary, and bathrooms all contribute to a sense of ease, though you still have cars, both parked and moving, to deal with.

And that hill you climbed? There's a nice payoff. A downhill that's potentially a screamer takes you back down to the water, and it's a flat, fairly empty ride back to the start.

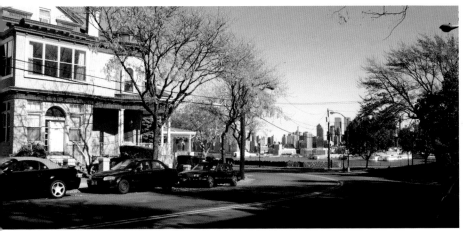

One of the reasons this place is so popular. So close yet so far.

Ride 54 - Weehawken Loop

Ride Log

0.0 Start in front of the Port Imperial ferry stop. Go right, then turn left to get out of the parking lot.

0.1 Turn left on Port Imperial Blvd.

1.2 Turn right on Baldwin Ave.

1.3 Turn right on J.F. Kennedy Blvd E.

2.0 Bear left. You're now riding along the palisades.

3.2 Turn right onto Anthony M. Defino Way.

3.7 Turn right onto Port Imperial Blvd.

4.8 Turn left into Port Imperial parking lot.

4.9 Finish at the start.

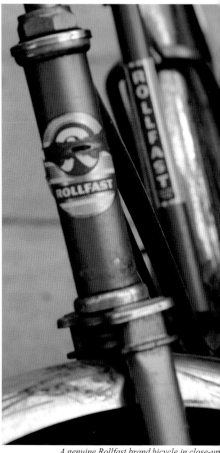

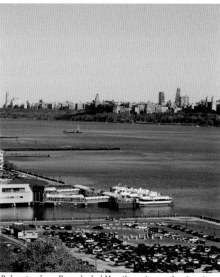

Below is where Burr dueled Hamilton. Across the river is a sight they never imagined.

A genuine Rollfast brand bicycle in close-up
Photo Matt Wittmer

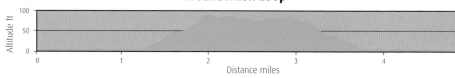

Weehawken Loop

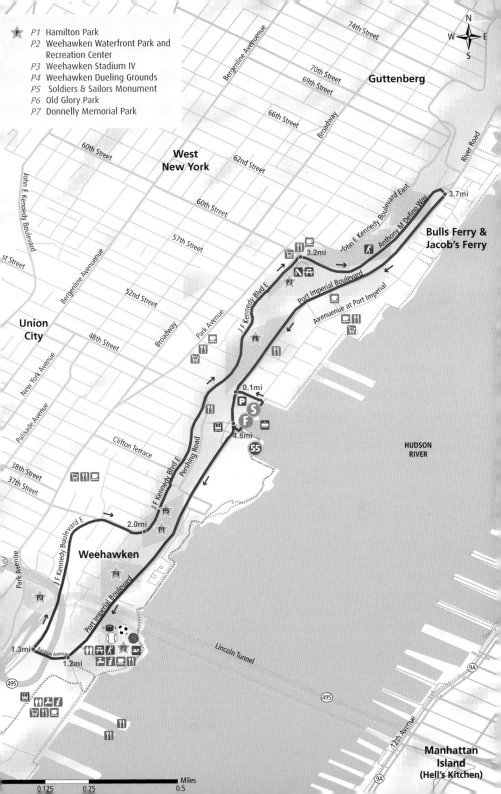

P P1 Hamilton Park
   P2 Weehawken Waterfront Park and
      Recreation Center
   P3 Weehawken Stadium IV
   P4 Weehawken Dueling Grounds
   P5 Soldiers & Sailors Monument
   P6 Old Glory Park
   P7 Donnelly Memorial Park

N
W   E
S

Guttenberg

74th Street
70th Street
69th Street
66th Street
62nd Street
60th Street
57th Street
60th Street
52nd Street
48th Street
38th Street
37th Street

West
New York

Bergenline Avenuenue
Broadway
Park Avenue
Bergenline Avenuenue
Broadway

River Road

John F. Kennedy Boulevard East
Anthony M Defino Way

3.7mi

Bulls Ferry &
Jacob's Ferry

J F Kennedy Blvd E
3.2mi
P7
Port Imperial Boulevard
Avenuenue at Port Imperial

P6

0.1mi

P
S
F
4.8mi
55

HUDSON
RIVER

Union
City

New York Avenue
Palisade Avenue
Clifton Terrace

John F. Kennedy Boulevard
st Street

J F Kennedy Boulevard E
Pershing Road

P5
2.0mi
P1

Weehawken

P4
P3
Park Avenue

Port Imperial Boulevard

1.3mi
Baldwin Avenue
1.2mi

P2

Lincoln Tunnel

495
495

(9A)

12th Avenue

Manhattan
Island
(Hell's Kitchen)

(9A)

0.125   0.25   Miles   0.5

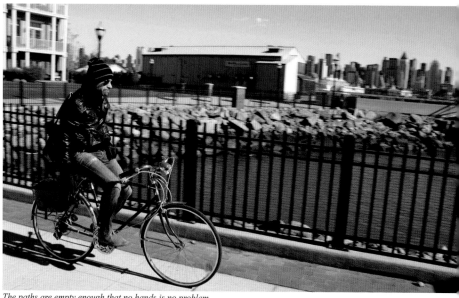

The paths are empty enough that no hands is no problem.

At a Glance

partially

Distance 5.5 miles **Elevation Gain** 120′

Terrain

Flat paths and roads the whole way.

Traffic

Light but mixed. Mostly on bike paths, so traffic will only be cyclists and pedestrians, but still keep your head up as you have to go onto regular roads.

How to Get There

You can take the New York Waterway ferry to the Newport Landing, the Hudson Bergen Light Rail to Newport or Hoboken N.J. Transit to Hoboken, and the PATH to Newport or Hoboken.

Food and Drink

No shortage of places along the water. If you can't fin what you're looking for, just go west to the main drag Washington Street, and you'll easily find succor.

Links to 54 56

Where to Bike Rating

 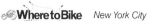

About...

Because of the book's format, where the rides are listed north to south in every section, it might not be obvious that this is the third segment of a three-part ride starting at Liberty State Park, going from Liberty into Jersey City, and then J.C. to Weehawken. Put them all together, and it's a 14-mile one-way ride, or a 28-mile round trip. Eventually, the three rides will be part of the Hudson River Waterfront Path that is slated to extend from Bayonne in the south to the George Washington Bridge.

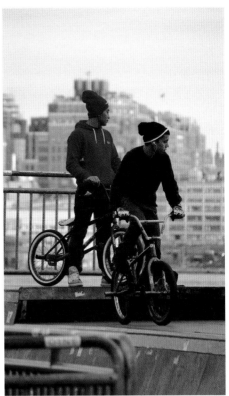

Freestyle BMX riders at Castle Point Skatepark.
Photo Matt Wittmer

The factoid everyone should know about Hoboken is that the land mass is one square mile. It used to be smaller, when it was an island separated from the rest of New Jersey. Today, in reality, it's 1.2 square miles, and if you include the water within its borders, it's two square miles. But the 1.2 number, combined with the 50,000 or so residents makes this a very densely populated place, in the running with neighboring Union City, West New York, and Gutenberg for the most densely populated municipal area in the country; it was fourth after the 2000 census, but that was when it had about 12,000 fewer residents. On this ride, you'll see a sizeable chunk of the new housing for those new Hobokeners.

Combine the density with the multitude of public transportation options—N.J. Transit terminal with six train lines, Hudson Bergen Light Rail, PATH trains going in multiple directions, and plenty of buses—Hobokenites have the highest rate of public transit use in the United States. So lots of people can get along fine without cars, just like in Manhattan across the river. They don't need bicycles, but with more and more bike paths, the riding is getting easier.

It's not a surprise that there would be busy public spaces along the water and a bike path to link them together. Hoboken is in the middle of this spin (we also cover Weehawken and Jersey City in other rides) and it offers you historic landmarks like the train terminal, Castle Point, and Elysian Park (home of Elysian Fields, site of the alleged first baseball game), modern parks, piers for relaxing and playing, and even a road to ride on. That road, Sinatra Drive, is named for Hoboken's most famous native. Maybe Pia Zadora will get a road someday, too.

On either end of the ride, are empty spaces. The first is shortly after you start in Jersey City. The second is just as you leave Hoboken. They'll probably eventually be filled in, we hope with park space, but right now, it gives the ride a 'work in progress' feel. Luckily, the rapidly evolving Weehawken section of the ride already has quite a passel of set aside parkland.

Ride 55 - Jersey City to Weehawken

Ride Log

P1 Erie-Lackawanna Park
P2 Hoboken World War Two Memorial
P3 Sinatra Park and Amphitheatre
P4 Castle Point Lookout
P5 Hoboken World War One Memorial
P6 Elysian Park
P7 Maxwell Place Park
P8 Hoboken Historical Museum
P9 Harborside Park
P10 Weehawken Waterfront Park and Recreation Center

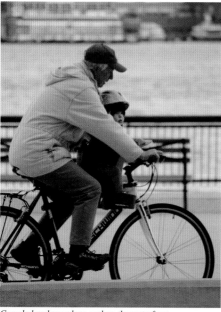

Grandad and grandson explore the waterfront.
Photo Matt Wittmer

0.0 New York WaterWays ferry dock at Newport Head west, following the Hudson River Waterfront Walkway. Keep the water on your right.

0.1 Turn right on River Dr.

0.5 Turn right to keep the Hudson Bergen Light Rail Terminal and then the Hoboken Train Terminal on your left.

0.8 Past the Hoboken terminal, keep the water on your right as you hug the shore.

0.9 Turn right to circumnavigate the first pier after the terminal.

1.2 Turn right on the bike path alongside Sinatra Dr.

1.5 Bike path ends. Keep going north on Sinatra Dr.

2.1 Turn right off of Sinatra to circumnavigate Maxwell Place Park.

2.3 Turn right onto Sinatra Dr.

2.6 Turn left to follow Sinatra Dr.

2.8 Turn right off of Sinatra onto bike path.

3.0 Turn right onto Park Ave.

3.3 Turn right onto 19th St.

3.4 Turn left onto Waterfront Terrace.

3.8 Ride straight to water and rejoin bike path. Follow path all the way to Port Imperial ferry terminal.

5.5 Arrive at Port Imperial ferry terminal.

Jersey City to Weehawken

Altitude ft — Distance miles

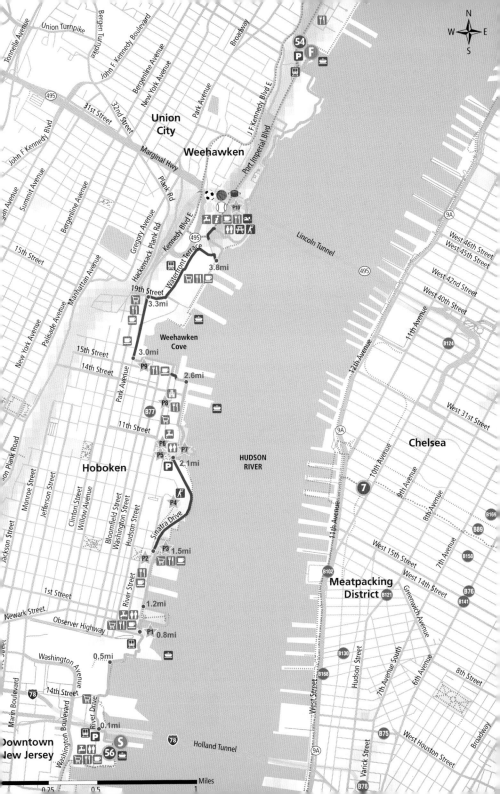

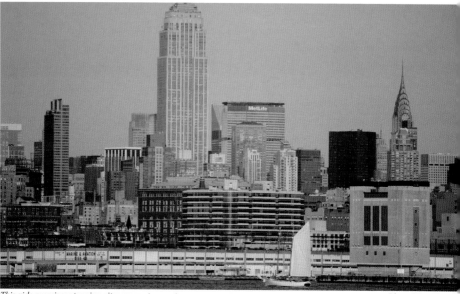

This ride promises stunning cityscapes at every turn.

At a Glance

Distance 3.2 miles   **Elevation Gain** 49′

Terrain

Flat. Pavement is mostly good, particularly on the multi-use paths.

Traffic

Mixed. Most everything is on a bike path, though some paths are on streets and some are dedicated.

How to Get There

If you're coming from the nearby Jersey waterfront, chances are you're near the Hudson Bergen Light Rail line and can take it to the ride, so long as you are going at non-peak hours. Go to the Liberty State Park stop. PATH trains will get you to the north end of the ride, the Newport stop, N.Y. Waterway ferries will get you to the ride in a few places as well, both by the start, Liberty Harbor dock, and the finish, Newport Landing.

Food and Drink

The ride down Grand seems to yield the most interesting places to stop, but there are also good food trucks on the street by the finish.

Side Trip

The Museum of Russian Art, just off the route, has a focus on Nonconformist Art. You'd be forgiven for thinking that all art is that; it is nonconformist in that it is art that wasn't made to conform to official Soviet art. But you shouldn't follow a crowd to visit the place.

Links to

Where to Bike Rating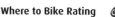

About...

This is an easy ride that highlights much of the revived Jersey City. It can be done in any number of ways; as a one-way ride, as a round-trip, or as part of a one, two, three, or even four-part trip, starting either at Liberty State Park to the south or Port Imperial in the north. In time, it will be easy to connect to the ride over the Bayonne Bridge south of here in the Staten Island section, or any of the rides from the George Washington Bridge in the north.

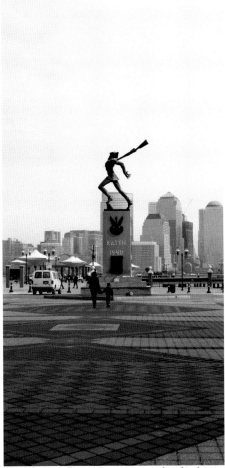

The Katyn Forest Massacre is remembered in the most gruesome monument in Jersey City.

The waterfront helped make Jersey City. Both the docks themselves and the proximity of those docks to factories and trains helped build this city for much of the 19th and 20th centuries. When those started dying, the city faced lean years. Now the waterfront is helping with the city's revival. Blue-collar industry seems not to be returning so much, but overflow from the city across the Hudson is helping grow the second-largest city in New Jersey.

Bohemians, business, and those thirsting for a little less city in their urban life have worked on separate tracks. Artists not interested in or unable to afford Brooklyn moved in and created their own scene. Office towers have been built along the water. And both new construction and old townhouses have given plenty of people a slightly slower pace of urban life.

There are bike lanes aplenty in Jersey City for many reasons. There's room for them. Car ownership is almost as low as it is in the place across the river, with around 40 percent choosing to live with an auto. And public transit use is high, rivaling both Hoboken and New York. The population is also young and median income is relatively low, so chances are people are healthy, not afraid of a little sweat, and a car can be a large expense.

This ride goes through older and newer Jersey City. It will be obvious what's what. Ironically, some of the oldest known European settlements in the city were located by Harsimus Cove, an area that is one of the most recently rebuilt.

While this ride has turns, you can pretty much do it without a map. Head for the Hudson River and when you get there, turn left. If you find yourself getting confused, then check the map. Rides of this length that have water limiting wrong turns, you can never get terribly, hopelessly lost, and detours are pretty short. J.C. is a good adventure; it is worth getting off the track.

Northern New Jersey

Ride Log

0.0 Start at end of Philip St and start of Jersey Ave on the edge of Liberty State Park and the end of Liberty Harbor.

0.4 Turn right onto Grand St.

1.3 Turn left onto Washington St.

1.4 Turn right onto Montgomery St.

1.6 At end of road, ride onto Pier and circumnavigate it counter clockwise and then head north along the water.

2.2 Turn left on Harborside Pl and then right onto Hudson St.

2.3 Turn left onto Second St.

2.5 Turn right onto Washington Blvd.

2.8 Turn right onto Town Square Pl.

3.0 Ride straight onto bike path.

3.2 Finish at NY Waterways Newport Ferry dock.

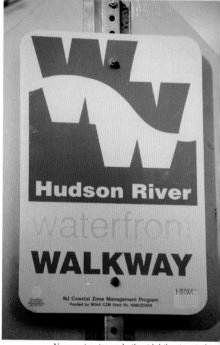

No worries, it was built with bikes in mind too
Photo Matt Wittme

 P1 Liberty State Park
P2 Jersey City Museum
P3 Museum of Russian Art
P4 Katyn Massacre Memorial
P5 J. Owen Grundy Park
P6 Hudson River Waterfront Walkway

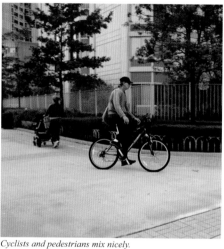

Cyclists and pedestrians mix nicely.

Jersey City Waterfront Ride

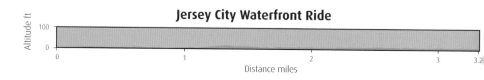

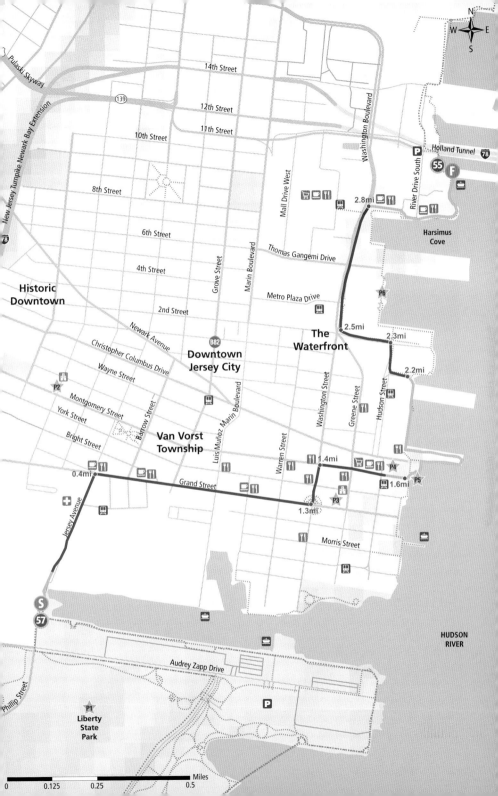

Liberty State Park Ride

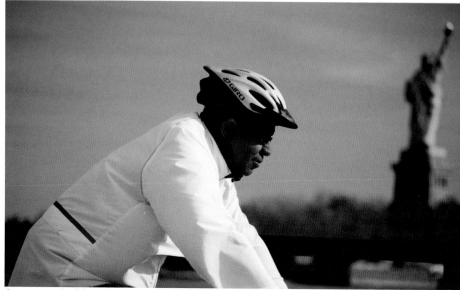

Just one example of this ride's continually splendid points of view.

Photo Matt Wittmer

At a Glance

Distance 5.2 miles   **Elevation Gain** 25′

Terrain

Flat paths and roads.

Traffic

Light. Over half the trip is on multi-use paths, so the traffic on them will be of the foot variety. The rest of the ride is on park roads and around parking lots, so the cars, if you encounter them, will be moving fairly slowly.

How to Get There

You can easily ride from anywhere in Jersey City, as well as take the HBLR to the Liberty State Park stop or the N.Y. Waterways ferry to Liberty Harbor. As there's ample parking, driving is also a possibility.

Food and Drink

If you stay within the confines of the park, there are few choices. You pretty much have the Liberty House

Restaurant and whatever truck or cart you find. The restaurant is working the gourmet food in a picturesque setting thing. A bit simpler is the Liberty Park Café (formerly Diner), which tries to hit points, café fare and comfort food. You can also easily ride into Jersey City, ride down Grand Street, and find lots of choices.

Side Trip

If you have kids, visit the Liberty Science Center, which specializes in hands-on education. It also has an IMAX movie screen for science-related or -themed movies.

Links to 56

Where to Bike Rating

About...

Timing is critical when riding here. If you go in the winter, around dawn, or dusk, you'll probably have the place to yourself and can maybe even get in a spirited training ride. But on a summer weekend, or a holiday, expect this to be a sightseeing ride or one for family. Luckily, you can add to the ride by taking all the paths and roads within the route laid out, as well as branching out to Philip Street, toward the western edge of the park.

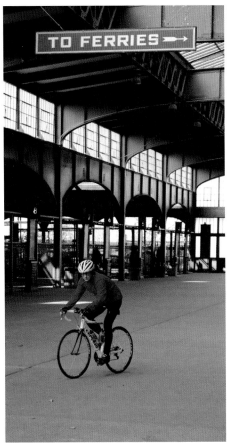

Ferry over, ride on. *Photo Matt Wittmer*

For all the talk about New York City's ties to Ellis Island and The Statue of Liberty, it is surprising to realize that both sites are not only far across the harbor, but only a stone's throw from New Jersey. Yes, people will joke about Lady Liberty turning her back on Jersey, but when people got off Ellis Island, they could easily ferry to New Jersey, settle in the thriving industrial cities of Newark, Jersey City, and Hoboken, or make their way deep into America. And most went west rather than east to the Big Apple, with at least 70 percent heading for the Central Rail Road of New Jersey, which had the closest terminal to the famed immigration point. CRRNJ is long gone, and the park is made up largely of the train company's old ground.

There are many things to recommend Liberty State Park; it seems underutilized; it's in great condition; and the view of Manhattan is amazing. There are several environments within the park, from the modern waterfront promenade to the monuments, to a restored railroad terminal, to a quiet key, to a salt marsh.

It's also another great example of reclaiming the waterfront out of industrial decay. The northern boundary of the park is the Big Basin of the Morris Canal, which once ran across the state to Phillipsburg, all the way on the Delaware River, to carry coal to the Hudson. Just to the south of the basin is the CRRNJ terminal, which once took immigrants into New Jersey to get to points beyond. The southeastern edge of the park was once Black Tom Island, which had a small role in the drama of World War I; sabotage caused a munitions depot to ignite, and the blast damaged the Statue of Liberty as well as homes as far as 25 miles away.

The salt marsh just north of Black Tom is a successful part of the reclamation effort. The big expanse is in the middle of being restored to some sort of natural habitat. While you can only see these from roads and bike paths, they limit the growth of popularity of the park and keep crowds down for bike riding.

Northern New Jersey

Ride 57 - Liberty State Park Ride

Ride Log

0.0 Start at the Liberty State Park building at the end of Morris Pessin Dr/Black Tom Rd. Start by following the Hudson River waterfront walk.

0.1 Turn left to follow the water.

1.7 Turn right before getting to Terminal Museum.

1.9 Turn left to keep water on right.

2.1 Turn left to keep water on right.

3.2 Turn left onto Phillip St.

3.3 Turn left onto Audrey Zapp Dr.

3.8 Turn right onto Freedom Way.

5.1 Turn left onto Morris Pessin Dr/Black Tom Rd.

5.2 Finish at start, Liberty State Park building at end of Morris Pessin Dr/Black Tom Rd.

 P1 US Flag Plaza
P2 Liberation Monument
P3 Liberty Island and The Statue of Liberty
P4 Liberty State Park Interpretative Center
P5 Waterfront Park Area
P6 Ellis Island
P7 Columbus Monument
P8 Train Shed
P9 Central NJ Railroad-Terminal Museum
P10 Liberty Science Center

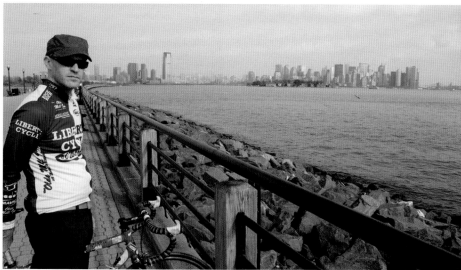

Cyclists come here for the sights as much as the riding.

Liberty State Park Ride

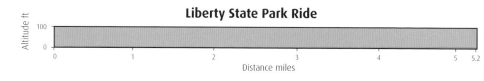

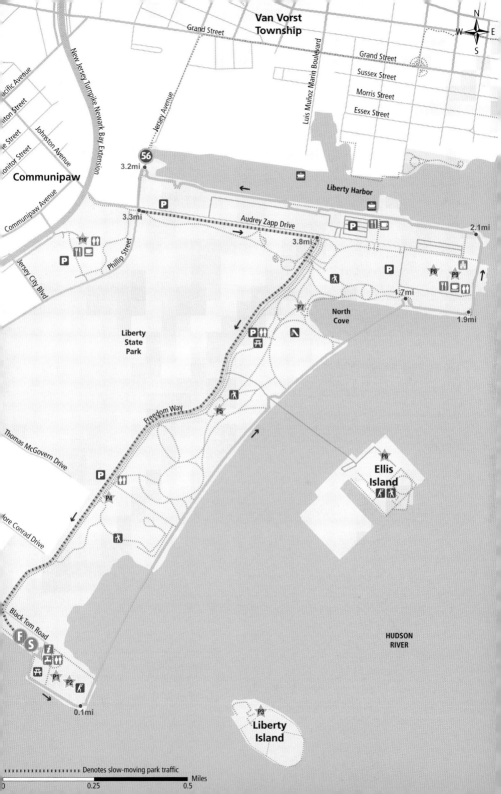

Lincoln Park

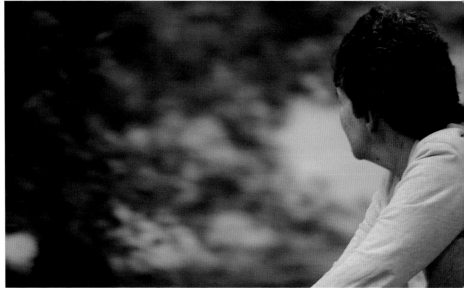

A wind-swept rider takes in Lincoln Park's greenery.

Photo Matt Wittmer

At a Glance

Distance 1.3 miles   **Elevation Gain** 40′

Terrain

Flat. Park roads in good condition.

Traffic

Light. You can ride here in the dark as well as through the day.

How to Get There

If you're using pubic transit, the Journal Square PATH station gets you pretty close. The West Side Avenue Hudson Bergen Light Rail Station is closer. And there is ample parking for those who want to drive.

Food and Drink

West Side Avenue offers plenty of choices. There is a gaggle of places to stop both north and south of the park. The north bunch feels more intimate while the south bunch has more parking.

Side Trip

If you like to combine your rides with scenic walks there is the Hackensack RiverWalk in the western sector of the park. It hugs the Hackensack River and will one day be part of a path stretching from Bayonne to the Meadowlands.

Where to Bike Rating

About...

Lincoln Park was the first park built in Hudson County. It dates from 1905. The space reflects both open space philosophies of then and now. From then, you'll find the park loop road, gazebos, a man made lake. From now, there are fields and courts galore (soccer, football, baseball, tennis, handball, paddleball, a running track) as well as playgrounds, a public golf course, and some space set aside as reclaimed nature.

While the ring road is pretty much never closed to car traffic, Lincoln Park is a great respite from those gas guzzling beasts, one of the few in this heavily urban area that is on a cramped peninsula that offers few easy escapes to more lush riding. Thanks to streetlights along the loop, it can be ridden day or night, in good weather or bad.

I first came to Lincoln Park as a teen, for early morning bike races at the tail end of winter. We remember it as always cold, windy, overcast, with leaf-less trees bending in the wind and faded green spaces lying dormant. It was a relief to reacquaint with the park when it was pretty and peaceful, and with only a light breeze. Never noticed the statuary before.

The park, like many open spaces in the area, is converted space. It was privately-owned swampland acquired by the county, drained, dried, and reimagined for a public yearning for a respite from urban ills, a precious idyll. Even though the space has been adjusted for more modern park users, there is still a lot of room for leisure. Picnics as well as bike riding.

What should prove interesting is what's going on in the western half of the park, aka Lincoln Park West, or the area that's over the bridge (you can ride it) and

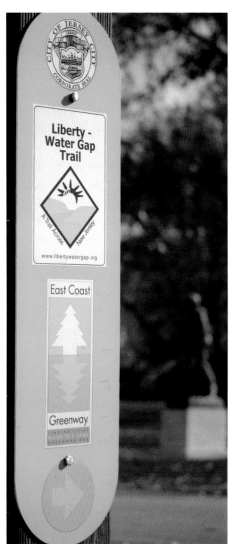

Try these trails for rides further afield.
Photo Matt Wittmer

beyond the highway. At one time, it was mostly wetlands, with facilities for nearby Saint Peter's College, now the golf course is being built. But beyond it is the Hackensack River and an ambitious effort to create a natural space on the banks. It would be great if they could make another paved loop around the golf course that takes you to the edges of the roads and river. Cycling is the next golf, after all.

Northern New Jersey

Ride Log

0.0 Start at Lincoln Park fountain. Follow park road around counter-clockwise.

1.3 Finish at Lincoln Park fountain.

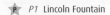 P1 Lincoln Fountain

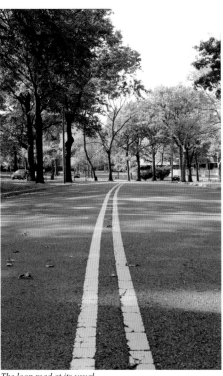

The loop road at its usual.

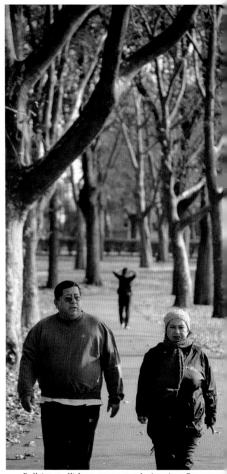

Roll (or stroll) here among stately American Sycamores
Photo Matt Wittmer

Lincoln Park

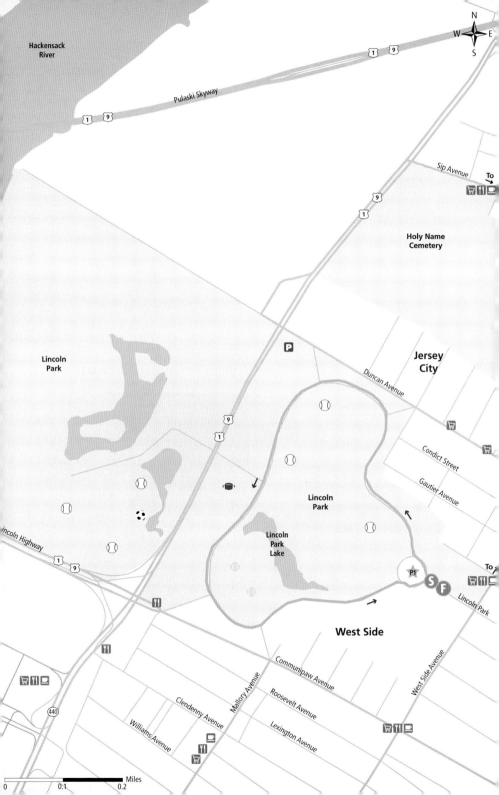

B1 Allendale Cycle
317 Franklin Turnpike, ALLENDALE, NJ
Tel: 201 825 0952
www.allendalecycle.com

B2 Bicycle Repairman Corporate
40-21a 35th Avenue, ASTORIA, NY
Tel: 718 706 0450
www.bikerepairman.com

B3 Bike Stop
37-19 28th Avenue, ASTORIA, NY
Tel: 718 278 2453

B4 Tony's Bicycles
35-01 23rd Avenue, ASTORIA, NY
Tel: 718 278 3355
www.tonysbicycles.com

B5 Eddy's Cycle City Inc
635 Broadway, BAYONNE, NJ
Tel: 201 339 3722

B6 Roberts Bicycles
33-13 Francis Lewis Blouvard, BAYSIDE, NY
Tel: 718 353 5432
www.robertsbicycles.net

B7 Arrow Cycle Inc
4055 White Plains Road, BRONX, NY
Tel: 718 547 2656
www.arrowcycleinc.com

B8 Bronx Bicycle Discount Center
912 E Gun Hill Road, BRONX, NY
Tel: 718 798 3242

B9 Castle Hill Bike Shop
3267 East Tremont Avenue, BRONX, NY
Tel: 718 597 2083

B10 Crosstown Bicycle
33 East 170th Street, BRONX, NY
Tel: 718 293 8837

B11 J D Custom Cycles Inc
1425 Blondell Avenue, BRONX, NY
Tel: 718 409 2994

B12 Neighborhood Cycle Inc
571 Van Cortlandt Avenue, BRONX, NY
Tel: 718 665 6031
www.neighborhoodcycle.com

B13 United Spokes
207 West 242 Street, BRONX, NY
Tel: 718 432 2453
www.unitedspokes.com

B14 Westchester Bicycle & Pro Shop
2611 Westchester Avenue, BRONX, NY
Tel: 718 409 1114
www.westchesterpro.com

B15 718 Cyclery
254 3rd Avenue, BROOKLYN, NY
Tel: 347 457 5760
www.718c.com

B16 9th Street Cycles *(Rentals available)*
375 9th Street, BROOKLYN, NY
Tel: 718 768 2453
www.bklynbikes.com

B17 Affinity Cycles
616 Grand Street, BROOKLYN, NY
Tel: 718 384 5181
www.affinitycycles.com

B18 Arnolds Bicycles & Trains
4220 8th Avenue, BROOKLYN, NY
Tel: 718 435 8558

B19 Bay Ridge Bicycle World
8916 Third Avenue, BROOKLYN, NY
Tel: 718 238 1118
www.bayridgebikes.com

B20 Bespoke Bicycles
64-b Lafayette Avenue, BROOKLYN, NY
Tel: 718 643 6816
www.bespoke-bicycles.com

B21 Bicycle Doctor
133 Grand Street, BROOKLYN, NY
Tel: 718 302 3145
www.brooklynbikedoctor.com

B22 Bicycle Habitat
476 5th Avenue, BROOKLYN, NY
Tel: 718 788 2543
www.bicyclehabitat.com

B23 Bicycle Station
171 Park Avenue, BROOKLYN, NY
Tel: 718 638 0300
www.bicyclestationbrooklyn.com

B24 Bike and Roll - Brooklyn Bridge Park
(Rentals)
Old Fulton Street, BROOKLYN, NY
Tel: 212 260 0400
www.bikeandroll.com

B25 Bike and Roll - Prospect Park *(Rentals)*
Grand Army Plaza, BROOKLYN, NY
Plaza Street And Eastern Parkway
Tel: 212 260 0400
www.bikeandroll.com

B26 Bike Life
56 Lincoln Road, BROOKLYN, NY
Tel: 347 789 5607

B27 Bikes On Myrtle
478 Myrtle Avenue, BROOKLYN, NY
Tel: 718 788 0478

B28 Bravo's Bike Repair
187 Wilson Avenue, BROOKLYN, NY
Tel: 718 602 5150

B29 Brooklyn Bicycle Centre
673 Coney Island Avenue, BROOKLYN, NY
Tel: 718 941 9095

B30 Brooklyn Bike and Board
560 Vanderbilt Avenue, BROOKLYN, NY
Tel: 347 295 2339
www.brooklynbikeandboard.com

 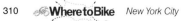

331 Brooklyn Heights Bike Shop
278 Atlantic Avenue, BROOKLYN, NY
Tel: 718 625 9633

332 B's Bikes
262 Driggs Avenue, BROOKLYN, NY
Tel: 718 349 1212

333 Carbon Negative
69 Guernsey Street, BROOKLYN, NY
Tel: 718 599 0440
www.carbonnegative.com

334 Dixon's Bicycle Shop *(Rentals available)*
795 Union Street, BROOKLYN, NY
Tel: 718 636 0067
www.dixonsbicycleshop.com

335 Ferrara Cycle Shop
6304 20th Avenue, BROOKLYN, NY
Tel: 718 232 6716

336 Fulton Bikes
1580 Fulton Street, BROOKLYN, NY
Tel: 718 778 2887

337 Graham Bicycle Discount Center
178 Graham Avenue, BROOKLYN, NY
Tel: 718 782 5741

338 Greenpoint Bikes
1078 Manhattan Avenue, BROOKLYN, NY
Tel: 718 389 3818
www.greenpointbikes.com

339 King Kog
453 Graham Avenue, BROOKLYN, NY
Tel: 347 689 2299
www.kingkog.com

340 Larry's Cycle Shop *(Rentals available)*
1854 Flatbush Avenue, BROOKLYN, NY
Tel: 718 377 3600
www.larryscycleshop.com

341 Mr C's Cycles
4622 7th Avenue, BROOKLYN, NY
Tel: 718 438 7283
www.mrccycles.com

342 Nelson's Bicycle Shop
251 Bushwick Avenue, BROOKLYN, NY
Tel: 718 821 4811

343 On the Move *(Rentals available)*
400 7th Avenue, BROOKLYN, NY
Tel: 718 768 4998
www.onthemovenyc.com

344 Post Bike Shop
257 Varet Street, BROOKLYN, NY
Tel: 718 599 7678
www.postbikes.com

345 R&A Cycles
105 5th Avenue, BROOKLYN, NY
Tel: 718 636 5242
www.racycles.com

346 Racer''s Edge Cycle & Fitnes
1970 Rockaway Parkway, BROOKLYN, NY
Tel: 718 531 3100

B47 Recycle-A-Bicycle - Brooklyn
35 Pearl Street, BROOKLYN, NY
Tel: 718 858 2972
www.recycleabicycle.org

B48 Red Hook Bike Shop
189 Richards Street, BROOKLYN, NY
Tel: 347 742 4816

B49 Ride Bike Pro Gear
4175 Bedford Avenue, BROOKLYN, NY
Tel: 718 552 0738
www.ridebikeprogear.com

B50 Ride Brooklyn *(Rentals available)*
468 Bergen Street, BROOKLYN, NY
718 857 7433
www.ridebrooklynny.com

B51 Rolling Orange
269 Baltic Street, BROOKLYN, NY
Tel: 718 935 0695
www.rollingorangebikes.com

B52 Roy's Sheepshead Cycle
2679 Coney Island Avenue, BROOKLYN, NY
Tel: 718 648 1440
www.roysbikes.com

B53 Spokes and Strings
140 Havemeyer Street, BROOKLYN, NY
Tel: 718 599 2409

B54 Terrific's Bikes & Videos
1547 Broadway, BROOKLYN, NY
Tel: 718 453 1575

B55 The Bike Shop - Brooklyn
514 Court Street, BROOKLYN, NY
Tel: 718 797 0326

B56 Time's Up
99 South 6th Street, BROOKLYN, NY
Tel: 212 802 8222
www.times-up.org

B57 Verrazano Bicycle Shop
7308 5th Avenue, BROOKLYN, NY
Tel: 718 680 6521
www.verrazanocycles.com

B58 Weber's Bicycle & Sewing Machines
4715 New Utrecht Avenue, BROOKLYN, NY
Tel: 718 871 4321

B59 Zukkies Bike Shop
279 Bushwick Avenue, BROOKLYN, NY
Tel: 718 456 0048

B60 Bicycle Shop NYC
349 W. 14th Street, CHELSEA, NY
Tel: 212 691 6149

B61 All-County Schwinn Cyclery
11 Homans Avenue, CLOSTER, NJ
Tel: 201 768 3086

B62 Almacen El Pedal
4722 Junction Boulevard, CORONA, NY
Tel: 718 426 7807

Bike Shops & Rentals

Where to Bike New York City 311

B63 Elias Bicycle Shop
39-24 108th Street, CORONA, NY
Tel: 347 776 6797

B64 Peak Mountain Bike Pro *(Rentals available)*
42-42 235th Street, DOUGLASTON, NY
Tel: 718 225 5119
www.peakmtnbike.com

B65 Steve's Moped & Bicycle World
40 Park Avenue, DUMONT, NJ
Tel: 201 384 7777
www.stevesmoped.com

B66 East Meadow Bikes
353 Merrick Avenue, EAST MEADOW, NY
Tel: 516 481 1637

B67 Century Bicycle Shop
14-18 150th Street, FLUSHING, NY
Tel: 718 358 0986

B68 Twin Bicycle & Sporting Goods
7520 Metropolitan Avenue, FLUSHING, NY
Tel: 718 326 7725
www.twinbicycles.com

B69 Spin City Cycle
110-50 Queens Boulevard, FOREST HILL, NY
Tel: 718 793 8850
www.spincitycycle.com

B70 Strictly Bicycles
2347 Hudson Terrace, FORT LEE, NJ
Tel: 201 944 7074
www.strictlybicycles.com

B71 Big City Bicycle
301 Nassau Boulevard, GARDEN CITY SOUTH, NY
Tel: 516 483 9266
www.longbeachbicycleny.com

B72 Bike and Roll - Governors Island *(Rentals)*
10 South St @ Whitehall Street
Governors Island, NY
www.bikeandroll.com

B73 Emey's Bike Shop
141 East 17th Street, GRAMERCY PARK, NY
Tel: 212 475 7409

B74 Bikeworks
7 Northern Boulevard, GREENVALE, NY
Tel: 516 484 4422

B75 Johns Mini Bike & Bicycle Shop
151 East Houston Street, GREENWICH VILLAGE, NY
Tel: 212 982 5310
www.johnsminibike.com

B76 Sixth Avenue Bicycles
546 Avenue Of Americas, GREENWICH VILLAGE, NY
Tel: 212 255 5100

B77 Flo On Wheel Cycles
1222 Washington Street, HOBOKEN, NJ
Tel: 201 798 5589

B78 Metro Bicycles - Canal Street Bicycles
(Rentals available)
75 Varick Street, New York, NY
Tel: 212 334 8000
www.metrobicycles.com

B79 Cigi Bicycle Shop - Jackson Heights
91-07 37th Avenue, JACKSON HEIGHTS, NY
Tel: 718 717 2377
www.cigibicycleshop.com

B80 Belittle Bicycles
169-20 Jamaica Avenue, JAMAICA, NY
Tel: 718 739 3795
www.bellbikes.com

B81 Hardware City
7906 Jamaica Avenue, JAMAICA, NY
Tel: 718 296 2000

B82 Grove Street Bicycles
365 Grove Street, JERSEY CITY, NJ
Tel: 201 451 2453
www.grovestreetbicycles.com

B83 Gray's Bicycles & Accessories
8234 Lefferts Blouvard, KEW GARDENS, NY
Tel: 718 441 9767

B84 Long Beach Bicycle & Fitness
755 East Park Avenue, LONG BEACH, NY
Tel: 516 432 9632
www.longbeachbicycleny.com

B85 LIC Bicycles *(Rentals available)*
25-11 Queens Plaza, LONG ISLAND CITY, NY
Tel: 718 472 4537
www.longislandcitybikes.wordpress.com

B86 Spokesman Cycles - Long Island City
(Rentals available)
49-4 Vernon Boulevard, LONG ISLAND CITY, NY
Tel: 718 433 0450
www.spokesmancycles.com

B87 Brickwell Cycling & Multisports
1463 Northern Blvd, MANHASSET, NY
Tel: 516 482 1193
www.brickwell.com

B88 Grand Bicycle Center
70-13 Grand Avenue, MASPETH, NY
Tel: 718 779 4691
www.grandbicycle.com

B89 A Bicycle Shop *(Rentals available)*
163 West 22nd Street, NEW YORK, NY
Tel: 212 691 6149
www.a-bicycleshop.com

B90 Adeline Adeline
147 Reade Street, NEW YORK, NY
Tel: 212 227 1150
www.adelineadeline.com

B91 Al's Cycle Solutions
693 10th Avenue, NEW YORK, NY
Tel: 212 247 3300
www.alscyclesolutions.com

392　bfold
224 E 13th Street, Unit #1, NEW YORK, NY
Tel: 212 529 7247
www.bfold.com

393　Bicycle Habitat
244 Lafayette Street, NEW YORK, NY
Tel: 212 431 3315
www.bicyclehabitat.com

394　Bicycle Heaven NY *(Rentals available)*
348 E 62nd Street, NEW YORK, NY
Tel: 212 230 1919
www.mybikeheaven.com

395　Bicycle Renaissance *(Rentals available)*
430 Columbus Avenue, NEW YORK, NY
Tel: 212 724 2350
www.bicyclerenaissance.com

396　Bicycles Plus 2nd Avenue
1690 2nd Avenue, NEW YORK, NY
Tel: 212 722 2201
www.bicyclesnyc.com

397　Bicycles Plus NYC
1400 3rd Avenue, NEW YORK, NY
Tel: 212 794 2929
www.bicyclesnyc.com

398　Bike and Roll - Battery Park *(Rentals)*
Battery Place And West Street, NEW YORK, NY
Tel: 212 260 0400
www.bikeandroll.com

399　Bike and Roll - Central Park - Columbus Circle
(Rentals)
Columbus Circle, NEW YORK, NY
Tel: 212 260 0400
www.bikeandroll.com

3100　Bike and Roll - Central Park - Tavern on Green
(Rentals)
West 67th Street, NEW YORK, NY
Tel: 212 260 0400
www.bikeandroll.com

3101　Bike and Roll - New York City *(Rentals)*
152 W.36th Street, Suite 801, NEW YORK, NY
Tel: 212 260 0400
www.bikenewyorkcity.com

3102　Bike and Roll - Pier 84 *(Rentals)*
557 12th Avenue, NEW YORK, NY
Tel: 212 260 0400
www.bikeandroll.com

3103　Bike and Roll - Riverside Park *(Rentals)*
Riverside Drive, NEW YORK, NY
Tel: 212 260 0400
www.bikeandroll.com

3104　Bike Rental Central Park *(Rentals)*
348 West 57th Street, NEW YORK, NY
Tel: 212 664 9600
www.bikerentalcentralpark.com

B105　Bike Works NYC
106 Ridge Street, NEW YORK, NY
Tel: 212 388 1077
www.bikecult.com

B106　Bikes By George
193 East 4th Street, NEW YORK, NY
Tel: 212 228 6641

B107　Busy Bee Bike
437 E 6th Street, NEW YORK, NY
Tel: 212 228 2347

B108　Central Park Bicycle Shop *(Rentals available)*
315 West, 57th Street, NEW YORK, NY
Tel: 646 399 7404
www.centralpark-newyorkcity.com

B109　Central Park Bike Tours
203 West 58th Street, NEW YORK, NY
Tel: 212 541 8759

B110　Champion Bicycles *(Rentals available)*
896 Amsterdam Avenue, NEW YORK, NY
Tel: 212 662 2690
www.championbicycles.com

B111　Chari & Co NYC
175 Stanton Street, NEW YORK, NY
Tel: 212 475 0102
www.chariandconyc.com

B112　Chelsea Bicycles *(Rentals available)*
130 West 26th Street, NEW YORK, NY
Tel: 646 230 7715
www.chelseabicyclesny.com

B113　City Bicycles and Hobbies *(Rentals available)*
315 W 38th Street, NEW YORK, NY
Tel: 212 563 3373

B114　CNC Bicycle Works Ltd
1101 First Avenue, NEW YORK, NY
Tel: 212 230 1919

B115　Conrad's Bike Shop
25 Tudor City Place, NEW YORK, NY
Tel: 212 697 6966
www.conradsbikeshop.com

B116　Continuum Cycles
199 & 207 Avenue B, NEW YORK, NY
Tel: 212 505 8785
www.continuumcycles.com

B117　Dah Shop
134 Division Street, NEW YORK, NY
Tel: 212 925 0155
www.dahshop.com

B118　Danny's Cycles
1690 2nd Avenue, NEW YORK, NY
Tel: 212 722 2201
www.dannyscycles.com

B119　Different Spokes
252 S 4th Street, Brooklyn, NY
Tel: 212 727 7278

B120 Eastern Mountain Sports - SoHo
      530 Broadway, NEW YORK, NY
      Tel: 212 966 8730
      www.ems.com

B121 Echelon Cycles *(Rentals available)*
      51 8th Avenue, NEW YORK, NY
      Tel: 212 206 7656
      www.echeloncyclesnyc.com

B122 Eddie's Bicycles *(Rentals available)*
      490 Amsterdam Avenue, NEW YORK, NY
      Tel: 212 580 2011
      www.eddiesbicycles.net

B123 Eduardo''s Bicycle Shop
      2131 2nd Avenue, NEW YORK, NY
      Tel: 212 722 2808

B124 Enoch's Bike Shop
      480 10th Avenue, NEW YORK, NY
      Tel: 212 582 0620
      www.enochsbikes.com

B125 Frank's Bike Shop *(Rentals available)*
      553 Grand Street, NEW YORK, NY
      Tel: 212 533 6332
      www.franksbikes.com

B126 Gotham Bikes Downtown *(Rentals available)*
      112 West Broadway, NEW YORK, NY
      Tel: 212 732 2453
      www.togabikes.com

B127 Harlem Bike Doctors
      2001 5th Avenue, NEW YORK, NY
      Tel: 917 428 3727

B128 Harlem Bike Doctors II *(Rentals available)*
      65 St Nicholas Avenue, NEW YORK, NY
      Tel: 919-518-4187

B129 Heavy Metal Bike Shop NY *(Rentals available)*
      2016 3rd Avenue, NEW YORK, NY
      Tel: 212 410 1144

B130 Hudson Urban Bicycles (HUB)
      139 Charles Street, NEW YORK, NY
      Tel: 212 965 9334
      www.hudsonurbanbicycles.com

B131 Innovation Bike Shop *(Rentals available)*
      105 W 106th Street, NEW YORK, NY
      Tel: 212 678 7130
      www.innovationbikeshop.com

B132 Jeff's Bicycles NYC
      1400 3rd Avenue, NEW YORK, NY
      Tel: 212 794 2929
      www.bicyclesnyc.com

B133 JR Bicycle Shop
      1820 Amsterdam Avenue, NEW YORK, NY
      Tel: 212 690 6511

B134 Landmark Bicycles *(Rentals available)*
      136 East 3rd Street, NEW YORK, NY
      Tel: 212 674 2343
      www.landmarkbicycles.com

B135 Liberty Bicycles
      846 9th Avenue, NEW YORK, NY
      Tel: 212 757 2418
      www.libertybikesny.com

B136 Manhattan Bicycles
      791 9th Avenue, NEW YORK, NY
      Tel: 212 262 0111

B137 Manhattan Velo *(Rentals available)*
      141 E 17th Street, NEW YORK, NY
      Tel: 212 253 6788
      www.manhattanvelo.com

B138 Mani's Bicycle Shop *(Rentals available)*
      8 Bennett Avenue, NEW YORK, NY
      Tel: 212 927 8501

B139 Master Bike Shop *(Rentals available)*
      225 West 77th Street, NEW YORK, NY
      Tel: 212 580 2355
      www.masterbikeshop.com

B140 Metro Bicycle Midtown *(Rentals available)*
      360 W 47th Street, NEW YORK, NY
      Tel: 212 581 4500
      www.metrobicycles.com

B141 Metro Bicycles - 6th Avenue *(Rentals available)*
      546 Avenue Of The Americas, NEW YORK, NY
      Tel: 212 255 5100
      www.metrobicycles.com

B142 Metro Bicycles - 88th Street *(Rentals available)*
      1311 Lexington Avenue, NEW YORK, NY
      Tel: 212 427 4450
      www.metrobicycles.com

B143 Lightwheels Bike and Boat Rental (*Rentals*)
      Meadow Lake, Flushing Meadows Park
      NEW YORK, NY
      Tel: 212 581 4500

B144 Metro Bicycles - New Rochelle *(Rentals available)*
      396 Main Street, NEW YORK, NY
      Tel: 914 633 6336
      www.metrobicycles.com

B145 Metro Bicycles - West Side Bicycles 96th Street
      (Rentals available)
      231 West 96th Street, NEW YORK, NY
      Tel: 212 663 7531
      www.metrobicycles.com

B146 MODSquad Cycles *(Rentals available)*
      2119 Frederick Douglass Boulevard, NEW YORK, NY
      Tel: 212 865 5050
      www.modsquadcycles.com

B147 My Bike Heaven
      348 E. 62nd Street, NEW YORK, NY
      Tel: 212 230 1919
      www.mybikeheaven.com

B148 New BoBo Toys
      96 Elizabeth Street, NEW YORK, NY
      Tel: 212 226 1668
      www.newbobotoys.com

B149 Newgen Bicycles
832 Ninth Avenue, NEW YORK, NY
Tel: 212 757 2418

B150 NYC Bicycle Shop
250 West 49th Street, NEW YORK, NY
Tel: 212 655 9629
www.nycbicycleshop.com

B151 NYC Velo *(Rentals available)*
64 2nd Avenue, NEW YORK, NY
Tel: 212 253 7771
www.nycvelo.com

B152 NYCeWheels *(Rentals available)*
1603 York Avenue, NEW YORK, NY
Tel: 212 737 3078
www.nycewheels.com

B153 Paragon Sports
867 Broadway At 18th Street, NEW YORK, NY
Tel: 212 255 8889
www.paragonsports.com

B154 Party Bike
570 Fashion Avenue, NEW YORK, NY
Tel: 212 398 2453

B155 Pedal Pusher Bike Shop *(Rentals available)*
1306 2nd Avenue, NEW YORK, NY
Tel: 212 288 5592
www.pedalpusherbikeshop.com

B156 Recycle-A-Bicycle - Manhattan
75 Avenue C, NEW YORK, NY
Tel: 212 475 1655
www.recycleabicycle.org

B157 Sid's Bikes - East Side
235 E. 34th Street, NEW YORK, NY
Tel: 212 213 8360
www.sidsbikes.com

B158 Sid's Bikes - West Side
151 W. 19th Street, NEW YORK, NY
Tel: 212 989 1060
www.sidsbikes.com

B159 Signature Cycles
80 W End Avenue, NEW YORK, NY
Tel: 212 706 0025
www.signaturecycles.com

B160 Spillway Bicycles and Accessories
163 Malcolm X Boulevard, NEW YORK, NY
Tel: 212 316 4753

B161 Spokesman Cycles - Union Square *(Rentals available)*
34 Irving Place, NEW YORK, NY
Tel: 212 995 0450
www.spokesmancycles.com

B162 Swim Bike Run (SBR) New York
203 West 58th Street, NEW YORK, NY
Tel: 212 445 1010
www.sbrshop.com

B163 The Hub Station
517 Broome Street, NEW YORK, NY
Tel: 212 965 9334

B164 Toga Bike Shop 1st Avenue
1153 First Avenue, NEW YORK, NY
Tel: 212 759 0002
www.togabikes.com

B165 Toga Bikes Westside
110 West End Avenue, NEW YORK, NY
Tel: 212 799 9625
www.togabikes.com

B166 Tread Bike Shop *(Rentals available)*
250 Dyckman Street, NEW YORK, NY
Tel: 212 544 7055
www.treadbikeshop.com

B167 Victor's Bike Repair *(Rentals available)*
4125 Broadway, NEW YORK, NY
Tel: 212 740 5137

B168 Waterfront Bicycle Shop *(Rentals available)*
391 West Street, NEW YORK, NY
Tel: 212 414 2453
www.bikeshopny.com

B169 Zen Bikes
134 West 24 Street, NEW YORK, NY
Tel: 212 929 2453
www.zenbikes.com

B170 Metro Bicycles - 14th Street *(Rentals available)*
332 E 14th Street, NEW YORK, NY
Tel: 212 228 4344
www.metrobicycles.com

B171 Nyack Bicycle Outfitters
72 N Broadway, NYACK, NY
Tel: 845 353 0268
www.nyackbike.com

B172 Veribike
210-23 Horace Harding Expressway
OAKLAND GARDENS, NY
Tel: 718 428 2545

B173 Campmor Inc
810 Route 17 North, PARAMUS, NJ
Tel: 201 445 5000
www.campmor.com

B174 The Bicycle II
736 North State Rt 17, PARAMUS, NJ
Tel: 201 632 0200
www.njbicycles.com

B175 Cyclesport
1 Hawthorne Avenue, PARK RIDGE, NJ
Tel: 201 391 5269
www.cyclesportonline.com

B176 Piermont Bicycle Connection
215 Ash Street, PIERMONT, NY
Tel: 845 365 0900
www.piermontbike.com

B177 Port Washington Cycles
999 Port Washington Boulevard,
PORT WASHINGTON, NY
Tel: 516 883 8243

Bike Shops & Rentals

B178 Cigi Bicycle Shop - Queens
42-20 111st Street, QUEENS, NY
Tel: 718 271 1473
www.cigibicycleshop.com

B179 Format
92-29 Queens Boulevard, QUEENS, NY
Tel: 718 887 2918

B180 Kissena Bicycle Center
45-70 Kissena Boulevard, QUEENS, NY
Tel: 718 358 0986

B181 Lightwheels Bike and Boat Rental
Meadow Lake, Flushing Meadows Park,
QUEENS, NY
Tel: 718 271 3005
www.lightwheels.com

B182 Metropolis Bicycles
92-64 Queens Boulevard, QUEENS, NY
Tel: 718 4783338
www.metropolisbicycles.com

B183 Spokesman Cycles - Atlas Park *(Rentals available)*
80-16 Cooper Avenue, QUEENS, NY
Tel: 718 366 0450
www.spokesmancycles.com

B184 Bicycle Barn
10734 Springfield Boulevard, QUEENS VILLAGE, NY
Tel: 718 479 3119
www.bicycle-barn.com

B185 ADT Bike & Skate
114-01 Jamaica Avenue, RICHMOND HILL, NY
Tel: 718 846 2099
www.adtbikes.com

B186 Ridgewood Cycle Shop
35 N Broad Street, RIDGEWOOD, NJ
Tel: 201 444 2553

B187 Laurelton Bicycle & Carriage Shop
23220 Merrick Boulevard,
SPRINGFIELD GARDENS, NY
Tel: 718 528 6886

B188 Bennett's Bicycles
517 Jewett Avenue, STATEN ISLAND, NY
Tel: 718 447 8652
www.bennettsbicycle.com

B189 Bike Shop of Staten Island
4026 Hylan Boulevard, STATEN ISLAND, NY
Tel: 718 948 4184

B190 The Bicycle Planet
300 Robbins Lane, SYOSSFT, NY
Tel: 516 364 4434
www.thebicycleplanet.com

B191 Bicycle Workshop
175 County Road, TENAFLY, NJ
Tel: 201 568 9372
www.bicycleworkshop.com

B192 Toga Bikes Nyack
530 North Highland Avenue, UPPER NYACK, NJ
Tel: 845 358 3455
www.togabikes.com

B193 Valley Stream Bicycle & Fitness
95 E Merrick Road, VALLEY STREAM, NY
Tel: 516 825 8181

B194 Brands Cycle & Fitness
1966 Wantagh Avenue, WANTAGH, NY
Tel: 516 781 6100
www.brandscycle.com

B195 Westwood Cycle
182 3rd Avenue, WESTWOOD, NJ
Tel: 201 664 1688
www.westwoodcycle.com

B196 South Shore Bicycles
1065-67 Broadway, WOODMERE, NY
Tel: 516 374 0606

B197 Bill's Cyclery
63-24 Roosevelt Avenue, WOODSIDE, NY
Tel: 718 335 1906
www.ubuybikes.com

B198 County Cycle Center
970 Mclean Avenue, YONKERS, NY
Tel: 914 237 8641

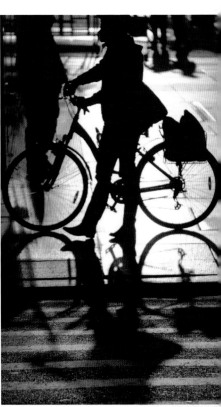

Photo Matt Wittme

Notes

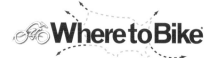 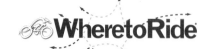
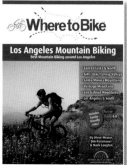
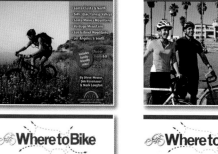
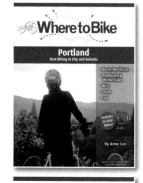
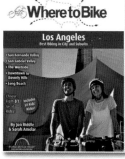
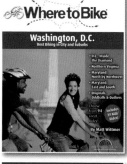
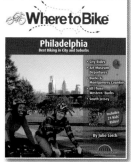
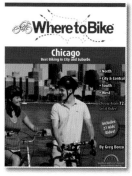
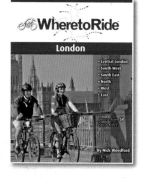
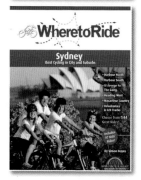

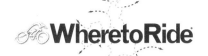 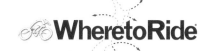
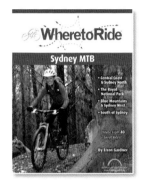 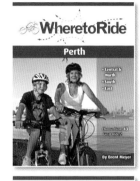 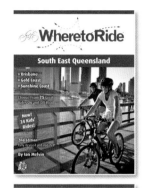
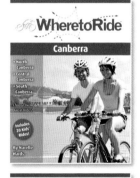 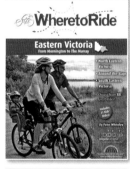 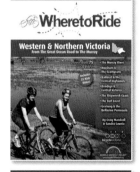
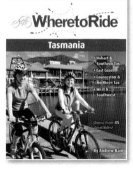 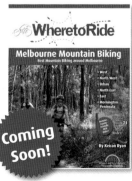 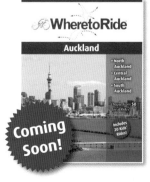

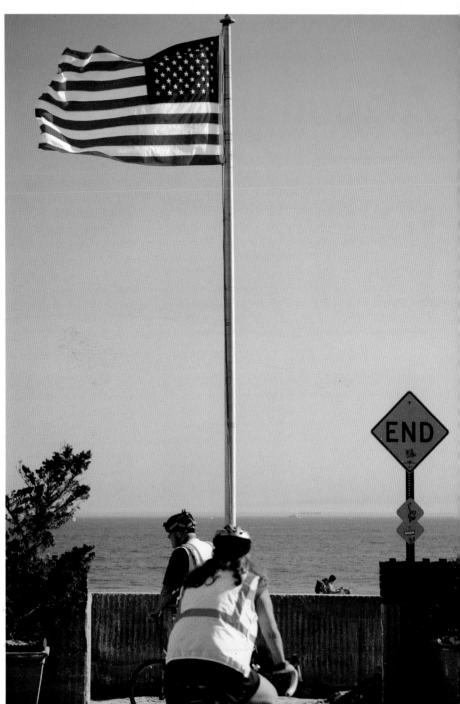

Photo Matt Wittmer